MSICU

Donated to
MSICU by
Heidi Pinnell RN

Managing Death in the ICU

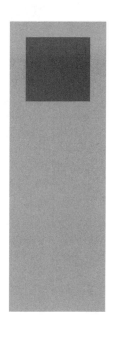

Managing Death in the ICU

The Transition from Cure to Comfort

Edited by

J. RANDALL CURTIS, M.D., M.P.H.

Associate Professor
Division of Pulmonary and Critical Care Medicine
University of Washington
Harborview Medical Center
Seattle, WA

GORDON D. RUBENFELD, M.D., M.Sc.

Assistant Professor
Division of Pulmonary and Critical Care Medicine
University of Washington
Harborview Medical Center
Seattle, WA

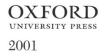

OXFORD
UNIVERSITY PRESS

2001

Oxford   New York
Athens   Auckland   Bangkok   Bogotá   Buenos Aires   Calcutta
Cape Town   Chennai   Dar es Salaam   Delhi   Florence   Hong Kong   Istanbul
Karachi   Kuala Lumpur   Madrid   Melbourne   Mexico City   Mumbai
Nairobi   Paris   São Paulo   Shanghai   Singapore   Taipei   Tokyo   Toronto   Warsaw

and associated companies in
Berlin   Ibadan

Published by Oxford University Press, Inc.
198 Madison Avenue, New York, New York, 10016

Oxford is a registered trademark of Oxford University Press

Library of Congress Cataloging-in-Publication Data
Curtis, J. Randall.
Managing death in the ICU : the transition from cure to comfort /
J. Randall Curtis, Gordon D. Rubenfeld.
p. ; cm.   Includes bibliographical references and index.
ISBN 0-19-512881-8
1. Intensive care units.   2. Terminally ill—Services for.
3. Terminally ill—Care.   4. Death—Psychology.
I. Rubenfeld, Gordon D.   II. Title.
[DNLM: 1. Intensive Care—psychology.   2. Adaptation, Psychological.
3. Attitude to Death.   4. Intensive Care Units.
5. Terminal Care—methods.
WY 154 C979m 2000]   RC86.7.C868 2000   362.1′75—dc21   00-022182

The science of medicine is a rapidly changing field. As new research and clinical experience
broaden our knowledge, changes in treatment and drug therapy do occur. The author and the
publisher of this work have checked with sources believed to be reliable in their efforts to provide information that is accurate and complete, and in accordance with the standards accepted at
the time of publication. However, in light of the possibility of human error or changes in the
practice of medicine, neither the author, nor the publisher, nor any other party who has been involved in the preparation or publication of this work warrants that the information contained
herein is in every respect accurate or complete. Readers are encouraged to confirm the information contained herein with other reliable sources, and are strongly advised to check the product
information sheet provided by the pharmaceutical company for each drug they plan to
administer.

9 8 7 6 5 4 3 2 1

Printed in the United States of America
on acid-free paper

Foreword

BERNARD LO, M.D.

An actual case study for managing death in the ICU goes like this: A young pregnant woman had metastatic melanoma. Against the recommendations of several physicians, she decided to carry her child to term. Late in the third trimester she developed respiratory failure because of progressive metastatic disease. Because her goal was to deliver a healthy child, she was intubated to allow the child to develop as fully as possible. After delivery, she became unresponsive.

Use of ICU technology saves many critically ill patients who would otherwise die. However, life-saving or life-prolonging interventions also lead to clinical and ethical dilemmas because some ICU patients do not recover despite intensive therapies. In the case sketched above, when was it appropriate for physicians to recommend that the goal be shifted to palliative care? Once the decision was made to do so, should sedation have been lightened in the hope that she might see her infant, or would that have caused her to suffer needlessly? How might clinicians have helped her husband and family say farewell and grieve? How should her final hours have been managed: should the endotracheal tube have been removed and intravenous lines disconnected? How could the nurses and physicians who had worked so hard to keep her alive until she delivered deal with their feelings of sadness?

Thirty years ago, dilemmas in ICUs concerned patients whose brain had ceased to function but whose ventilation and circulation were maintained. Were such patients dead or alive? Was it appropriate to discontinue ventilatory support? Was it ethically permissible to use the organs of such patients for transplantation? Although these questions now have answers, the ethical dilemmas now are more pervasive and broader in scope. In addition to deciding whether to withdraw or withhold medical interventions, physicians also need to consider how to relieve suffering and help the patient and family achieve closure at the end of life.

Care at the end of life is difficult in any setting, but particularly so in the ICU. First, the goal of care when patients are admitted to the ICU is to prolong life through the provision of medical technologies. Thus palliative care almost always requires a change in goals. Over several days to weeks of ICU care, the patient may not respond to therapy, an unfavorable medical prognosis may become clear, or a series of complications may create a downward spiral. Such an interval may not provide the ICU team or the family with sufficient time to renounce the original goal of care. Second, most ICU patients near the end of life are no longer able to make decisions about their medical care. Surrogate decision making is often more complex and controversial than decision making by competent patients. There may be no surrogate, or family members may disagree over what the patient would want or what is best for the patient. Third, the expense of ICU care and the need to restrain the ever-rising cost of health care place pressure on ICU physicians to allocate scarce resources prudently. As ICU bed supply is increasingly constrained, physicians may want to withhold or withdraw ICU interventions before the family is ready to shift to palliative care. Fourth, because ICUs are organized to provide invasive medical technology, they seem a cold and dehumanized setting for a patient's last days.

This book fills several important needs for physicians, nurses and other health care professionals who care for critically ill patients. First, it articulates a new role: caring for patients who do not recover from their illness or injury. For years, critical care specialists have been responsible for decisions to forego life-sustaining interventions such as mechanical ventilation and for relieving physical symptoms during the dying process. This book shows how these clinicians also need to relieve psychosocial suffering in patients and families, as well as help them to achieve closure at the end of life. Second, the book provides practical and specific advice on how to fulfill the goals of palliative care in an ICU setting. This book presents the knowledge that clinicians need to provide effective palliative care for ICU patients, with emphasis on what is different from outpatient or hospice care. Third, this book addresses the interpersonal and emotional aspects of providing palliative care in the ICU, which is interdisciplinary and collaborative. Care is regularly transferred from one attending physician to another. Health care professionals may have different opinions on when a palliative emphasis is appropriate or how to implement it. The ICU providers spend long hours providing care to restore a patient to health and may find it difficult to accept that a patient is dying. In the vignette described earlier, physicians, nurses, and respiratory therapists experienced a medley of strong feelings: pride that the woman's life had been prolonged so that her baby was delivered at term, but also sadness that they could not do more, and grief that her time with her child was so short. As all who work in ICUs know, the work is often draining. At the same time, there are opportunities to make connections with dying patients and their families and to learn from their experiences as they confront death. Dying in the ICU need not be viewed as a failure of the original goals of ICU care, nor as a failure of the medical system that allowed a dying patient to be cared for in the ICU. Instead, patients, families, and caregivers can find meaning in a patient's life and final days. In the case vignette, the ICU team fretted over how they could help the patient's husband cope with her death. In the end, they did not need to solve his problems for him. Before the ventilator was withdrawn, he brought his guitar to her room and said farewell by playing her favorite songs. Those who listened and watched realized that providing palliative care allows health care workers to be enriched by the courage and wisdom of patients and their families.

The editors dedicate this book to Dr. Leonard D. Hudson for his commitment to the care of critically ill patients and their families and to the education of a generation of critical care clinicians. Dr. Hudson embodies the principles of compassionate caring that we have tried to incorporate in this book and, in his role as a mentor, provided us with the inspiration and support for the work that lead to this book. For this, and much more, we thank him.

This book was supported by a conference grant provided by the Robert Wood Johnson Foundation.

Contents

Contributors

DEREK C. ANGUS, M.D., M.P.H.
Critical Care Medicine
University of Pittsburgh Medical Center
Pittsburgh, PA

ANTHONY BACK, M.D.
Department of Oncology
VA Puget Sound Health Care System
University of Washington
Seattle, WA

SUSAN D. BLOCK, M.D.
Chief of Adult Psychosocial Oncology
  Unit
Dana Farber Cancer Institute
Department of Psychiatry
Brigham and Women's Hospital

NANCY CHAMBERS, M.Div.
Pastoral Care and Education
Harborview Medical Center
Seattle, WA

DEBORAH J. COOK, M.D.,
  F.R.C.P.C., M.S. (Epid.)
Associate Professor of Medicine and
  Clinical Epidemiology
McMaster University
St. Joseph Hospital
Hamilton, Ontario, Canada

STEPHEN CRAWFORD, M.D.
Pulmonary and Critical Care Division
University of California San Diego
  Medical Center
San Diego, CA

J. RANDALL CURTIS, M.D.,
  M.P.H.
Associate Professor of Medicine
Division of Pulmonary & Critical Care
  Medicine
University of Washington
Harborview Medical Center
Seattle, WA

BARBARA J. DALY, Ph.D., R.N.,
  F.A.A.N.
Associate Professor
School of Nursing
Case Western Reserve University
Co-Director, Clinical Ethics
University Hospitals of Cleveland
Cleveland, OH

MARION DANIS, M.D.
Department of Clinical Bioethics
Clinical Center
National Institutes of Health
Bethesda, MD

MALCOLM FISHER, M.B.Ch.B.,
M.D., F.A.N.Z.C.A., F.R.C.A.
Clinical Professor
Departments of Medicine and Anesthesia
University of Sydney
Royal North Shore Hospital of Sydney
St. Leonards, NSW, Australia

KATHLEEN FOLEY, M.D.
Co-Chief, Pain & Palliative Care Service
Memorial Sloan-Kettering Cancer Center
New York, NY

JOHN E. HEFFNER, M.D.
Professor and Vice-Chair
Department of Medicine
Division of Pulmonary and Critical Care
Medicine
Medical University of South Carolina
Charleston, SC

MARSHALL B. KAPP, J.D.,
M.P.H.
Professor, Departments of Community
Health and Psychiatry
Wright State University School of
Medicine
Dayton, OH

MARIN H. KOLLEF, M.D.
Pulmonary and Critical Care Division
Washington University School of Medicine
St. Louis, MO

MITCHELL M. LEVY, M.D.
Pulmonary, Sleep, and Critical Care
Medicine
Brown University School of Medicine
Rhode Island Hospital
Providence, RI

JOHN M. LUCE, M.D.
Professor of Medicine and Anesthesiology
University of California, San Francisco
Division of Pulmonary and Critical Care
Medicine
San Francisco General Hospital
San Francisco, CA

STEVEN H. MILES, M.D.
Associate Professor
University of Minnesota, Center for
Biomedical Ethics
Minneapolis, MN

RICHARD A. MULARSKI, M.D.
Pulmonary Diseases and Critical Care
Medicine
Oregon Health Sciences University
Portland, OR

JUDITH E. NELSON, M.D., J.D.
Associate Professor, Department of
Medicine
Division of Pulmonary and Critical Care
Medicine
Associate Director, Medical Intensive
Care Unit
Mount Sinai School of Medicine
New York, NY

DAVID M. NIERMAN, M.D.
Clinical Associate Professor of Medicine
and Surgery
Director, Medical Intensive Care Unit
Mount Sinai School of Medicine
New York, NY

MOLLY L. OSBORNE, M.D.,
Ph.D.
Associate Professor and Associate Dean
Pulmonary Section and Critical Care
Medicine
Oregon Health Sciences University
Portland, OR

DONALD L. PATRICK, Ph.D.,
M.S.P.H.
Professor and Director of Social and
Behavioral Sciences
Department of Health Services
University of Washington School of
Medicine
Seattle, WA

THOMAS J. PRENDERGAST, M.D.
Chief, Pulmonary Section
Veterans Administration Medical Center
White River Junction, VT

PETER PRONOVOST, M.D., Ph.D.
Department of Anesthesiology and
  Critical Care Medicine,
Surgery, and Health Policy and
  Management
Johns Hopkins University
Baltimore, MD

KATHLEEN A. PUNTILLO, R.N.,
  D.N.Sc.
Associate Professor of Nursing
Department of Physiological Nursing
University of California at San Francisco
San Francisco, CA

WALTER M. ROBINSON, M.D.,
  M.P.H.
Pulmonary Division
Children's Hospital
Division of Medical Ethics
Harvard Medical School
Boston, MA

MARK J. ROSEN, M.D.
Chief, Pulmonary and Critical Care
  Medicine
Beth Israel Medical Center
Professor of Medicine
Albert Einstein College of Medicine
New York, NY

GORDON D. RUBENFELD, M.D.,
  M.Sc.
Assistant Professor
Division of Pulmonary & Critical Care
  Medicine
University of Washington
Harborview Medical Center
Seattle, WA

JONATHAN SACKNER-BERNSTEIN,
  M.D., F.A.C.C.
Associate Chief
Division of Cardiology
Director, Heart Failure Program
St. Luke's-Roosevelt Hospital Center
New York, NY

SARAH E. SHANNON, Ph.D.,
  R.N.
Research Assistant Professor
Biobehavioral Nursing and Health
  Systems
University of Washington
Seattle, WA

JOAN M. TENO, M.D., M.S.
Associate Professor of Community
  Health
Brown University School of Medicine
Associate Medical Director, Hospice Care
  of Rhode Island
Providence, RI

EELCO F.M. WIJDICKS, M.D.,
  Ph.D., F.A.C.P.
Professor of Neurology
Mayo Medical School
Director, Neurology-Neurosurgery ICU
Consultant, Department of Neurology
Mayo Foundation and Mayo Clinic
Rochester, MN

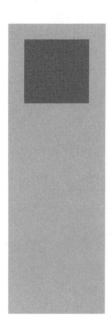

Part I

The Changing Landscape of Death in the ICU

Chapter 1

Introducing the Concept of Managing Death in the ICU

J. RANDALL CURTIS
GORDON D. RUBENFELD

*I*n the medical professions and among the lay public, there is growing concern that excessive resources are used to provide unwanted life-sustaining medical care for patients at the end of their lives. Many authors have criticized the high cost of dying in our society and have proposed solutions to decrease the cost of end-of-life care,[1] while others have questioned whether changing the way we provide care at the end of life will save money.[2] Several well-conceived and carefully executed interventions to decrease costs and improve the quality of end-of-life care have been unsuccessful.[3-5] While the general public has expressed increasing concern that medical care at the end of life is poor and that death will be unnecessarily prolonged by technological, invasive, and impersonal treatment,[6] patients and providers are worried that managed care may limit access to potentially life-saving, but expensive, treatments.[7] In this complex and contradictory environment, clinicians are struggling to provide the highest quality medical care for many dying patients in intensive care units around the world.

The ICU is an important focus in discussions on improving the quality of end-of-life care because the mortality there is high and it is a common location where clinicians, patients, and families make the transition from attempting to cure disease and prolong life to providing comfort and allowing death with dignity.[8] For some patients, the best way to improve ICU care at the end of life is to avoid intensive care altogether. However, even under ideal circumstances of excellent communication and accurate prognostication, many patients and families will choose intensive care that ultimately will not work. In fact, with an aging population and advances in medical technology, it seems likely that, unless elderly patients are willing to completely forego effective life-prolonging treatments such as organ transplantation and heart surgery, decisions to shift from curing disease to maximizing comfort will occur even more frequently in the ICU than they do now. Critical care clinicians will continue to face the clinical and emotional challenges of redirecting their efforts from cure to comfort and, when death seems inevitable, of providing for the highest quality death possible. The challenge to clinicians and educators in this area is to span two cultures: the rescue culture of critical care and the hospice culture of palliative medicine. Currently, limited resource materials are available that review the topic and provide specific, practical clinical advice on caring for critically ill, dying patients.

This book reviews the state of the art in caring for patients dying in the ICU; it is organized into four sections. In the first section, death in the ICU is discussed in the context of recent changes in medical care. Several important studies that have attempted but failed to improve the quality of end-of-life care are described, and the changing epidemiology and ethics of death in the ICU are reviewed. This section also provides some insight into the role that end-of-life care plays in the lives of the critical care clinician. The second section of the book reviews the initial step in the transition from cure to comfort: the decision to limit life-sustaining treatments. This section includes chapters on the role of outcome prediction, the effect of bias in decision making, and the role that quality of life should play in these decisions. In this section, the role of advance directives and advance care planning in end-of-life care in the ICU is also reviewed. In the third section, the authors present the practical skills needed to provide the highest quality of care to patients dying in the ICU. These skills include communicating with patients and families, managing pain and other symptoms, the principles and mechanics of withdrawing life-supporting therapies, and the essential roles that nurses and palliative care specialists play in the ICU. This section also reviews the importance of helping clinicians cope with the large numbers of dying patients they care for and examines the role of spirituality in end-of-life care in the ICU. In the fourth section, important societal issues concerning death in the ICU are examined, including the role of race, ethnicity, religion, and socioeconomic status, the influence of economics, and the role of organizational change in improving end-of-life care in the ICU. This section also reviews legal issues of relevance to clinicians working in the ICU and provides an international perspective on dying and death in the ICU. In the final section, the authors describe issues unique to the care of patients with some of the more common diseases that precipitate a death in the ICU. Care for members of special populations, namely infants and children and the elderly, is also discussed.

Most of the contributors to this book are not only clinicians with experience in caring for patients in the ICU. but are also researchers and writers who have struggled to find ways to improve the care we provide for patients dying in the ICU. Their common goal is to provide practical advice to clinicians who care for patients dying in the ICU. In some cases, although there were insufficient data to make evidence-based treatment guidelines, the authors collected the available evidence and incorporated their experience and expertise to make specific recommendations to the reader. The primary audience for this book is the broad range of clinicians who provide care to critically ill patients: surgeons, pulmonologists, cardiologists, anesthesiologists, pediatricians, critical care nurses, nurse specialists, and respiratory therapists. The book is also intended as a resource for pastoral care personnel, nutritionists, pharmacists, and other ICU clinical staff who work with dying patients on a regular basis. We also hope that this book will provide useful information on critical illness for palliative care specialists who want to be a resource in the ICU. Finally, medical directors of ICUs and managed care organizations who are charged with improving the quality of care for dying patients may find this book useful in directing efforts toward this goal.

The difficult decisions accompanying the transition from aggressive life-sustaining therapy to equally aggressive comfort care will never be easy. We hope that the material presented here will inform and improve the care provided to patients dying in the ICU and to all critically ill patients. When the book is found, dog-eared and scribbled on, at ICU nurses' stations and physicians' workrooms, then we will have contributed to this difficult goal..

References

1. Callahan D. The Troubled Dream of Life: Living with Mortality. New York: Simon & Schuster, 1993.
2. Emanuel EJ, Emanuel LL. The economics of dying: the illusion of cost savings at the end of life. *N Engl J Med* 1994;330:540–544.
3. The SUPPORT Principal Investigators. A controlled trial to improve care for seriously ill hospitalized patients: the Study to Understand Prognoses and Preferences for Outcomes and Risks of Treatments (SUPPORT). *JAMA* 1996;274:1591–8.
4. Danis M, Southerland LI, Garrett JM, et al. A prospective study of advance directives for life-sustaining care. *N Engl J Med* 1991;324:882–888.
5. Schneiderman LJ, Kronick R, Kaplan RM, Anderson JP, Langer RD. Effects of offering advance directives on medical treatment and costs. *Ann Intern Med* 1992; 117:599–606.
6. Fein EB. Talking around death; chronicling the end for 20: hard choices are harder when wishes go unsaid. *New York Times* March 5, 1997: B5.
7. Cowley G, Turque B. Critical condition: from the capital to kitchen tables, and from frustration with HMOs to worries about cost, health care is topic A. *Newsweek* November 8, 1999:58–61.
8. Pendergast TJ, Luce JM. Increasing incidence of withholding and withdrawal of life support from the critically ill. *Am J Respir Crit Care Med* 1997;155:15–20.

Chapter 2

The Changing Ethics of Death in the ICU

RICHARD A. MULARSKI

MOLLY L. OSBORNE

 echnology drives bioethics when new treatments are used clinically before their ethical implications have been considered. The intensive care unit is a major arena where technology propels and focuses the ethics of death and dying. Many of the health care systems in the United States and elsewhere are faced with increasing demand for expensive health care services coupled with limited financial resources and competing societal needs.[1] The following example illustrates some of the choices now available for managing death in the ICU: should an elderly patient who has metastatic cancer and has requested no heroic measures be intubated during an endoscopy procedure for an acute upper gastrointestinal hemorrhage? Which choice offers greater comfort? The analysis presented here will trace the major historical and contextual events that have influenced the ethics of dying in the practice of critical care medicine (Table 2–1).

Historical Background

Technology was welcomed by doctors throughout the early half of the 20th century as a means of moving past the realm of charlatans and sorcerers to positively effecting morbidity and mortality. At the same time in Western medicine, ethical behavior was governed by the Hippocratic tradition, with principles stemming from the application of nature as the predominant guide to healing. Out of the statement "be of benefit and do no harm," which was a minor comment nested within a treatise attributed to Hippocrates on the topic of fever, grew the principles of nonmaleficence and beneficence.[2] Nonmaleficence, the edict of *primum non nocere*, states that no harm should be inflicted

Table 2–1. Bioethics in the 20th century

Principle	*Reference*
Toward Autonomous Decisions	
From paternalism to autonomy	Karen Ann Quinlan case (1976)[10]
The "right to die"	Nancy Cruzan case (1990)[20,21]
Autonomy by surrogate (substituted judgment)	American Thoracic Society Bioethics Task Force (1991)
Truth-Telling	
From purple dots to DNR orders	*New York Times* (1986)
Sham codes deemed unethical	*New York Times* (1986)
Honest prognostication	Patient Self-Determination Act (1990)
Clarifying Confusing Distinctions	
Heroic<>ordinary: ethically indistinguishable	American Thoracic Society
Withhold<>withdraw: ethically indistinguishable	Bioethics Task Force (1991)
Killing<>let die, active euthanasia or withdrawing life support: distinctly different	
Overruling Autonomy	
Allocation of scarce resources in medical decision making	American Thoracic Society Bioethics Task Force (1997)[23]
The Oregon experience with physician-assisted suicide	The Oregon Health Division (Chin et al. 1998)[22]
Futility in medical decision making	Schneiderman et al. (1990)[29]

on another person. Beneficence states that beyond avoidance of harm, there exists an obligation to do good. In the practice of medical ethics this implies a balance of maximal benefit and minimum harm.

As the use of technology in medicine increased, the field of ethics was compelled to change from being a philosophical and scholarly pursuit in the mid-20th century to becoming a practical discipline. The field of bioethics emerged from a multidisciplinary effort in the 1950–60s to respond to technology that posed dilemmas at individual and societal levels. The roots of bioethics still lay in philosophy, evolving from Western tradition and principles ascribed to Hippocratic tradition, and deriving early leadership from Judaic and Christian moral theologies and the developing school of secularism. Secularism encompassed the attempt to delineate and apply universally intrinsic human truths, usurping societal and intellectual concepts that themselves were in response to technology. In *How Medicine Saved the Life of Ethics*, Stephen Toulmin developed the technology-driven thesis, based on his years of experience on the National Commission for the Protection of Human Subjects of Biomedical and Behavioral Research (1974–1978), extolling the transition from theoretical inquiries to casuistry—e.g., case-based ethics and practical application.[3]

Toward Autonomous Decisions

From paternalism to autonomy

The ability of medicine to treat critically ill people occurred in an environment of evolving bioethical principles of respect for persons, autonomy, and self-determination. No longer was the physician's beneficence conclusive. Competent individuals or their declared representatives were determined to have both the right and capability to deliberate about personal goals and to act under the direction of such deliberation. The recognition and establishment of self-determination, the legitimacy of individuals' opinions and choices, and respect for confidentiality all led to new patterns of practice in the ICU. The last principle that became applicable to the emerging bioethics included justice, the social concept founded in distributive philosophy and fairness. This concept requires that benefits and burdens be distributed fairly and equitably without regard to gender, age, social status, economic status, religion, or ethnicity.

The goals of intensive care medicine remain the same as the age-old tenets for all of traditional medicine: (1) restore health (save the salvageable—provide aggressive care to allow the patient who can to heal and regain strength) and (2) relieve suffering (facilitate a peaceful and dignified death—do not prolong the process of dying, use sensitivity and compassion in addressing the needs of the family, and help them process grief).[4] The use of technology transformed the ICU as the technique of cardiopulmonary resuscitation was applied to patients with anticipated imminent death. Society's trust in technological advances increased our utilization of health care especially at the end of life, and led to the institutionalization of dying. As Dan Callahan has written, ". . . we will live longer lives, be better sustained by medical care, in return for which our deaths in old age are more likely to be drawn out and wild."[5] Technology devoid of humanism risks indignity. Hence, ethics in critical care may be viewed as a response to humanity acknowledging the limitations of technology and, implicitly, the inevitability of death.

The right to die

Self-determination recognizes that each person has a fundamental right to control his or her own body and to be protected from unwanted intrusions. The Society for the Right to Die cites a very early U.S. Supreme Court case that wrote, "No right is held more sacred or is more carefully guarded by the common law than the right of every individual to the possession and control of his own person, free from all restraints or interference by others, unless by clear and unquestionable authority of law."[6] The legal right and ethical premise of self-determination are frequently cited in legal and ethical cases in which the authority to determine end of life is contested, as in the 1914 case Schloendorff v. New York Hospital: "Every human being of adult years and sound mind has a right to determine what will be done with his own body."[7]

Self-determination has evolved into a bioethical principle of autonomy, which is now the ruling principle when dissonance occurs in ethical principles applied to an individual case.[1] Although society is beginning to set limits on the application of technology at end-of-life care, many individuals are ill-prepared to accept death at the onset of critical illness, and appropriate utilization of intensive care remains at the cusp of current ethical challenges.[8] Willingness to undergo intensive care is not influenced by age, severity of critical illness, length of stay, or charges for care. Of patients studied who were 55 years or older, all with prior ICU stays, 70% of patients and families said they would be willing to undergo ICU care even for as little as a 1-month survival benefit. Only 8% were unwilling to undergo ICU care to achieve any prolonged survival.[9] Eighty-two percent of preferences were uncorrelated with functional status or quality of life.[9]

Autonomy by surrogate (substituted judgement)

Karen Ann Quinlan, the 22-year-old woman whose case was adjudicated in 1976, has become a symbol of the evolution of autonomy and its legal precedence. Ms. Quinlan was maintained in a coma thought to be due to the ingestion of drugs and alcohol. She had not met the criteria for brain death that were established by the Harvard committee, but had a prognosis limited to a persistent vegetative state. Although her father was appointed as her legal guardian in an attempt to remove her from the ventilator, her physicians refused to honor this request. Physicians still have exaggerated concerns about the morality and liability of complying with the wishes of their patients, despite reported cases where doctors were held liable for *not* respecting patient autonomy. Judicial activism has nonetheless upheld the principle of autonomy, and in this landmark case, surrogacy and quality of life were linked with this principle. The New Jersey Supreme Court made a distinction between a "biological vegetative existence" and a "normal functioning, integrated existence." Determination of the possibility of a reasonable return to "a cognitive and sapient life" was felt to be a medical decision that required ethical considerations and involved discussion with the patient and/or the family. In the Quinlin case, the conflict between physician and family was resolved on the ground of the constitutional right to privacy, which upheld autonomy. In the absence of the individual exerting her right to self-determination, a surrogate could carry out her choice and prevail over the physician's judgement.[10]

Although Ms. Quinlan was removed from the ventilator, she remained in a coma for a decade. The fate of Karen Ann Quinlan brought the issue of the rights to die and to refuse treatment into the American courtroom and to national attention. When the New Jersey Supreme Court granted Ms. Quinlan's father the power to have her life support terminated, the concepts of advanced directives and withdrawal of treatment were introduced. The case required the creation of definitions that attempt to delineate the gray boundary where lifesaving treatments yield to death-prolonging interventions. The ethics of death were questioned, and substituted judgment, surrogate decision making, and standards of the patient's best interest were introduced into bioethics. The concept of one person being able to substitute judgment for another was novel. This extension of autonomy is a foundation of our current approach to decision making. All 50 states provide statutory authority of some form of advance directive and all but 3 states authorize living wills and durable power of attorney for health care decisions.[11]

Truth-Telling

From purple dots to do-not-resuscitate orders

Resuscitation in the event of a cardiopulmonary arrest is an accepted standard of care in the United States.[12] Yet patients have an absolute right to refuse any form of medical treatment. Guidance for patients, their family members, and doctors and nurses regarding resuscitation in the event of a cardiopulmonary arrest is relatively new. The ethical principles underlying formal do-not-resuscitate (DNR) orders and proscribing sham codes are respect for individuals and the importance of truth-telling.

There has been a history of "confused medical ethics and secretive practices on the emotionally charged issue of saving the lives of terminally ill or hopeless comatose patients."[13] For example, in 1983 a grand jury investigation found that physicians at La Guardia Hospital in Queens, New York had ordered that small purple dots be stuck to the charts of terminally ill patients, indicating that they were not to be resuscitated in the event they suffered cardiopulmonary arrests. This clearly violated professional obligations to patients and their families, and prevented medically appropriate decision making.[14]

Slow codes

Similarly, some hospital staff have unofficially "slow coded" patients.[14] *Slow codes*, also known as *partial, show, light blue*, or *Hollywood codes*, are cardiopulmonary resuscitative efforts that involve a deliberate decision against an aggressive attempt to bring a patient back to life.[15] Under this practice, doctors and nurses use delaying tactics to ensure that any resuscitation efforts will fail, but that still allow the staff to tell survivors that everything had been done to save the patient. Hospitals have nonetheless required that virtually every patient who suffered cardiac or respiratory arrest be resuscitated. Concerns have been raised that some patients were denied resuscitation without their consent, yet other patients were inappropriately resuscitated and forced to endure unnecessary suffering because hospitals and physicians feared lawsuits or criminal prosecution.

The bioethical consideration of this topic has been strong and remonstrative. The American College of Physicians Ethics Manual considers such "halfhearted resuscitation efforts" to be unethical.[16]

Honest prognostication

Although the laws requiring discussion of advance care planning for medicare reimbursement are almost 10 years old, the recognition of patient autonomy and right to self-determination occurred several years earlier. In 1983 the President's Commission for the Study of Ethical Problems in Medicine and Biomedical and Behavioral Research released a report delineating conclusions on foregoing life-sustaining treatments, reaffirming patient autonomy, and right of self-determination (as laid out in its earlier document, *Making Health Care Decisions*), even if the outcome is death. In the first page of the report's introduction, several observations are enumerated that continue to have relevancy and yet have led to little progress in the care of the dying:[12,17]

> Death is less of a private matter than it once was. Today, dying more often than not occurs under medical supervision, usually in a hospital or nursing home.

> Patients dying in health care institutions today typically have fewer of the sources of nonmedical support, such as family and church, that once helped people in their final days.

> Also important . . . are the biomedical developments of the past several decades. Without removing the sense of loss, finality, and mystery that have always accompanied death, these new developments have made death more a matter of deliberate decision.

> Dramatic breakthroughs . . . have made it possible to retard and even to reverse many conditions that were once regarded as fatal. Matters once the province of fate have now become a matter of human choice.

> Moreover, medical technology often renders patients less able to communicate or to direct the course of treatment.

Clarifying Confusing Distinctions

The 1983 report by the President's Commission for the Study of Ethical Problems in Medicine (*Deciding to Forego Life-Sustaining Treatment*) is one of the strongest of the many reports released by the Commission. It clarifies several traditional moral distinctions that continue to be pivotal benchmarks for bioethics policy development and legal discourse. The Commission reached the conclusions outlined below.

Heroic < > *ordinary*

- The determination of "ordinary" verses "extraordinary" should not determine whether a patient may accept or decline but rather proportionality of benefit and burden of an intervention.

Withhold < > *withdraw*

- The distinction between failing to initiate therapy and stopping therapy, that is, withholding versus withdrawing treatment, is not itself of moral importance because a justification that is adequate for not commencing a treatment is sufficient for ceasing it.
- Actions that suggest administration of a pain medicine that may hasten a patient's death are justified by the benefits expected to exceed the negative consequences as long as the sole purpose is not to poison or kill a patient (the double effect).
- In the absence of an overt determination of legally acceptable wishes, surrogates should make use of proportionate treatment, testing the balance between the burden and benefits of therapy.

The proportionate treatment test became a frequently cited benchmark in legal proceedings, as in a California case addressing withdrawal of life support in the ICU.[18] In 1981, Clarence Herbert, a 55-year-old man, sustained a postoperative myocardial infarction with evidence of significant central nervous system injury. His family and physicians concurred that treatment should be withdrawn, based on comments made that the patient would not wish to be kept alive artificially. Two days after the event, mechanical ventilation was removed but he continued living; 2 days later, IV fluid and nutrition were withheld and the patient died a week later. In 1983, two physicians in the case were charged with murder by the Los Angeles District Attorney. The California Superior Court dismissed the charges, citing proportionality as the key criterion to be used in deciding whether to withdraw life support. The case also ruled that hydration and nutrition given by artificial means were medical procedures and evaluated in the same means as other procedures and interventions. Although physician concerns of liability continue, there are no reported cases in which a doctor is held liable for complying with the wishes of their patients.[19] The ethical equivalence of withholding versus withdrawing treatment has evolved in a similar manner and now is a major premise in end-of-life care.

The case of Nancy Cruzan broadened the means of terminal support from life support alone to life-extending and ordinary care. This was the first case adjudicated by the U.S. Supreme Court on the "right-to-die" doctrine. As a result of a 1983 auto accident this young women sustained injuries that left her in a vegetative state. Her family applied not to have a ventilator discontinued but to stop the tube feedings on which her survival depended. The Missouri Supreme Court held that refusal of treatment was a personal decision and could not be exercised by a surrogate without "clear and convincing evidence" that Cruzan herself rejected such care.[20] The case was appealed to the United States Supreme Court and in 1990 became the first case the high court heard involving the right to refuse life-sustaining treatment. The Court split on the ruling by five to four, and characterized the case as essentially one involving the right to die. Chief Justice Rehnquist wrote that the "United States Constitution would grant a competent person a constitutionally protected right to refuse lifesaving hydration and nutrition [based not on the right of privacy but rather on the right to liberty in the 14th Amendment]."[21] However, the Court upheld the state's legitimate interest in sufficient proof that this was the person's expressed decision while competent, on the basis that the decision is deeply personal, that abuses can occur in the absence of loving surrogates, and that the state may simply assert an unqualified interest in the preservation of human life. Although the Supreme Court did not set any standards, it introduced the concept that no rational distinction can be made between ordinary and extraordinary treatment.

Killing < > let die, active euthanasia or withdrawing life support

The approval of physician-assisted suicide in Oregon is the most recent development in the changing ethics of end-of-life and furthers our discussion of patient autonomy in the face of terminal illness.[22] As is clear from the 15 deaths due to assisted suicide that occurred in 1998, patient autonomy is an overriding force in decision making at the end of life.

Overruling Autonomy

Allocating scarce resources

Health care providers caring for critically ill patients commonly make decisions regarding the fair allocation of ICU resources.[23] Because ICU resources are expensive, comprising 15%–20% of hospital costs, the extraordinary expenditure of resources for marginal gains can unfairly compromise a basic minimum level of health care services for all. As pointed out by the American Thoracic Society Bioethics Task Force in 1997, however, theories of justice have proven notoriously unhelpful in providing practical answers to the most difficult questions that involve imposing limits on beneficial care.[24] A summary of principles for fair allocation of ICU resources is given in Table 2–2. Often the actual situation faced by a clinician has a range of morally permissible alternatives, and understanding prognoses and patient preference is surprisingly difficult.[25] Perhaps a public approach to reaching consensus on this issue, one that would reflect broad cultural values, represents the most promising solution.[23] An example of a public-based approach to the potential benefits of technology is the revised Oregon Medicaid Plan, which restricts access to certain medical inter-

Table 2–2. Principles for fair allocation of ICU resources

Principle 1	Each individual's life is valuable and equally so.
Principle 2	Respect for patient autonomy, as represented by informed consent, is a central tenet for providing health care, including ICU care.
Principle 3	Enhancement of the patient's welfare, by providing resources that meet an individual medical needs and that the patient regards as beneficial, is the primary duty of health care providers.
Principle 4	ICU care, when medically appropriate, is an essential component of a basic package of health care services that should be available for all.
Principle 5	The duty of health care providers to benefit an individual patient has limits when doing so unfairly compromises the availability of resources needed by others.

Data from Bioethics Task Force (1997).[23] American Thoracic Society.

ventions that have been judged by a public body with community input to be marginally beneficial relative to cost.[8,26]

Futility

The pendulum has shifted as health care providers question the appropriateness of initiating intensive care at the same time that autonomy and the patient's right to die have become ingrained in the psyche of medical decision makers. Such concerns were addressed by the American College of Chest Physicians/Society of Critical Care Medicine (ACCP/SCCM) consensus panel in 1990,[27] which asserted that it is better not to initiate intensive care measures "if there is a reasonable medical certainty of a nonsalvageable condition." The concept of futility is avoided in the ACCP/SCCM document and continues to be debated in terms of definition and application. Indeed, the term futility is often misapplied to situations in which the quality of life is what is really at stake. The ACCP/SCCM panel contends that in the presence of reasonable doubt or uncertainty about irreversibility of the patient's medical condition, it is appropriate to initiate intensive care. The bias should be "in favor of treatment" but frequent queries and reappraisals should be made with realistic and honest medical advice and family input on decisions to terminate and withdraw treatment as appropriate.

With the advent of increased societal requests for and legislative legitimacy to physician-assisted dying, palliative measures have been extended to a balance of treatment and alleviation of pain in terminal patients. In the case of *Washington v. Gulcksberg* involving physician-assisted suicide and its fundamental liberty, Justice O'Connor, commented that "a patient who is suffering from a terminal illness and who is experiencing great pain has no legal barriers to obtaining medication, from qualified physicians, even to the point of causing unconsciousness and hastening death."[28] This affirmation of the 'double effect' emphasizes that relief of suffering is paramount to preservation of life, both legally and ethically. Issues such as the moral, ethical, and legal right of physician-assisted suicide form the future of the evolving ethics in the ICU. Other pertinent issues include the right to aggressive care in cases of futility, utilization of scarce resources, and whether sound medical decisions can be used to withhold treatment from unrealistic patients. Studies such as SUPPORT (the Study to Understand Prognosis and Preferences for Outcomes and Risks of Treatments), although illustrative in their demonstration of the difficulty in studying and modifying practices in terminal care, suggest that the family and society are at the forefront of decision-making on intensive care in the years to come.[25]

Conclusion

Changes in bioethics have occurred in concert with the technological breakthroughs of this century. Since World War II in particular, we have moved from paternalism to autonomy; from charts with purple dots to advance care planning and honest prognostication; from unquestioned measures to sustain life to withholding and withdrawing life support; and finally, to legalization of physician-assisted suicide in the state of Oregon. Our responsibility as health care providers is to continue to keep the use of technology within the broad confines of bioethical principles.

References

1. American Thoracic Society Bioethics Task Force. Withholding and withdrawing Life Sustaining Therapy. *Ann Intern Med* 1991;115:478–485.
2. Beaucamp TL, Childress JF. Principles of Biomedical Ethics. New York: Oxford University Press, 1994, p. 269.
3. Toulmin S. How medicine saved the life of ethics. In: Bioethics: An Introduction to the History, Methods, and Practice (Jecker NS, Jonsen AR, Pearlman RA, eds.). Sudbury, MA: Jones and Bartlett Publishers, 1997, pp. 101–109.
4. Raffin TA. Ethical and legal aspects of forgoing life-sustaining treatments. In: Principles and Practice of Medical Intensive Care. Carlson RW, Geheb MA, (eds.). Philadelphia: W.B. Saunders, 1993, pp. 1731–1740.
5. Callahan D. The Troubled Dream of Life: In Search of a Peaceful Death. New York: Simon and Schuster, 1993, p. 53.
6. *Union Pacific Railway Co v. Botsford,* 141 U.S. 250, 251 (1891). In: The Physician and the Hopelessly Ill Patient, publication of The Society for the Right to Die, 1985.
7. *Schloendorff v. New York Hospital,* 211 N.Y. 125, 129, 105 N.E. 92, 93 (1914).
8. Hadorn, DC. Setting health care priorities in Oregon: cost-effectiveness meets the rule of rescue. *JAMA* 1991;265:2218–2225.
9. Danis M, Patrick DL, Sourherland LI, Green ML. Patients' and families' preferences for medical intensive care. *JAMA* 1988;260:797–802.
10. *In re Quinlan,* 355 A2d 647 (JN), 429 US 922 (1976).

stin LO. Deciding life and death in the courtroom. *JAMA* 199ı

resident's Commission for the Study of Ethical Problems in Meu.
medical and Behavioral Research. Deciding to Forego Life-sustaining
Report on the Ethical, Medical, and Legal Issues in Treatment Decisions
ton DC: U.S. Government Printing Office, 1983.

13. *The New York Times*, August 13, 1987;
14. *The New York Times*, April 20, 1986;
15. Gazelle G. The slow code—should anyone rush to its defense? *N Engl J Me* 1998;338:467–469.
16. American College of Physicians Ethics Manual, 3rd ed. *Ann Intern Med* 1992;117:747–960.
17. President's Commission for the Study of Ethical Problems in Medicine and Bio-medical and Behavioral Research. Making Health Care Decisions: A Report on the Ethical and Legal Implications of Informed Consent in the Patient-Practitioner Relationship. Washington DC: U.S. Government Printing Office, 1982.
18. *Barber v. Superior Court,* 195 Cal Rptr 484 (Ct App 1983).
19. Gostin LO. Drawing a line between killing and letting die. *J Law Med Ethics* 1993;21:71–78.
20. *Cruzan v. Director, Missouri Dept of Health,* 497 US 261 (1990).
21. Annas GJ. Nancy Cruzan and the right to die. *N Engl J Med* 1990;323:670–673.
22. Chin AE, Hedberg K, Higginson GK, Fleming DW. Legalized physician-assisted suicide in Oregon—the first year's experience. *N Engl J Med* 1999;340:577–583.
23. American Thoracic Society Bioethics Task Force. Fair allocation of intensive care unit resources. *Am J Respir Crit Care Med* 1997;156:1282–1301.
24. Gold JA. Global budgeting in the real world. *J Clin Ethics* 1997;5:342.
25. SUPPORT Principle Investigators. A controlled trial to improve care for seriously ill hospitalized patients: the Study to Understand Prognoses and Preferences for Outcomes and Risks of Treatments. *JAMA* 1995;274:1591–1598.
26. Eddy DM. What's going on in Oregon. *JAMA* 1991;266:417–420.
27. ACCP/SCCM consensus panel. Ethical and moral guidelines for the initiation, continuation, and withdrawal of intensive care. *Chest* 1990;97:949–958.
28. *Washington v. Gulcksberg,* 117 SCt 2258 (1997).
29. Schneiderman LJ, Jecker NS, Jonsen AR. Medical Futility: Its meaning and ethical implications. Ann Intern Med 1990;112:949–54.

Chapter 3

The Changing Nature of Death in the ICU

JOHN M. LUCE

THOMAS J. PRENDERGAST

*I*ntensive care units proliferated in the United States and other developed countries in the 1950s, 1960s, and 1970s alongside advances in medical knowledge, improvements in artificial ventilation, the introduction of cardiac monitoring, and the need for prolonged support following complex surgeries. This proliferation was influenced by physician demands that new technologies be made available for their patients and by willingness on the part of hospitals to meet these demands. Such willingness stemmed from the need to remain competitive, the desire to attract the best physicians and their patients—by providing state-of-the-art treatment—and the fact that hospitals and physicians alike were reimbursed on a fee-for-service basis. In the mid-1980s, over 90% of all American acute care hospitals had at least one ICU, and U.S. expenditures for critical care approached $15 billion, or 11% of all acute care costs.[1] By 1998, it was estimated that ICUs consumed up to 34% of hospital budgets, and that critical care expenditures amounted to over $62 billion.[2]

For most of their history, ICUs have reported death rates of approximately 10% to 20%, depending on the types of patients treated there.[3,4] Furthermore, we have observed that, until recently, most of the patients who have died in the ICU have done so despite full life support, including attempted cardiopulmonary resuscitation (CPR). The wishes of patients and their surrogates regarding support have rarely been solicited in our experience, and do-not-resuscitate (DNR) orders have seldom been used to limit treatment. This practice has been consonant with the belief, held by health professionals and the public alike, that the ICU and its technologies have the obligation to preserve life whenever possible regardless of human and economic costs.

In recent years, however, the obligation of the ICU has been challenged, just as its expenses have been scrutinized. For example, clinical research has revealed that many patients, including those with severe respiratory failure and such underlying conditions as advanced hematological malignancies,[5] solid tumors,[6] and acquired immunodeficiency syndrome,[7] rarely leave the ICU alive, or do so only after prolonged pain and suffering. Furthermore, these and other survivors of critical illness frequently die shortly after being transferred out of the ICU, thereby minimizing its apparent benefits.[8,9] As the clinical limitations of intensive care have become recognized, physicians[10] and hospital administrators have questioned whether the economic resources used to finance ICUs should be used for other, more beneficial medical purposes, especially in our era of capitation and managed care. And although patients and their surrogates seldom pay the ICU bill directly, they nevertheless have come to question the value of intensive care in all instances and to seek ways to refuse it if they so desire.

The right of patients and their surrogates to refuse treatment and have it withdrawn, over the objections of physicians and hospitals if necessary, was first legally affirmed on a state level in the cases of Karen Ann Quinlan in 1976 and Joseph Barber in 1983. In the case of Nancy Cruzan in 1990, the U.S. Supreme Court reaffirmed this right on the part of patients who can participate in medical decisions, but allowed states to require evidence of patients' wishes regarding termination of life support. The federal Patient Self-Determination Act of 1991 was passed to encourage the expression of patients' wishes by requiring that caregivers at health care facilities ask hospitalized patients if they have advance directives and help them prepare such directives if they do not.

Although the Patient Self-Determination Act and the legal cases that preceded it support patient and surrogate autonomy, more recent cases have involved physicians and hospitals that sought to restrain autonomy. For example, in the case of Helen Wanglie in 1991, the Hennepin County Medical Center asked a district court to replace a surrogate because he insisted on continued mechanical ventilation for his wife, a therapy Mrs. Wanglie's physicians considered not beneficial because it would not heal her lungs or end her unconsciousness. In this case, the court decided that the husband was the appropriate surrogate.

Similarly, in the case of Catherine Gilgunn, the Massachusetts General Hospital and several of its physicians were sued for writing a DNR order for Mrs. Gilgunn and removing mechanical ventilation from her over the objections of her daughter. In 1995, a Suffolk County Superior Court jury absolved the physicians and the hospital of liability, apparently because they believed that further treatment was futile despite the possibility that Mrs. Gilgunn might have wanted to be kept alive.[11]

In parallel with these legal cases from *Quinlan* to *Gilgunn*, presidential commissions,[12] individual authors,[13] institutional ethics committees,[14] and professional societies[15-18] have supported patient and surrogate autonomy while also spelling out circumstances in which futile care should be foregone. At the same time, the advent of medical cost-consciousness related to managed care has restrained the application of therapies that merely prolong death with little hope of long-term cure.[19] The legal, ethical, and economic consensus that has resulted from these developments has in turn reinforced a trend toward limitation of ineffective treatments, which is currently reflected in the changing nature of death in the ICU. Whereas critically ill patients previously died despite full support and attempted CPR, such patients are more likely to die today during the withholding and withdrawal of life support with DNR orders in place. Thus, physicians, with the implicit or explicit approval of the hospitals in which they practice, increasingly have become involved in managing death in the ICU, just as they manage cardiovascular decompensation and respiratory failure.[20]

How Death Is Managed

The first major observational study[21] of how critically ill patients die was conducted by our group over the academic year 1987–1988 in two medical-surgical ICUs at hospitals affiliated with the University of California, San Francisco (UCSF). During a 1-year period, 224 (13%) of the 1719 patients admitted to the ICUs died. Of the 224 patients who died, 114 (51%) did so after a decision had been made to limit treatment; 22 patients had life support, including CPR, withheld, and 92 had life support withdrawn. Of the 114 patients who were not supported, 89 died in the ICU, and 15 died after they were transferred to other areas of the hospitals, with the provision that they would not be readmitted to the ICU if they decompensated. None of the 114 patients received attempted CPR, and DNR orders were written for 109 of them.

Only 5 of the 114 patients for whom therapy was limited were considered capable of making medical decisions by their physicians, and none had executed advance directives. Surrogates were involved in the decision to withhold and withdraw life support from 102 of the 109 patients judged incapable of decision making, but for the remaining 7 patients, surrogates could not be found; physicians made decisions for these patients. Physicians recommended that treatment be limited either because the patient was brain-dead (18 patients) or because of a poor prognosis (96 patients). Contributing reasons included the futility of continued intervention (in 29 patients), extreme suffering (in 8), and a request by the patient or a surrogate (in 6). All but two of the surrogates agreed with the course of therapy limitation recommended by physicians, either immediately or within a few days. Full support was administered to the two patients whose surrogates insisted upon it until the patients died.

Over the academic year 1992–1993, 5 years after our first study, we conducted a similar investigation[22] in the same medical-surgical ICUs affiliated with UCSF. During this second period, 200 (13%) of the 1711 patients admitted to the ICUs died, the same proportion as previously. A decision was made to withhold or withdraw life support from 179 (90%) of the 200 patients who died, compared with 51% in the first study in the second study, life support was withheld from 27 of the 179 patients and was withdrawn from 140 of them. 12 patients had only CPR withheld. Of the 179 patients, 162 died in the ICU and 17 died after transfer. None of the 179 patients received attempted CPR, and most had DNR orders.

In the second study, only six patients were judged by their physicians to be competent to make treatment decisions, compared with five patients in the first study. Eight patients had completed advance directives; none had done so in the first study. Surrogates were unavailable for 11 patients, for whom physicians made decisions, but surrogates were involved in making decisions for the remaining 168. Physicians recommended that treatment be terminated for 25 of the 179 patients because they were brain-dead. Life support was withheld or withdrawn for 21 patients at the request of the patients or their surrogates, compared with only 6 patients in the previous study.

In the cases of 133 patients (74% of the 179), the futility of further treatment was decisive in physicians' recommendations to limit care; assessments of what constituted futility differed widely, and the term "futility" was probably a substitute for "poor prognosis" in many instances. In eight cases, the surrogates of incompetent patients refused to accept a recommendation to withhold or withdraw life support, compared with two patients in the first study. As was true of the two patients in 1987 and 1988, all eight patients continued to receive ICU care. However, in one instance support was withheld without consent, and in five others DNR orders were written without consent. Two patients had CPR attempted despite physician recommendations to the contrary, and neither patient survived.

These two studies clearly document an evolution in medical practice toward a more active role in managing the deaths of critically ill patients in the two ICUs at hospitals affiliated with UCSF. Indeed, these studies suggest that physicians, patients, and surrogates increasingly take steps to limit treatment in many such patients. This change is reflected not only in the increased incidence of the withholding and withdrawal of life support but also in the increased use of advance directives on the part of patients and the increased number of requests by patients and surrogates that treatment be limited. Finally, we observed an increased willingness on the part of physicians to write DNR orders without patient or surrogate consent, a practice demonstrated in a recent survey of critical care physicians.[23]

Our data do not explain why managing death has become more commonplace in the two ICUs. However, the finding was not due to differences in overall in-unit mortality or patient mix. We believe that the changing manner of death in the ICU most likely reflects changes in professional and public attitudes regarding the propriety of limiting treatment that is unlikely to benefit patients. We also speculate that the evolution we observed has occurred in other units, although we only studied the two medical-surgical ICUs in hospitals affiliated with UCSF. This speculation is supported by a number of studies[24-31] documenting changes in terminal care management at other institutions.

To determine the generalizability of our observations, we contacted the directors of all American postgraduate training programs in critical care medicine and asked them to categorize prospectively all patients who died in their ICUs over a 6-month period in 1994 and 1995 into one of five mutually exclusive categories. The national survey of end-of-life care[32] that resulted from this effort involved 131 ICUs from 110 institutions in 38 states. A total of 74,502 patients were admitted to these ICUs during the 6-month study period, 6303 of whom died (9% mortality in the units). Of the 6303 patients who died, 1544 (20%) did so despite full ICU support including attempted CPR, 1430 (24%) did so after receiving full support but not attempted CPR, 794 (14%) had life support withheld, 2139 (36%) had life support withdrawn, and 393 (6%) were brain-dead. Thus, of the 5910 patients who died in the ICU and were not brain-dead, 4366 (74%) received less than full support. This percentage probably would have been higher had we included patients who died shortly after being transferred out of the ICU with no provision for readmission, as we did in our two previous studies at UCSF.

One striking finding described in the national survey was the wide variation in end-of-life care: the range of proportions of death preceded by failed CPR was 4% to 79%, for DNR status the range was 0 to 83%, and for withholding or withdrawal of life support the range was 0% to 67%, and 0% to 79%, respectively. This variation could not be explained by the types of ICUs (medical, surgical, medical-surgical, neurosciences, and other), hospital types (university, community, public, veterans, and other), or geographic regions of the hospitals. However, a pattern was observed in the two states with strict legal standards for care limitation by surrogates: ICUs in New York and Missouri had lower proportions of deaths preceded by withdrawal of support than did the mid-Atlantic and Midwest regions in which these states are located.

Although the national survey did not demonstrate changes in ICU deaths over time, it did suggest that limits to life support have become so commonplace in the United States as to represent a de facto standard of end-of-life care for critically ill patients. Nevertheless, the extreme variation in the categories of ICU death underscores the absence of a true consensual approach to end-of-life care. A first step in creating consensus would be for all hospitals to track their own end-of-life practices. A second would be for critical care specialists to develop guidelines for limiting treatment, as will be discussed later in this chapter.

How Do-Not-Resuscitate Orders Are Written

Corroboration of the changing epidemiology of ICU deaths has come from recent studies of the increased frequency of the use of DNR orders. Koch et al.[33] reviewed the medical records of 237 consecutive patients who received such orders in a medical ICU at the University of Florida and found that DNR orders were written twice as often before ICU death in 1988 than 4 years earlier. In a larger study, Jayes and associates[34] compared data from 42 ICUs in 40 U.S. hospitals with more than 200 beds from 1988 to 1990 with similar data collected at 13 of the 40 hospitals from 1979 to 1982. The investigators reported that DNR orders were written more frequently for ICU patients (9%) admitted during the latter period than during the former (5%) and preceded 60% of all in-unit deaths in 1988 to 1990 compared with only 39% in 1979 to 1982. Do-not-resuscitate orders also were written sooner (for 3.6% vs. 2.0% of patients on day 1 in the ICU), and patients with DNR orders remained in the ICU longer in 1988 to 1990 (2.8 vs. 1.4 days) than in 1979 to 1982.

In a subsequent investigation, Jayes and colleagues[35] explored variations in the use of DNR orders in the same 42 ICUs. They found that the frequency of ICU DNR orders could be predicted on the basis of individual risk factors such as age, severity of physiological abnormalities, and prior health status. Nevertheless, after adjusting for patient characteristics, there was still large variation in the frequency of DNR orders in their national sample. For example, DNR orders were written significantly less frequently than predicted in 5 of the 42 ICUs and more frequently than predicted in 3 of them. Nonwhite patients had significantly fewer DNR orders after adjustment for other variables. The investigators found no relationship between risk-adjusted DNR order frequency and adherence to published guidelines. They speculated that variation in DNR use may be due to unmeasured differences, including surrogate attitudes regarding life support, or physician behavior.

Variations in Physician Behavior

The importance of physician variability has been underscored by two studies from the medical ICU at Barnes-Jewish Hospital in St. Louis. This ICU functions as a closed unit in terms of day to day patient management, but private attending physicians maintain ultimate responsibility for their patients and make major decisions, including those involving limitations of care. For patients without private attending physicians, the ICU attendings who are full-time critical care practitioners serve as attendings of record. In the first study, Kollef[36] retrospectively analyzed patient deaths during a 12-month period in 1994. In the second study, Kollef and Ward[37] performed similar prospective analysis during a 5-month period in 1996. Because both studies came to similar conclusions and the more recent study is also the more complete one, it is reviewed here.

Of the 501 patients admitted to the ICU during the study period in 1996, 60% had private attending physicians and 40% did not. On average, the private attending physicians, who were general internists or specialists such as oncologists, cared for 2 patients over the 5 months, whereas a typical full-time critical care faculty member cared for 40. The patients treated by the two types of attending physicians did not differ in terms of their indications for ICU admission, although admission diagnoses were quite different. Patients with private attendings were more likely to have an underlying diagnosis of malignancy, immunosuppression, end-stage organ failure, a greater severity of illness, higher predicted mortality, and advance directives than patients without private attendings. They were also more likely to be white and to have health insurance.

The overall hospital mortality rate was 23% among patients in this study; patients with private attending physicians had a mortality of 29% compared to 13% for patients without private attendings. When nonsurvivors were analyzed according to their attending status, no differences in severity of illness, predicted mortality, or DNR status were observed. However, the patients with private attending physicians had greater lengths of stay in the ICU, longer durations of mechanical ventilation, and more ICU and hospital charges. Although they had a greater hospital mortality, patients with private attending physicians presumably had a lesser ICU mortality, given that they were less likely to undergo the withdrawal of life-sustaining therapies in the unit prior to death (30% vs 81% for patients without private attendings). Patients with underlying malignancies were also less likely to undergo withdrawal if they had private attendings (32% vs. 100%). Finally, among the patients who had private attendings and who actually underwent withdrawal of support, over half had withdrawal initiated not by their private attending physicians but by one of the critical care physicians.

Certainly clinical differences between the patients who had private attending physicians and those who did not may have been overlooked by Kollef and Ward in their study, despite the large amount of data they collected. The patients' surrogates may also have differed in some regard, although no mention was made of this possibility. Yet such differences, if they existed, were probably less significant than the differences among attending physicians in determining which patients had life support withheld or withdrawn. Assuming that the limitation of life-supporting therapy is beneficial, to reduce unnecessary suffering as well as health care costs, Kollef and Ward have demonstrated that patients who have higher socioeconomic status, health insurance, and hence access to private attendings at their institution, are disadvantaged relative to patients with lower economic status. This disadvantage probably results from the private patients receiving more extensive but not necessarily more efficacious care.

Of course, the most likely advantage of patients without private attending physicians in this study was not their lack of sponsorship but the fact that they were managed by critical care physicians. In this regard, the study was less an indictment of "private" attendings than an endorsement of ICU specialists. The investigators argued that such physicians have more experience, are more available in the unit to make decisions, provide more appropriate care for dying patients, and are more comfortable in withholding and withdrawing support. That intensivists did not underuse potentially beneficial treatments was supported by the observation that the ratio of actual to predicted mortality was lower among patients cared for by intensivists than among patients cared for by nonintensivists in the Barnes-Jewish Hospital ICU.

Future Management of Death

We believe that critical care specialists will care for most, if not all, ICU patients in the future. We base this belief not only on Kollef and Ward's finding that intensivists are more likely to limit treatment but also on studies[2,38] demonstrating that "closed" units in which such specialists direct care are associated with better risk-adjusted mortality, shorter length of stay, and more appropriate use of resources. Given that death has been and remains commonplace in ICUs (the mortality rate was 9% in our national end-of-life care study), specialists who care for critically ill patients in the future must also become specialists in the management of death in the ICU.

To help ourselves and our colleagues manage death, we must learn how death is managed in our units and whether it is managed well. The Study to Understand Prognoses and Preferences for Outcomes and Risks of Treatment (SUPPORT)[39] suggested that physicians do not communicate adequately with patients and surrogates and that patients suffer greatly as they die, at least in the ICUs studied. Further research is needed to determine whether the SUPPORT findings are generalizable and what measures are useful in improving the quality of death. From such research should come practice guidelines to accompany current recommendations[40] regarding compassionate care.

In addition to research, critical care specialists require clinical training in death management. In particular, we need better education in how to prognosticate for ICU patients and how to access and use the large data sets that increasingly make prognostication a scientific process. We also need training in communication and conflict resolution, skills that commonly are called for with our patients and their surrogates. Finally, we need to develop a curriculum in death management for intensivists that befits the changing nature of death in the ICU.

References

1. Kelley MA. Critical care medicine—a new specialty? *JAMA* 1988;318:1613–1617.
2. Multz AS, Chalfin DB, Samson IM, Dantzger DR, Fein AM, Steinberg HN, Niederman MS, Scharf SM. A "closed" medical intensive care unit (MICU) im-

proves resource utilization when compared with an "open" MICU. *Am J Respir Crit Care Med* 1998;157:1468–1473.

3. Thibault GE, Mulley AG, Barnett GO, Goldstein RL, Reder VA, Sherman EL, Skinner ER. Medical intensive care: indications, interventions, and outcomes. *N Engl J Med* 1980;302:938–942.

4. Knaus WA, Draper EA, Wagner DP, Zimmerman JE. An evaluation of outcome from intensive care in major medical centers. *Ann Intern Med* 1986;104:410–418.

5. Rubenfeld GD, Crawford SW. Withdrawing life support from mechanically ventilated recipients of bone marrow transplants: a case for evidence-based guidelines. *Ann Intern Med* 1996;125:625–633.

6. Schapira DV, Studnicki J, Bradham DD, Wolff P, Jarrett A. Intensive care, survival, and expense of treating critically ill cancer patients. *JAMA* 1993;269:783–786.

7. Wachter RM, Luce JM, Safrin S, Berrios DC, Charlebois E, Scitovsky AA. Cost and outcome of intensive care for patients with AIDS, *Pneumocystis carinii* pneumonia, and severe respiratory failure. *JAMA* 1995;273:230–235.

8. Seneff MG, Wagner DP, Wagner RP, Zimmerman JE, Knaus WA. Hospital and 1-year survival of patients admitted to intensive care units with acute exacerbation of chronic obstructive pulmonary disease. *JAMA* 1995;274:1852–1857.

9. Chelluri L, Pinsky MR, Donahoe MP, Grenvik A. Long-term outcome of critcially ill elderly patients requiring intensive care. *JAMA* 1993;269:3119–3123.

10. Luce JM. The changing physician-patient relationship in critical care medicine under health care reform. *Am J Respir Crit Care Med* 1994;150:266–270.

11. *Gilgunn v. Massachusetts General Hospital*, Mass Sup CT, No. 92–4820, verdict 21, (1995).

12. President's Commission for the Study of Ethical Problems in Medicine and Biomedical and Behavioral Research. Deciding to Forego Life-sustaining Treatment: A Report on the Ethical, Medical, and Legal Issues in Treatment Decisions. Washington, DC: Government Printing Office, 1983.

13. Luce JM. Ethical principles in critical care. *JAMA* 1990;263:696–700.

14. Ruark JE, Raffin TA, Stanford University Medical Center Committee on Ethics. Initiating and withdrawing life support: principles and practice in adult medicine. *N Engl J Med* 1988;318:25–30.

15. Council on Ethical and Judicial Affairs, American Medical Association. Decisions near the end of life. *JAMA* 1992;267:2229–2233.

16. American Thoracic Society. Withholding and withdrawing life-sustaining therapy. *Am Rev Respir Dis* 1991;144:726–731.

17. Task Force on Ethics of the Society of Critical Care Medicine. Consensus report on the ethics of foregoing life-sustaining treatments in the critically ill. *Crit Care Med* 1990;18:1435–1439.

18. Council on Ethical and Judicial Affairs, American Medical Association. Medical futility in end-of-life care: report of the Council on Ethical and Judicial Affairs. *JAMA* 1999;281:937–941.

19. Cher DJ, Lenert LA. Method of Medicare reimbursement and the rate of potentially ineffective care of critically ill patients. *JAMA* 1997;278:1001–1007.

20. Karlawish JHT, Hall JB. Managing death and dying in the intensive care unit. *Am J Respir Crit Care Med* 1997;155:1–2.

21. Smedira NG, Evans BH, Grais LS, Cohen NH, Lo B, Cooke M, Schecter WP,

Fink G, Epstein-Jaffe E, May C, Luce JM. Withholding and withdrawal of life support from the critically ill. *N Engl J Med* 1990;322:309–315.

22. Prendergast TJ, Luce JM. Increasing incidence of withholding and withdrawal of life support from the critically ill. *Am J Respir Crit Care Med* 1997;155:15–20.

23. Asch DA, Hansen-Flaschen J, Lanken PN. Decisions to limit or continue life-sustaining treatment by critical care physicians in the United States: conflicts between physicians' practices and patients' wishes. *Am J Respir Crit Care Med* 1995; 151:288–292.

24. Eidelman LA, Jakobson KJ, Pizov R, Geber D, Leibovitz L, Sprung CL. Foregoing life-sustaining treatment in an Israeli ICU. *Intensive Care Med* 1998;24:162–166.

25. Keenan SP, Busche KD, Chen LM, McCarthy L, Inman KJ, Sibbald WJ. A retrospective review of a large cohort of patients undergoing the process of withholding and withdrawal of life support. *Crit Care Med* 1997;25:1324–1331.

26. Turner JS, Michell WL, Morgan CJ, Benatar SR. Limitation of life support: frequency and practice in a London and a Cape Town intensive care unit. *Intensive Care Med* 1996;22:1020–1025.

27. Koch KA, Rodeffer HD, Wears RL. Changing patterns of terminal care management in an intensive care unit. *Crit Care Med* 1994;22:233–243.

28. Vernon DD, Dean JM, Timmons OD, Banner W Jr, Allen W-EM. Modes of death in the pediatric intensive care unit: withdrawal and limitation of supportive care. *Crit Care Med* 1993;21:1798–1802.

29. Vincent JL, Parquier JN, Preiser JC, Brimioulle S, Kahn RJ. Terminal events in the intensive care unit: review of 258 fatal cases in one year. *Crit Care Med* 1989;17:530–533.

30. Bedell SE, Pelle D, Maher PL, Cleary PD. Do-not-resuscitate orders for critically ill patients in the hospital. How are they used and what is their impact? *JAMA* 1986;256:233–237.

31. Younger SJ, Lewandowski W, McClish DK, Juknialis BW, Coulton C, Bartlett ET. 'Do not resuscitate' orders. Incidence and implications in a medical-intensive care unit. *JAMA* 1985;253:54–57.

32. Prendergast TJ, Claessens MT, Luce JM. A national survey of end-of-life care for critically ill patients. *Am J Respir Crit Care Med* 1998;158:1163–1167.

33. Koch KA, Rodeffer HD, Wears RL. Changing patterns of terminal care management in an intensive care unit. *Crit Care Med* 1994;22:233–243.

34. Jayes RL, Zimmerman JE, Wagner DP, Draper EA, Knaus WA. Do-not-resuscitate orders in intensive care units: current practices and recent changes. *JAMA* 1993;270:2213–2217.

35. Jayes RL, Zimmerman JE, Wagner DP, Knaus WA. Variations in the use of do-not-resuscitate orders in ICUs: findings from a national study. *Chest* 1996;110:1332–1339.

36. Kollef MH. Private attending physician status and the withdrawal of life-sustaining interventions in a medical intensive care unit population. *Crit Care Med* 1996; 24:968–975.

37. Kollef MH, Ward S. The influence of access to a private attending physician on the withdrawal of life-sustaining therapies in the intensive care unit. *Crit Care Med* 1999;27:2125–2132.

38. Carson SS, Stocking C, Podsadecki T, Christenson J, Pohlman A, MacRae S, Jordan J, Humphrey H, Siegler M, Hall J. Effects of organizational change in the medical

intensive care unit of a teaching hospital: a comparison of 'open' and 'closed' formats. *JAMA* 1996;276:322–328.

39. Desbiens NA, Wu AW, Broste SK, Wenger NS, Connors AF, Lynn J, Yasui Y, Phillips RS, Fulkerson W, for the support investigators. Pain and satisfaction with pain control in seriously ill hospitalized adults: findings from the SUPPORT research investigations. *Crit Care Med* 1996;24:1953–1961.

40. Brody H, Campbell ML, Faber-Langendoen K, Ogle KS. Withdrawing intensive life-sustaining treatment—recommendations for compassionate clinical management. *N Engl J Med* 1997;336:652–657.

Chapter 4

Making a Personal Relationship with Death

MITCHELL M. LEVY

*G*iven how frequently patients die in the ICU, one would think that talking with patients and families about death would come easily for critical care clinicians. Unfortunately for our patients, the irony is that just because we see death all the time we are not necessarily comfortable with it. Death, grief, and the prospect of loss remain issues that raise the same anxiety and discomfort for caregivers as for patients and their families. Why is it that every time we sit down to speak with a patient or family about death and that moment of silence starts, we panic? Why do we think that we have to fill the space as soon as someone exhibits grief, or rage, or simply discomfort? Why does that silence seem so interminable that we feel compelled to have something technical or wise to say? We see people die all the time, and yet at times we act as if we were strangers to the process of dealing directly with death and loss.

How have we arrived at this point? First, as clinicians, we are not trained to feel comfortable with death. It is true that we can be very articulate about the need to help patients "die with dignity" and the responsibility of caregivers to respect the wishes of patients with regard to end-of-life care. In addition, as do-not-resuscitate (DNR) orders become more commonplace in the ICU, the process of talking with patients and families about end-of-life care has become a matter of routine. And yet, when confronted directly with the emotional intensity that surrounds the dying process, most critical care clinicians recoil. Despite our best intentions to provide more humane and compassionate end-of-life care, the prospect of death, along with the silence that punctuates a family discussion about death and the feeling of desolation and hopelessness that death evokes, still makes most caregivers physically and emotionally uncomfortable. This discomfort combined with our lack of training in good communication skills results in difficult times for dying patients and their loved ones in the ICU. Can we do our job better? After all this talk about death and dying, have we evolved as clinicians? What are the foundations of compassionate end of life care and how can we learn to be comfortable with death?

As caregivers for critically ill patients, it is our responsibility to begin to contemplate the answers to these difficult questions. As the development and use of technology proliferate, so does our daily experience of frustration and futility in the ICU. Compared with 10, even 5 years ago, we now are better able to prolong the lives of our patients in the presence of inevitably fatal disease. More sophisticated techniques in mechanical ventilation and dialysis, improved infection surveillance, and aggressive resuscitation are some of the interventions that are available for critically ill patients. Yet each day we are confronted with the inevitability of death. In many critical illnesses, such as acute respiratory distress syndrome (ARDS), mortality rates are declining. Despite this, we routinely see our patients succumb to long battles with devastating illness. Each day we are asked to comfort patients and their loved ones through the process of facing death. Our approach to that process and the skills we apply in those situations should be no less sophisticated and carefully conceived than those applied during other types of care in the ICU.

Defining Good End-of-Life Care

To use a tired cliché, good end-of-life care is like art: it is difficult to define, but you know it when you see it. Perhaps that is why it has been so difficult to teach end-of-life skills to nurses, physicians, and other caregivers-in-training. Perhaps educators have not introduced formal end-of-life care training into medical education for so long because the task of defining excellent end-of-life care is daunting. Whatever the reason, educational programs for training in end-of-life care skills are still woefully inadequate. Although many medical and nursing schools offer ethics of death and dying courses, these courses are for the most part conceptual; formal training in practical end-of-life care skills is not routinely offered in many postgraduate training programs. Learning these skills is a matter of on-the-job training for most caregivers. Yet the impact of end-of-life care on patients and their families may not only be profound but also just as important as making the right diagnosis. Simply put, it is not possible to match the therapeutic intervention with the wishes of patients and families if clinicians are uncomfortable talking about death.

Case Study

T.R. was a 38-year-old woman with a history of metastatic breast carcinoma. She presented with difficulty breathing 4 weeks after autologous bone marrow transplant and rescue chemotherapy. She had known liver and bone metastases and it was unclear whether infiltrates seen on her chest X-ray were due to new metastatic disease, an opportunistic infection, or both. It was clear to the ICU team after discussions with the patient and her very large, devoted family that she was a "fighter" who was determined to "beat this disease" and survive so that she might watch her children, ages 5, 7, and 9, grow up. The ICU team also knew that her oncologist had been unable or unwilling to inform the patient of the likely outcome of her disease. She and the family made it clear to the team that "everything should be done" for the patient, including all necessary resuscitative measures.

After several days and multiple diagnostic tests and procedures, including a bronchoscopy, she was found to have both metastatic disease and bilateral influenza A pneumonia. For the first several days in the ICU, although she was severely dyspneic, she steadfastly declined intubation. She did not refuse intubation, but asked the team to delay "putting in the tube" until absolutely necessary. Despite her obvious difficulty breathing, she remained stoic and insisted that she was doing fine. She was able to avoid intubation by lying still, but was clearly uncomfortable and short of breath while speaking.

Despite worsening dyspnea during the fourth and fifth hospital days, she again requested that intubation be delayed. On the sixth hospital day, her oxygen saturation was consistently 85%–88%. She now had great difficulty speaking and was no longer able to take anything by mouth because of her severe dyspnea. It is now clear that she required intubation, and because of her underlying disease and the severity of her bilateral pneumonia, she was unlikely to survive.

Just prior to intubation, the patient and the ICU attending physician discussed intubation. The physician described to the patient her underlying disease, current condition, and probable outcome. The patient was cognizant and oriented and clearly able to understand and appreciate the dismal prognosis she faced. The patient made clear her wish that all aggressive measures be continued, including intubation.

At this point, rather than immediately proceed with intubation, the physician discussed one more option with the patient. In a conversation that included only the patient, the bedside critical care nurse, and the ICU attending physician, the ICU attending made clear his opinion that, once intubated, the patient would most likely not recover and would not be able to speak with her family again. He supported her decision to be intubated, but given his opinion on the likely outcome, asked whether the patient would like some time to gather her children and family so that she could speak with them during the next several hours. The patient eagerly accepted this plan. With the permission of the patient, this information and plan were shared with the patient's husband and mother. They were told that in the opinion of the critical care team, despite continuation of all aggressive therapy and resuscitative measures, this would probably be the last opportunity for the family to talk with the patient and hear her voice.

The critical care team was initially concerned about the possible reaction of the family. Would they see this plan as a subtle way of giving up? Surprisingly, rather than viewing this suggestion as undermining the patient's hope or willingness to fight, the family welcomed this opportunity, brought the patient's children to her, and spent the next 4 hours visiting together.

After 4 hours, the family was asked to leave and the patient was intubated and placed on mechanical ventilation. Over the next 3 days, the patient deteriorated rapidly and developed ARDS, requiring large doses of sedatives and analgesics to maintain adequate oxygenation. She went on to develop septic shock from a nosocomial bacterial pneumonia, became unresponsive to pressor therapy, and died, with full resuscitative measures, 1 week after initial intubation.

After her death, in the midst of their grief, the family expressed their deep appreciation for the last several hours spent with the patient prior to intubation. The patient's mother told the critical care team that their compassion for her daughter was evident to the entire family and had provided them with an important measure of strength, which helped the family enormously. They were especially grateful that her children had a chance to say good-bye to their mother.

Where Do We Start?

What is the basis for effective, compassionate end-of-life care? The main starting point is simple: a caregiver must be willing to have "the conversation." This means taking the time to sit down with the patient and/or family to create the proper environment and communicate in an open, genuine manner about the truth of a patient's illness. One must be honest and direct. But in order to embark on this journey, a clinician must first feel comfortable with death. This does not mean to suggest that death is good and that as clinicians we should welcome it. But the opposite view is also a foolish approach. Death does not have to be viewed as good or bad, welcome or unwelcome. It is inevitable for all of us, and for some, particularly those with terminal illness, it arrives sooner rather than later. This is not to suggest that clinicians should underestimate the pain and sorrow that accompany death, but rather to accept, as human beings, the reality of death and the pain of suffering. In this way, we can appreciate the anxiety and sadness that surround the process of dying, as well as our own reaction as caregivers, as normal, healthy responses. Death need not be hidden, smoothed over, avoided, or even softened. Grief and sadness are healthy responses to meeting death, and as caregivers we can learn to be comfortable with the intensity of those feelings and try not to cover them up or make them go away

Dealing with Uncertainty

Why is it so difficult for caregivers to feel comfortable about death and the process of dying? Making a personal relationship with death and the process of dying depends on the ability of the caregiver to deal with uncertainty—the uncertainty of prognosis, of illness progression, of death itself. Without question, the dosing of pain medication, the response of various family members, the wishes of patients, and even the process of death itself all involve some degree of uncertainty. For a caregiver, one of the most fundamental challenges is to develop some degree of comfort with uncertainty—to be able to deal with uncertainty in a confident, reasoned fashion. The all-too-frequent caregiver response to uncertainty, whether it arises from the caregiver or the patient, is to resort to avoidance. The discomfort of the caregiver faced with uncertainty may be one of, if not *the* major obstacle to outstanding end-of-life care.

Looking at Our Own Mortality

In critical care, we spend a lot of our working hours in close proximity to death, but we often avoid making a personal relationship with the dying process. Both personally and professionally, death makes us uncomfortable. We tend not to contemplate our own mortality; we do not ask ourselves how we feel about our own death or the loss of a loved one. Many caregivers shrink from the feelings associated with grieving and dying. Not infrequently, and quite naturally, the primary response to any contemplation or discussion of death is anxiety and discomfort. How we respond to this anxiety and discomfort in our own lives will dramatically shape our end-of-life skills. It is hard to conceive of how we might make patients feel more comforted during the process of dying if we are frightened by the prospect of our own. How can we ask a family member to come to grips with the potential loss of a loved one if we cannot bear to consider the same reality in our own lives? How can we offer comfort to a patient who is in a panic at the prospect of dying and not being around to see his or her children grow up, when we ourselves cannot bear to think of such a thing?

If our usual response to uncertainty is avoidance, then good end-of-life care is difficult. If the caregiver is ultimately uncomfortable or unfamiliar with the emotions that arise during a person's dying, it becomes almost impossible to listen to patients and families in any meaningful way during end-of-life discussions.

The Discomfort of Dealing with Death

To return to the case presented earlier, during discussions among the critical care team, members expressed the feeling that if this were a member of their family, they would want one last chance to speak with their loved ones and hear them respond—even if it meant raising an alarm for the entire family that the patient was imminently dying. The reason why the family was gathered by the critical care team prior to intubation of the patient is simple: the team did not avoid the sadness and grief expressed by the patient's family. Instead, the team was willing to deal with the uncertainty and emotional turmoil. Thus to some extent, the team made the decision from the view of a family member, rather than as clinicians. More than anything, this communicated to the patient and family a deep sense of caring, which provided sustenance at a very difficult moment.

Being at Ease with Death

The first step in developing good end-of-life skills is becoming comfortable with death. Patients feel comforted and nurtured by a caregiver who is at ease with the dying process, who does not automatically shrink back from honest, direct expression of grief, loss, and uncertainty, and who can present steadiness in the face of a patient's fear and anxiety about dying. This first step, having the confidence to deal with death in an honest and straightforward manner, is also the most difficult for many caregivers.

The ability to deal with uncertainty without resorting to avoidance is a skill that can be learned. For some caregivers, this process is intuitive and appears to come naturally. For many others, this is not the case. The good news for patients and caregivers is that these skills are trainable. For patients, these skills may arise from having no choice about dying. For caregivers, it is a matter of appreciating the importance of developing a comfortable relationship with death. We owe it to ourselves and to our patients to contemplate our feelings about death, to know intimately our thoughts and feelings on the process of dying, and to consider the possibility of our own death. One of the fundamental qualities of a good end-of-life caregiver is that this person is, first and foremost comfortable with the process of dying.

What does compassionate end-of-life care look like? First, a caregiver does not avoid the discomfort and uncertainty of dealing with death, and talks honestly with patients. A concerned caregiver also offers advice to help a family feel good about a difficult decision. Finally, a patient and family feel cared for and respected during a time when this type of kindness and attention is most needed. This kind of care looks very simple. Patients and caregivers should expect and receive nothing less.

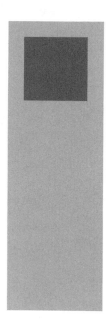

Part II

The Decision to Limit Life Support in the ICU

Chapter 5

Outcome Prediction in the ICU

MARIN H. KOLLEF

$\mathcal{T}$he major goals of intensive care can be simplified as the following: to save the lives of salvageable patients with reversible medical conditions and to offer the dying a peaceful and dignified death.[1,2] Prognostic information can be viewed as a tool for accomplishing and facilitating these primary goals. This may occur, in part, by enabling clinicians to provide understandable information to patients and their families to facilitate decision-making processes regarding the level of desired medical support. The accurate prediction of patient-specific outcomes is, and will continue to be, an important area of clinical research that has the real potential to influence medical practices. Physicians, nurses, patients and their families, health care administrators, government agencies, and health insurance companies all require accurate and assessible data on which to base their decision-making processes. Within ICUs, with their large quantity of clinical data (e.g., ventilator alarms, laboratory reports, family questions and concerns, medication infusions, hemodynamic monitoring data), refinements in our ability to identify important data, collect and process that data accurately and inexpensively, and use it to guide medical decision-making at the bedside will be the necessary focus of future research efforts. To effectively achieve the major goals of intensive care, especially as they relate to the management of the dying patient, we may need to develop new strategies for the delivery of health care at the end of life.

This chapter will attempt to formulate answers to several important questions regarding outcome prediction in the ICU setting. First, why are objective probability estimates important? Second, do objective measures of risk change clinical decision making? Third, should such objective measures of risk or outcome be utilized for clinical decision making, including end-of-life issues? Fourth, can futility be objectively defined so that it can be practically employed as a decision-making tool for critically ill patients? Lastly, what clinical situations fit into an objective definition of futility? The complete answers to these questions are currently unavailable. This chapter will attempt to offer a general framework for establishing answers to these questions in order to assist clinicians involved in the care of dying, critically ill patients.

Why Are Objective Probability Estimates Important?

The ability to accurately and objectively predict patient outcomes in the ICU is generally considered to be an important aspect of critical care,[3] as Feinstein noted: "The omission of prediction from the major goals of basic medical science has impoverished the intellectual content of clinical work since a modern clinician's main challenge in the care of patients is to make predictions."[4] Medical decision making, especially decisions based on perceived patient prognosis, can be distorted in several ways. First, processing of multiple data elements by the clinician in the ICU can be difficult, especially in terms of identifying the elements most likely to influence patient outcomes. Second, individual clinician biases can erode objective decision making. This may be most important when lack of prior personal experience with a specific problem or issue leads to uncertainty. This often forces the clinician to make adaptations in reasoning and to take mental shortcuts (heuristics) that may lead to errors in judgment and inaccurate estimates of probability.[3,5] Lastly, most physicians are not accustomed to making clinical decisions based on numerical probability estimates. They rely instead on clinical likelihoods, which may be biased by personal experience and can often be vaguely expressed with phrases such as "a likely low risk of death," "a high risk of complications," or "probable survival." For these reasons, formal objective prognostic tools have been viewed as a mechanism for improving clinical decision making in the ICU.[6]

At the present time, there are two general types of prognostic instruments for clinical application in the ICU. Categorical prediction rules assign patients to risk categories based on specific identifiable characteristics. Examples of these instruments include commonly employed weaning criteria for identifying patients who are likely to be liberated from mechanical ventilation, Child's criteria for patients with liver disease, and Ranson's criteria for patients with pancreatitis.[7-9] Mathematic prediction models that provide numerical estimates of outcome are the other major category of prediction instruments, including prediction models such as the Acute Physiology and Chronic Health Evaluation (APACHE) and the Mortality Prediction Model (MPM).[1] These models offer continuous probability estimates based on regression models that provide an estimate of outcome (i.e., mortality as the dependent variable) using previously identified predictor variables or risk factors (i.e., independent variables that make up the prediction model). At present, it appears that both types of instruments are complimentary to each another in terms of the clinical information they provide.[8,9]

Do Objective Measures of Risk Change Clinical Decisions?

Objective validated measures of outcome can be viewed as tools for changing clinician behavior that are based on scientifically sound data. In general, the simple availability of data, in the form of objective measures of risk or outcome, is not usually adequate to change or influence clinical decision making.[10,11] Such measures typically require systematic application in the form of a practice guideline, protocol, or institutional treatment policy to be effective instruments of change. To illustrate the importance of this process, I will compare two clinical studies evaluating the influence of objective risk measures on clinician behaviors and patient outcomes. The first, the Study to Understand Prognoses and Preferences for Outcome and Risks of Treatments (SUPPORT), was aimed at improving end-of-life decision making in an attempt to reduce the frequency of a mechanically supported, painful, and prolonged process of dying.[12] The second study is a prediction model that identifies patients at low risk for complications following hospital admission for upper gastrointestinal hemorrhage and examines the influence of a clinical practice guideline on reducing variation in practices while improving patient outcomes.[13] Although these two examples focus on different groups of patients and different disease processes, the strategies with which they were clinically employed will serve to illustrate the potential benefits and limitations of objective scoring systems as tools for modifying physician behaviors.

The SUPPORT investigators developed an intervention aimed at improving clinical communication and decision making by providing timely and reliable prognostic information, eliciting and documenting patient and family preferences and their understanding of disease prognosis and treatment, and providing a skilled nurse to help facilitate needed discussions, convene meetings, and bring relevant information to patients, their families, and health care providers.[12] The main elements of this intervention strategy are outlined in Table 5–1. The intervention nurse was free to shape her role so as to achieve the best possible patient care and clinical outcomes. A total of 9105 adults hospitalized with one or more of nine life-threatening diagnoses were evaluated, with an observed 6-month mortality rate of 47%.

During its observational first phase, SUPPORT documented shortcomings in communication, frequency of aggressive treatment, and the characteristics of hospital death. Only 47% of physicians knew when their patients preferred to avoid cardiopulmonary resuscitation (CPR); 46% of do-not-resuscitate (DNR) orders were written within 2 days of death, and 38% of patients who died spent at least 10 days in an ICU. During the second phase of the study when intervention was applied, no improvement in patient–physician communication (37% of control patients and 40% of intervention patients discussed CPR preferences) or in the five targeted outcomes (incidence or timing of written DNR orders, physicians' knowledge of their patients' preferences not to be resuscitated, number of days spent in the ICU and receiving mechanical ventilation while comatose before death, or level of reported pain occurred). The investi-

Table 5–1. Comparison of SUPPORT and Cedars-Sinai Medical Center investigations of acute upper gastrointestinal hemorrhage

	SUPPORT Study	*CSMCPI Study*
Use of validated scoring system	Yes (APACHE III, TISS)	Yes (CSMCPI)
Outcome estimated	Hospital mortality 6-month survival Functional status	Life-threatening complication
Intervention	Physician feedback of risk estimates Nurse facilitator to assist in physician– patient communications	Physician feedback of risk estimates
Delivery mode of risk estimates	Written progress notes in chart Verbal discussions	Written progress notes in chart Verbal discussions
Agent for communication of risk estimates	Nurse	Physician
Single or multimodality behavior-modifying strategies	Single modality	Multimodality
Behavior-modifying strategies employed	Concurrent feedback	Education Concurrent feedback Active participation by physician opinion leader
Disease process	Complex	Simple
Emotional backdrop of issues	High	Low

SUPPORT, Study to Understand Prognoses and Preferences for Outcome and Risks of Treatments; CSMCPI, Cedars-Sinai Medical Center Predictive Index; APACHE, Acute Physiology and Chronic Health Evaluation; TISS, Therapeutic Intervention Scoring System.

gators concluded that opportunities for more patient–physician communication, although advocated as a major method for improving patient outcomes, may have been inadequate to change established practices even when using objective estimates of patient outcomes. In this study, APACHE III was used to provide objective estimates of severity of illness and SUPPORT 6-month survival estimates were used to provide the likelihood of mortality.

Although the SUPPORT intervention was unsuccessful, this study documented serious problems in the care of hospitalized patients near the end of life. It also demonstrated that the mere accessibility of computer-based projections of survival and functional status to physicians was not adequate in changing clinical behaviors and practices for the dying patient. The SUPPORT investigators suggested that several important processes probably needed to occur for a prognostic scoring system to influence clinical decision making for end-of-life care. These processes included improving the quality of discussions between physicians and patients, improving patients' understanding of their prognoses, increasing physicians' appreciation of patients' preferences for life support measures including CPR, and enhancing physicians' respect for patients' informed refusals of interventions (e.g., writing a DNR order for a patient not wanting CPR).[14]

Hay and colleagues at Cedars-Sinai Medical Center employed a retrospectively validated scoring system using four independent variables (hemodynamics, time from bleeding, comorbidity, and esophagogastroduodenoscopy findings) to objectively predict patient risk for life-threatening complications when presenting to the hospital with upper gastrointestinal tract hemorrhage.[13] The intervention consisted of structured messages posted on patients' charts and by structured telephone interactions by a study physician with patients' attending physicians. Guideline compliance was defined as patient discharge from the hospital within 24 hours of achieving low-risk status. Providing real-time quantitative risk information was associated with an increase in guideline compliance from 30% to 70% ($P < 0.001$) and a decrease in mean hospital length of stay from 4.6 ± 3.5 days to 2.9 ± 1.3 days ($P < 0.001$). No differences in complications, patient health status, or patient satisfaction were found.

Both SUPPORT and the Cedars-Sinai study employed objective measures to estimate patient risk for specific outcomes (e.g., low-risk status following upper gastrointestinal hemorrhage, prolonged ICU stays) (Table 5–1). The Cedars-Sinai study provided categorical risk information as low, intermediate, and high for life-threatening complications in patients with a specific disease process as opposed to the continuous probability risk data provided in SUPPORT. The Cedars-Sinai study was successful in achieving a practice change whereas SUPPORT was not. In general, the use of combination methods for achieving behavior modification is superior to using single element implementation strategies.[15] Both studies employed concurrent feedback of risk estimates (regarding patient outcomes in SUPPORT and likelihood for adverse events in the Cedars-Sinai study) to the treating physician. However, SUPPORT attempted to alter physician practices used in a complex process (i.e., care of the dying patient) that is often confounded by high-intensity emotions of the health care providers, the patients, and their families. The care of patients with acute gastrointestinal hemorrhage can be more objectively defined and should be associated with less emotional turmoil than in end-of-life decision making. The Cedars-Sinai study directly employed physician leaders to be involved in the behavior-modifying process, whereas this did not occur in SUPPORT. Additionally, the Cedars-Sinai study provided guideline-directed clinical management suggestions, in addition to risk information, that were developed and validated at the institution. These latter two properties may have been the most important differences between these two interventions. Other investigations have shown the importance of having physician leaders, local opinion setters, or other "champions" of the change process involved in order to optimize its likelihood for success.[16,17]

In summary, these two investigations offer insight on how best to design interventions aimed at changing clinician behaviors. Changes in hospital culture, physician practices, and societal expectations will be required to successfully change the care of dying patients.[14] Unfortunately, scoring systems and prediction models alone will be unable to achieve this goal. Nevertheless, they may be used as aids in clinical decision making and act as a check for avoiding serious errors in clinical judgement.[1,2,18] Additionally, validated objective prediction models can be used as education tools, as was done in the Cedars-Sinai study, to educate physicians on the best practices for their patients. Finally, behavior-modifying strategies appear necessary, along with the use of prediction instruments, to develop effective interventions for improving the care of hospitalized patients. The Cedars-Sinai study suggests that a multimodality approach to behavior modification (e.g., education of health care providers, regular concurrent feedback on practice, use of a local leader to facilitate behavior changes) is the most likely one to succeed.

Should Objective Measures of Risk Change Behaviors for the Care of Dying Patients?

Objective measures of risk should be employed to standardize specific aspects of medical care, especially for patients with serious medical conditions requiring complex decision making and invasive interventions. However, such risk estimates need to be part of a systematic approach or process whose main goal is to improve patient outcomes and the process of providing medical care. Improving the quality of care usually requires some change in the organization and culture of the hospital with the active support of hospital leaders. Without such change and support, objective measures of risk will be ineffective in promoting practice changes. Objective scoring systems should be simply viewed as tools to help facilitate the improvement process and to validate its success or failure. The importance of having a cooperative culture within the hospital to facilitate change has recently been reviewed.[19] Such a spirit of cooperation may partially explain the success of the intervention at Cedars-Sinai Medical Center, which has a long history of establishing protocols and standardized approaches for the management of various medical processes. Physicians who perceive change as threatening their self-esteem, sense of competence, or autonomy will generally oppose a change initiative.[15]

Figure 5–1 offers a general outline of how objective scoring systems can be integrated into a model for improving the care of dying patients. This is based, in part, on similar models used to enhance customer satisfaction in the business world.[20] A fundamental principal of such change or improvement models is to have a continuous process in place for the identification and testing of improvement concepts. Therefore, if a Plan-Do-Study-Act (PDSA) cycle is used to improve patient–physician discussions of DNR orders, for example,

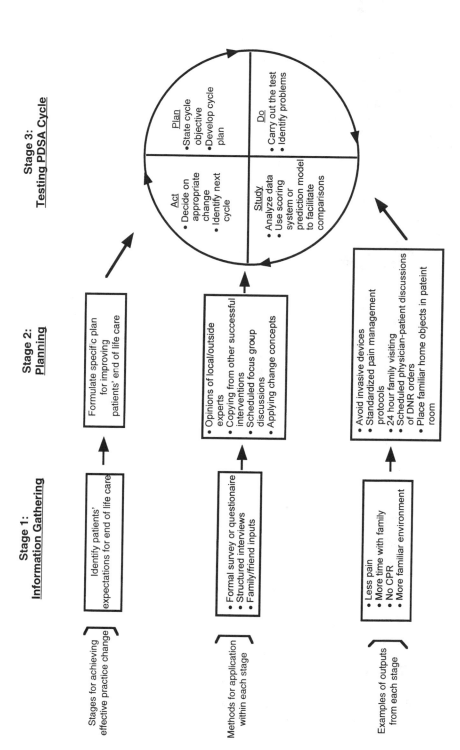

Figure 5-1. A potential roadmap for improving end-of-life care in the ICU setting. CPR, cardiopulmonary resuscitation; DNR, do-not-resuscitate; PDSA, Plan-Do-Study-Act.

Table 5–2. Processes for improving medical care near the end of life that are aided by formalized scoring systems

---

1. Identifying patients who are likely near the end of life through severity-of-illness models such as APACHE, SAPS, PRISM, and MPM as well as through models aimed at identifying organ system failures
2. Comparing data for patients at different institutions and individual ICUs, for patients treated by different attending physicians, or according to exposure to a specific practice or intervention to identify variations in practices (e.g., use of DNR orders, withdrawal of life support)
3. To set automatic thresholds for review or intervention. For example, an ICU could establish an end-of-life team that would automatically review the care of patients with specific severity-of-illness scores and organ failure scores.
4. To assess the impact of an end-of-life intervention on the use of futile therapy in the ICU setting

---

APACHE, Acute Physiology and Chronic Health Evaluation; SAPS, Simplified Acute Physiology Score; PRISM, Pediatric Risk of Mortality; MPM, Mortality Prediction Model.

then the next cycle is immediately planned to further improve this issue or to address another related issue.[21,22]

In terms of end-of-life issues, the use of objective scoring systems should be able to enhance institutional processes aimed at improving end-of-life care. They should be used as a means of validating clinical decision making and facilitating the improvement process rather than attempting to be the sole stimulus for change. Table 5–2 provides a framework for improving the care of patients near the end of life through the use of formal prediction instruments. At a minimum, objective predictors of outcome can be used to compare patients at different time periods or institutions to more objectively assess the influence of variations in practice patterns on clinical outcomes for these groups of patients.

Using severity of illness models to identify patients near the end of life

Severity-of-illness models or prognostic scoring systems can be used by clinicians to identify patients who are likely to be near the end of life. This offers the opportunity to tailor the care of such patients in a way that is more consistent with their poor prognosis. For example, painful or uncomfortable interventions could be limited in these patients while comfort measures become the top priority. Many prognostic models have been developed in an attempt to achieve the above stated aim. For illustrative purposes, I will describe two prediction models that focus primarily on multiple organ dysfunction.

Marshall and co-workers developed a Multiple Organ Dysfunction Score based on six organ systems (respiratory, renal, hepatic, cardiovascular, hematologic, and central nervous system).[23] Descriptions for each organ system were developed, and each was assigned a score from 0 to 4, with 4 indicating the greatest degree of organ dysfunction. For both the development set of patients and the validation set of patients, a score of >20 was associated with a 100%

mortality. Therefore, it can be strongly argued that patients with a Multiple Organ Dysfunction Score of >20 are receiving futile care in the ICU setting.

Kollef and Allen have prospectively validated a previously developed two-factor model as a predictor of mortality for medical ICU patients requiring abdominal surgery.[24,25] Patients having an APACHE II score >18 and three or more acquired organ system derangements had a hospital mortality rate >60%. Although not a perfect marker of mortality, these data suggest that patients meeting the above criteria are the least likely to benefit from surgery. Additionally, early identification of such patients could allow the establishment of therapeutic limits leading to the withdrawal of life-sustaining interventions either before or after surgery. Similarly, Bosscha and colleagues demonstrated that a combination of two objective scoring systems (APACHE II and the Mannheim Peritonitis Index [MPI]) could be used to define futility in patients with abdominal surgery.[26] In this study, all patients with an APACHE II score >20 and an MPI >27 died in the hospital.

Using objective scoring systems for patient comparisons

Objective prediction tools can also be used to compare practices and clinical outcomes between medical institutions, individual ICUs, and different time periods in order to identify variations in practice that relate to outcome differences. Such comparisons offer the possibility of identifying individual practices associated with more desirable outcomes, which could potentially be incorporated into settings having less desirable clinical outcomes. Variability in medical practices is used as a natural experiment to link practices to outcomes.[1]

The variability that currently exists in medical practices related to end-of-life decision making is another powerful argument for introducing some objective measures into the decision-making process. Keenan and colleagues evaluated 160 patient deaths in six Canadian community hospitals and 292 patient deaths in three teaching hospitals.[27] They found a difference in the distribution of the mode of death between these classes of hospitals: a greater proportion of patients died as a result of withholding life support in community hospitals than in teaching hospitals (11.9% vs. 3.8% respectively, $P = 0.004$). Kollef and Ward prospectively examined 501 consecutive admissions to a medical ICU.[28] There were 113 (22.6%) deaths, with 87 (77%) of the dying patients having a private attending physician and 26 (23%) having no access to a private attending physician. Despite a similar severity of illness, patients with a private attending physician were significantly less likely to have life-sustaining therapies withdrawn prior to death than were patients without access to a private attending physician (29.9% vs. 80.8%; $P < 0.001$). Multivariate analysis also demonstrated that access to a private attending physician was independently associated with white race, private health insurance (fee-for-service or capitated health insurance), severity of illness according to APACHE II, and the presence of advance directives.

Identification of specific practice differences between hospitals and physicians were demonstrated in the above two studies examining end-of-life practice.[27,28] Objective scoring systems can help to compare patient populations to determine if severity of illness or some other categorical variable accounts for such observed practice differences. More importantly, objective scoring systems may subsequently be implemented in concert with interventions aimed at modifying or reducing the variability of such practices as was attempted in the SUPPORT study.[12]

Use of prediction instruments to set automatic thresholds for review or intervention

Scoring systems have been advocated as tools for setting objective measures or triggers for specific interventions or lack of interventions. Most efforts to date have focused on the identification of low-risk patients, through use of these methods, to allow triage of these patients to less intensive hospital areas, allowing ICU resources to be spared for patients requiring a higher level of care.[29,30] The Cedars-Sinai study demonstrated that such scoring systems, when linked to a structured patient care plan or intervention, can be successful in reducing the use of ICU resources for low-risk patients. Unfortunately, the use of similar triggers (i.e., objective scoring systems) for effecting the care of patients near the end of life has not been clearly demonstrated. The SUPPORT trial attempted to accomplish this using formal risk estimates of outcome, but it was unsuccessful.

Although no successful examples of using objective scoring systems proactively to limit futile intensive care at the end of life can be identified, these types of systems hold some promise for the future. This may be especially true for specific subgroups of patients, such as those with underlying malignancies that are generally associated with poor outcomes. Several groups of investigators have suggested that formal prediction models or outcome models can be employed to assist clinicians in objectively discussing limits to medical care for patients with advanced malignancies or malignancies not responding to therapies.[31,32]

Using formal scoring systems to assess the impact of end-of-life interventions

Objective scoring systems may also be used to assess the impact of an end-of-life intervention in terms of its successful limitation of invasive therapies. Field and Campbell and colleagues have reported the results of the Comprehensive Supportive Care Team (CSCT) at the Detroit Receiving Hospital. This team was developed to offer supportive care as an alternative to traditional ICU management for patients who were hopelessly ill.[33-35] The team was composed of a clinical nurse specialist experienced in critical care, a staff physician who was in critical care or internal medicine, a chaplain, social worker, respiratory therapist, and the patient's primary nurse. Care was designed to address the physical, psychological, and spiritual needs of the patient and the family by eliminating invasive monitoring and procedures; relieving pain, giving analgesies, sedatives, and music therapy; relieving dyspnea, fever, and anxiety; and providing unrestricted visiting, counseling, and support to families. While these studies do not report any satisfaction measures, they do report significant decreases in clinical interventions and in Therapeutic Intervention Scoring System (TISS) points from 17 to 11 ($P < 0.001$).[34] Additionally, these investigators demonstrated that critically ill patients receiving "comfort-only" care can be effectively managed outside of the ICU setting.[35]

These investigations suggest that objective measures or scoring systems could be used to facilitate clinical practices aimed at improving patient care near the end of life. Instead of simply being predictors of death or some other outcome, these scoring systems should be part of a systematic approach to dealing with the dying patient (Figure 5–1). Changes in clinical behavior will most likely occur when changes in hospital culture and physician behaviors are undertaken.[15] Scoring systems may assist in this process in several important ways, as shown in Table 5–2. By providing unbiased risk estimates of outcome, scoring systems can be used to more objectively monitor clinical practices and help select interventions that have a demonstrated ability to improve patient outcomes.

Can Futility Be Objectively Defined?

A simple definition of futility in terms of medical care would be performing treatments that have no reasonable chance of achieving a therapeutic benefit for the patient.[36] Unfortunately, this definition does not provide an exact quantitative measurement of a "reasonable chance." In attempting to provide a quantitative definition of futility, Schneiderman and colleagues have proposed that when physicians conclude (either through personal experience, experiences shared with colleagues, or consideration of reported empiric data) that in the last 100 cases a medical treatment has been useless, they should regard that treatment as futile.[36,37] Determining that a treatment is futile obligates the physician to communicate this information to the patient and family to aid in decision making. Several authors have suggested that under some circumstances, physicians are professionally obligated to resist initiating futile treatments and to withdraw treatments determined to be futile.[38,39]

Opponents to quantifying futility have argued that few treatments can be judged futile on the basis of having a less than 1 in 100 chance of success and that more stringent criteria based on well-designed clinical trials are required.[39-41] Unfortunately, well-defined scoring systems that are both clinically relevant and easy to apply have not been forthcoming for addressing the issue of medical futility. Nevertheless, several initial attempts have been made to objectively define futility. Mechanical ventilation following bone marrow transplantation and CPR for hospitalized patients will be briefly discussed as examples of conditions for which quantitative thresholds exist to help define potentially futile medical practices.

Bone marrow transplant patients

Rubenfeld and Crawford have studied extensively the bone marrow transplant patient population at the Fred Hutchinson Cancer Research Center in Seattle, Washington.[42-44] They have identified a set of objective risk factors that define medical futility for this patient population.[44] In their experience, patients undergoing bone marrow transplantation who developed respiratory failure requiring mechanical ventilation and who either required more than 4 hours of vasopressor support or had sustained hepatic and renal failure had no chance of survival. Among a cohort of 398 patients meeting these criteria, they found no survivors.[44] Therefore, this prediction rule would fall within the parameters of less than 1 in 100 chance of survival, the above-noted definition of futility. These clinical criteria (e.g., mechanical ventilation, vasopressor support, sustained hepatic and renal failure) should be easily identifiable, making this a relatively simple scoring system to apply. However, despite the presence of such a prediction rule, it appears that physicians are not yet effectively utilizing mortality prediction data in their clinical decision making to either withhold or withdraw life support from this specific group of patients.[45] This experience is similar to that noted by the SUPPORT investigators—objective measures of patient outcome did not appear to influence the administration of life sustaining therapies to dying patients.[12]

Cardiopulmonary resuscitation

The use of CPR raises many ethical issues, especially in the ICU setting. Murphy and colleagues determined the success rate of CPR in 503 consecutive elderly patients aged 70 years and over in five Boston health care institutions (two acute care hospitals, two chronic care hospitals, one long-term care institution).[46] Of 503 patients, 112 (22%) survived initially, but only 19 (3.8%) survived to hospital discharge. The poorest outcomes were for patients with unwitnessed arrests (1 of 116 survived), terminal arrhythmias such as asystole and electromechanical dissociation (1 of 237 survived), or CPR lasting longer than 15 minutes (1 of 360 survived). Outcomes were poor regardless of whether the cardiopulmonary arrest was in-hospital (17 of 259 survived) or out-of-hospital (2 of 244 survived). Similarly, Karetzky et al. found that over a 3-year period and among 668 hospitalized patients, CPR was successful in only 12 (3.3%) patients in intensive care and 43 (14.0%) patients not in intensive care.[47] These authors concluded that futile resuscitative efforts are routinely performed, in part because physicians and patients are unaware of outcome results and factors influencing survival.

Cardiopulmonary resuscitation in surgical/trauma patients has also been examined to determine potentially futile care. Rosemurgy et al. found that among 12,462 trauma patients cared for by prehospital services, 138 (1.1%) underwent CPR at the scene or during transport.[48] None of those patients survived, and their aggregate medical care costs was $871,186. In 11 cases (8%), tissue for transplantation was procured (only corneas). The authors concluded that the infrequent organ procurement did not seem to justify the cost (primarily borne by hospitals) among this class of patients receiving futile medical care. Smith and colleagues demonstrated that a small number of surgical ICU patients underwent CPR (55 of 5237 patients [1.1%]).[49] Among patients having CPR, 16 (29%) survived longer than 24 hours after CPR but died in the hospital, and 7 (13%) survived to discharge. No patient with a worsening Glasgow Coma Scale, acute physiology score from APACHE II, or any acute organ failure survived, whereas survival was 32% for patients with a stable or improving acute physiology score ($P < 0.001$).

Given the cost and invasiveness of CPR as demonstrated by the above studies, coupled with its lack of overall effectiveness, it seems reasonable to limit this intervention in patients with expected poor outcomes. Withholding or withdrawing CPR from such hospitalized patients (i.e., medical patients with an unwitnessed cardiac arrest, surgical patients with organ failure or worsening acute physiology scores) may be reasonable if it is considered to be futile.

Finally, it is important to note that treatments for some clinical conditions can be characterized as futile without a prognostic scoring system.[37] For example, certain congenital conditions (e.g., anencephaly), chromosomal abnormalities, neurologic degenerations, and advanced organ systems diseases that are incompatible with life and for which organ transplantation is not a feasible option represent futile conditions for medical intervention. The anatomical and physiologic character of these disorders precludes any effective treatment. For such disorders, physicians recognize that treatment is futile according to professional standards of care. However, even for such conditions, variability in the practices of health care providers can be found.[50] This suggests that the opinions of health care providers should be secondary to the wishes of the patient, since individual patients' desires with regard to end of life should take precedence (i.e., ethical principle of autonomy).

Which Clinical Situations Exemplify an Objective Definition of Futility?

For a clinical situation to best fit under the category of medical futility, it needs to be clearly defined and reproducible. The bone marrow transplant patient who develops respiratory failure and septic shock requiring prolonged vasopressor support is an example of a clearly defined clinical situation that can be readily identified as a clinical situation that will most likely result in death.[44] This situation can be easily determined by clinicians at the bedside who should be able to identify all of its elements (e.g., bone marrow transplant, respiratory failure, prolonged vasopressor administration). Similarly, the criteria for futility in a 75-year-old patient with widespread malignancy and progressive septic shock complicated by multiorgan failure (respiratory failure, renal failure, obtundation) can be readily identified.[51,52] Clinical situations in which the prognosis is not as clearly defined are less likely to fit into an objective definition of futility. The situation of a 20-year-old woman with presumed viral encephalitis who requires tracheal intubation for airway protection but shows no recovery after 1 week of obtundation is less clear with regard to futility because of the patient's age and the lack of accurate prognostic information on her encephalopathy to guide the clinicians caring for her.

Clinical situations judged to be futile should ideally be based on sound data. The examples of the bone marrow transplant patient and the patient with widespread malignancy would fulfill this criterion. However, there are many clinical situations for which published data or outcomes are not available for substantiating a determination of futility. For those clinical situations in which adequate clinical data are lacking, the use of a consensus panel that includes patients, public representatives from society as a whole, and physicians may be used to determine clinical situations that are futile.[53] Additionally, outcomes studies should be generated to make such decision making more objective. It is also important to formalize the definition of futility to the extent possible. Curtis and colleagues found that medical residents had grave misunderstandings of the concepts of both quantitative and qualitative futility.[54] They suggested that education about futility be incorporated into medical education to facilitate changes in practices.

Additional criteria for determining clinical situations that fit futility include the treating physicians having adequate experience for the clinical situation at hand, and readily defined outcomes. It would be difficult for a physician with little or no experience in treating lung transplant patients who develop respiratory failure secondary to graft rejection to make a determination of medical futility. Similarly, it would be unreasonable to expect a physician who infrequently treats critically ill patients to make accurate assessments regarding individual prognoses and determination of futility. Thus experienced physicians, with expertise in critical care medicine, should make these types of determinations.[55,56] In terms of having clearly defined outcomes for establishing medical futility, those outcomes other than mortality should be considered in medical decision making (e.g., functional status, quality of life) as was done in SUPPORT. These specific outcomes, which should be discussed with patients, can have a great impact on decisions to withhold or withdraw life-sustaining medical care.[57] Finally, open discussions about patients' prognoses and preferences, available medical interventions and their limitations, and opinions of the medical care providers are important components of good-quality medical care regardless of whether objective criteria for medical futility are met.

Potential Downside of Limiting Futile Care

Although limiting ineffective care in critically ill patients is a reasonable goal, it should not be sought at the expense of potentially beneficial care. Cher and Lenert demonstrated that a total of 3914 (4.8%) of 81,494 Medicare patients experienced potentially ineffective care in California.[58] Potentially ineffective care was defined as the occurrence of in-hospital death or death within 100 days of hospital discharge, and resource use (total hospital costs) above the 90th percentile. The occurrence of potentially ineffective care was significantly less likely among health maintenance organization (HMO) members than for non–HMO members (adjusted odds ratio, 0.75; 95% confidence interval, 0.65 to 0.87). However, HMO members were not more likely to experience in-hospital death and were only slightly more likely to experience death by 100 days after hospital discharge. The authors concluded that HMO practices may be better at limiting or avoiding injudicious use of critical care near the end of life. However, another interpretation of these findings was that there was an 8% increase in 100-day mortality and a 9% increase in mortality 1 year after hospitalization for HMO members.[59] One potential explanation for this finding is that managed care may also have limited potentially effective care, resulting in the observed mortality difference.

Another consideration with regard to futility models is that they may not result in significant cost savings, especially if elaborate administrative structures are required to support their implementation. Teno and co-workers examined the impact of prognosis-based futility guidelines on survival and hospital length of stay in a cohort of seriously ill adults in the five SUPPORT hospitals.[60] Of 4301 patients, 115 (2.7%) had an estimated probability of surviving 2 months that was ≤1%. These 115 patients had total hospital charges of $8.8 million. By using the 1% futility guideline, 199 of 1688 (10.8%) of hospital days would have been forgone, with an estimated savings of $1.2 million in hospital charges. Nearly 75% of the savings would have resulted from stopping treatment for 12 patients, 6 of whom were under 51 years old. Implementation of a strict, prognosis-based futility guideline using probability estimates would have resulted in only a modest cost savings. Therefore, cost savings per se should not be viewed as the primary impetus for initiating such guidelines. Rather, limiting patient suffering and discomfort during the dying process should be seen as the goal of such interventions.

Summary

Objective scoring systems and prediction models for the prediction of clinical outcomes in the ICU setting should be viewed as tools to be employed by clinicians caring for the critically ill. These tools should be used to identify patients at risk for a specific outcome (e.g., mortality, poor long-term functional status). By themselves, these methods cannot be expected to alter clinical practices. This requires having a multidisciplinary approach to the care of critically ill patients that includes a cooperative culture having as one of its aims the continuous improvement of patient care and the processes associated with that care. In this way, general scoring systems like APACHE or more disease-specific models like the bone marrow transplant model may be used to improve the care of dying patients. At least one community-based initiative to define and limit futile and inappropriate care is developing a definition of futility on the basis of organ failure scoring methods.[61]

References

1. Kollef MH, Schuster DP. Predicting intensive care unit outcome with scoring systems. Underlying concepts and principles. *Crit Care Clin* 1994;10:1–18.
2. Luce JM, and Wachter RM. The ethical appropriateness of using prognostic scoring systems in clinical management. *Crit Care Clin* 1994;10:229–241.
3. Watts CM, Knaus WA. The case for using objective scoring systems to predict intensive care unit outcome. *Crit Care Clin* 1994;10:73–89.
4. Feinstein AR. An additional basic science for clinical medicine: I. The constraining fundamental paradigms. *Ann Intern Med* 1983;99:393–397.
5. Dawson NV, Arkes HR. Systematic errors in medical decision making: judgement limitations. *J Gen Intern Med* 1987;2:183–187.
6. Knaus WA, Wagner DP, Lynn J. Short-term mortality predictions for critically ill hospitalized adults: science and ethics. *Science* 1991;254:389–394.
7. Rabeneck L, Feinstein AR, Horwitz RI, Wells CK. A new clinical prognostic staging system for acute pacreatitics. *Am J Med* 1993;95:61–70.
8. Singh N, Gayowski T, Wagener MM, Marino IR. Outcome of patients with cirrhosis requiring intensive care unit support: prospective assessment of predictors of mortality. *J Gastroenterol* 1998;33:73–79.
9. Seneff MG, Zimmerman JE, Knaus WA, Wagner DP, Draper EA. Predicting the duration of mechanical ventilation. The importance of disease and patient characteristics. *Chest* 1996;110:469–479.
10. Conway AC, Keller RB, Wennberg DE. Partnering with physicians to achieve quality improvements. *Jt Comm J Qual Improv* 1995;21:619–626.
11. Gimshaw JM, Hutchinson A. Clinical practice guidelines—do they enhance value for money in health care? *Br Med Bull* 1995;51:927–940.
12. The SUPPORT Principal Investigators. A controlled trial to improve care for seriously ill hospitalized patients. The Study to Understand Prognoses and Preferences for Outcome and Risks of Treatments (SUPPORT). *JAMA* 1995;274:1591–1598.
13. Hay JA, Maldonado L, Weingarten SR, Ellrodt AG. Prospective evaluation of a clinical guideline recommending hospital length of stay in upper gastrointestinal tract hemorrhage. *JAMA* 1997;278:2151–2156.
14. Lo B. Improving care near the end of life. Why is it so hard? *JAMA* 1995;274:1634–1636.
15. Clemmer TP, Spuhler VJ. Developing and gaining acceptance for patient care protocols. *New Horizons* 1998;6:12–19.

16. Blumenthal D. Total quality management and physicians' clinical decisions. *JAMA* 1993;269:2775–2778.
17. Lomas J, Enkin M, Anderson GM, Hannah WJ, Vayda E, Singer J. Opinion leaders vs. audit and feedback to implement practice guidelines: delivery after previous cesarean section. *JAMA* 1991;265:2202–2207.
18. Koperna T, Schultz F. Prognosis and treatment of peritonitis. Do we need new scoring systems? *Arch Surg* 1996;131:180–186.
19. Clemmer TP, Spuhler VJ, Berwick DM, Nolan TW. Cooperation: the foundation of improvement. *Ann Intern Med* 1998;128:1004–1009.
20. Langley GJ, Nolan KM, Nolan TW, Norman CL, Provost LP. The Improvement Guide. A Practical Approach to Enchancing Organizational Performance. *San Francisco:* Jossey-Bass Publishers, 1996, pp. 50–73.
21. Rainey TG, Kabcenell A, Berwick DM, Roessner J. Reducing Costs and Improving Outcomes in Adult Intensive Care. Boston: Institute for Healthcare Improvement, 1998, pp. 28–39.
22. Brock WA, Nolan K, Nolan T. Pragmatic science: accelerating the improvement of critical care. *New Horizons* 1998;6:61–68.
23. Marshall JC, Cook DJ, Christou NV, Bernard GR, Sprung CL, Sibbald WJ. Multiple Organ Dysfunction Score: a reliable descriptor of a complex clinical outcome. *Crit Care Med* 1995;23:1638–1652.
24. Kollef MH, Allen BT. Determinants of outcome for patients in the medical intensive care unit requiring abdominal surgery. A prospective, single-center study. *Chest* 1994;106:1822–1828.
25. Kollef MH, Allen BT. Outcome in medical intensive care unit patients requiring abdominal surgery: prospective validation of a risk classificaion system. *South Med J* 1997;90:405–412.
26. Bosscha K, Reijnders K, Hulstaert PF, Algra A, van der Werken C. Prognostic scoring systmes to predict outcome in peritonitis and intra-abdominal sepsis. *Br J Surg* 1997;84:1532–1534.
27. Keenan SP, Busche KD, Chen LM, Esmail R, Inman KJ, Sibbald WJ. Withdrawal and withholding of life suport in the intensive care unit: a comparison of teaching and community hospitals. *Crit Care Med* 1998;26:245–251.
28. Kollef MH, Ward S. The influence of access to a private attending physician on the withdrawal of life-sustaining therapies in the intensive care unit. *Crit Care Med* 1999;27:2125–2132.
29. Wagner DP, Knaus WA, Draper EA. Identification of low-risk monitoring admissions to medical-surgical ICUs. *Chest* 1987;92:423–428.
30. Henning RJ, McClish D, Daly B, Nearman H, Franklin C, Jackson D. Clinical characteristics and resource utilization of ICU patients: implications for organization of intensive care. *Crit Care Med* 1987;15:264–269.
31. Jackson SR, Tweeddale MG, Barnett MJ, Spinelli JJ, Sutherland HJ, Reece DE, Klingemann HG, Nantel SH, Fung HC, Toze CL, Phillips GL, Shepherd JD. Admission of bone marrow transplant recepients to the intensive care unit: outcome, survival and prognostic factors. *Bone Marrow Transplant* 1998;21:697–704.
32. Escalante CP, Martin CG, Elting LS, Rubenstein EB. Medical futility and appropriate medical care in patients whose death is thought to be imminent. *Support Care Cancer* 1997;5:274–280.
33. Field B, Devich LE, Carlson RW. Impact of a comprehensive supportive care team

on management of hopelessly ill patients with multiple organ failure. *Chest* 1989;96:353–356.

34. Campbell ML, Field BE. Management of the patient with do no resuscitate status: compassion and cost containment. *Heart Lung* 1991;20:345–348.

35. Campbell ML, Thill-Baharozian M. Impact of the DNR therapeutic plan on patient care requirements. *Am J Crit Care* 1994;3:202–207.

36. Schneiderman LJ, Jecker NS, Jonsen AR. Medical futility: its meaning and ethical implications. *Ann Intern Med* 1990;112:949–954.

37. Schneiderman LJ, Jecker NS, Jonsen AR. Medical futility: response to critics. *Ann Intern Med* 1996;125:669–674.

38. Luce JM. Withholding and withdrawal of life support: ethical, legal and clinical aspects. *New Horizons* 1997;5:30–37.

39. Jecker NS, Schneiderman LJ. Medical futility: the duty not to treat. *Cambridge Q Healthcare Ethics* 1993;2:151–159.

40. Guidelines for cardiopulmonary resuscitation and emergency cardiac care. Emergency Cardiac Care Committee and Subcommittees, American Heart Association. Part VIII: ethical considerations in resuscitation. *JAMA* 1992;268:2282–2288.

41. Brody BA, Halevy A. Is futility a futile concept? *J Med Philosy* 1995;20:123–144.

42. Crawford SW, Schwartz DA, Petersen FB, Clark JG. Mechanical ventilation after marrow transplantation. Risk factors and clinical outcome. *Rev Respir Dis* 1988;137:682–687.

43. Crawford SW, Petersen FB. Long-term survival from respiratory failure after marrow transplantation. *Am Rev Respir Dis* 1992;145:510–514.

44. Rubenfeld GD, Crawford SW. Withdrawing life support from mechanically ventilated recipients of bone marrow transplants: a case for evidence-based guidelines. *Ann Intern Med* 1996;125:625–633.

45. Crawford SW. Using outcomes research to improve the mangement of blood and marrow transplant recipients in the intensive care unit. *New Horizons* 1998;6:69–74.

46. Murphy DJ, Murray AM, Robinson BE, Campion EW. Outcomes of cardiopulmonary resuscitation in the elderly. *Ann Intern Med* 1989;111:199–205.

47. Karetzky M, Zubair M, Parikh J. Cardiopulmonary resuscitation in intensive care unit and non-intensive care unit patients. Immediate and long-term survival. *Arch Intern Med* 1995;155:1277–1280.

48. Rosemurgy AS, Norris PA, Olson SM, Hurst JM, Albrink MH. Prehospital traumatic cardiac arrest: the cost of futility. *J Trauma* 1993;35:468–473.

49. Smith DL, Kim K, Cairns BA, Fakhry SM, Meyer AA. Prospective analysis of outcome after cardiopulmonary resuscitation in critically ill surgical patients. *J Am Coll Surg* 1995;180:394–401.

50. Cook DJ, Guyatt GH, Jaeschke R, Reeve J, Spanier A, King D, Molloy DW, William A, Streiner DL. Determinants in Canadian healthcare workers of the decision to withdraw life support from the critically ill. *JAMA* 1995;273:703–708.

51. Ewer MS, Ali MK, Atta MS, Morice RC, Balakrishnan PV. Outcome of lung cancer patients requiring mechanical ventilation for pulmonary failure. *JAMA* 1986;256:3364–3366.

52. Schuster DP, Marion JM. Precendents for meaningful recovery during treatment in a medical intensive care unit: outcome in patients with hematological malignancy. *Am J Med* 1983;75:402–408.

53. Alpers A, Lo B. When is CPR futile? *JAMA* 1995;273:156–158.
54. Curtis JR, Park DR, Krone MR, Pearlman RA. Use of a medical futility rationale in do-not-resuscitation orders. *JAMA* 1995;273:124–128.
55. Carsson SS, Stocking C, Podsadecki T, Christenson J, Pohlman A, MacRae S, Jordan J, Humphrey H, Siegler M, Hall J. Effect of organizational change in the medical intensive care unit of a teaching hospital: a comparison of 'open and 'closed' formats. *JAMA* 1996;276:322–328.
56. Multz AS, Chalfin DB, Samson IM, Dantzker DR, Fein AM, Steinberg HN, Nierderman MS, Scharf SM. A 'closed' medical intensive care unit (MICU) improves resource utilization when compared with an 'open' MICU. *Am J Respir Crit Care Med* 1998;157:1468–1473.
57. Weeks JC, Cook EF, O'Day SJ, Peterson LM, Wenger N, Reding D, Harrell FE, Kossin P, Dawson NV, Connors AF Jr, Lynn J, Phillips RS. Relationship between cancer patients' predictions of prognosis and their treatment preferences. *JAMA* 1998;279:1709–1714.
58. Cher DJ, Lenert LA. Method of Medicare reimbursement and the rate of potentially ineffective care of critically ill patients. *JAMA* 1997;278:1001–1026.
59. Curtis JR, Rubenfeld GD. Aggressive medical care at the end of life. Does capitated reimbursement encourage the right care for the wrong reason? *JAMA* 1997;278:1025–1026.
60. Teno JM, Murphy D, Lynn J, Tosteson A, Desbiens N, Connors AF Jr, Hamel MB, Wu A, Phillips R, Wenger N. Prognosis-based futility guidelines: does anyone win? *J Am Geriatr Soc* 1994;42:1202–1207.
61. Murphy DJ, Barbour E. GUIDe (Guidelines for the use of intensive care in Denver): a community effort to define futile and inappropriate care. *New Horizons* 1994;2:326–331.

Chapter 6

Transdisciplinary Research to Understand the Role of Bias and Heuristics

DEBORAH J. COOK

*R*esults from biomedical, social science, and psychological studies of end-of-life decision making are just beginning to be integrated into care for patients in the ICU. Concurrent with this trend are qualitative investigations into decision making at the end of life,[1,2] an increasing understanding of the ICU as a social world,[3,4] and calls to assess the ethical[5] and social[6] influences of the use of life support technologies. In this chapter the use of these methods toward understanding end-of-life care in the ICU will be discussed by means of examples from the critical care literature and through a transdisciplinary perspective.

Multidisciplinary research typically involves different investigators studying a given health problem from their own disciplinary perspectives; the product is usually multiple discipline-specific analyses that may mesh well with each other and are usually understood by people within those particular disciplines. Much of the critical care end of life research is multidisciplinary, involving physicians, biostatisticians, and sometimes nurses and others. Interdisciplinary research, however, is a more coordinated effort to investigate a given health problem conjointly from several disciplinary perspectives. This research is still discipline guided, although the process usually yields a hybrid perspective on the same problem. Many critical care research programs studying activity clinimetrically or evaluating health care team behavior, are interdisciplinary. Transdisciplinary research, however, requires investigators from various disciplines to jointly research a problem and strive to understand it from a common, synthetic framework, as opposed to discrete disciplinary perspectives. This challenging type of investigation is well suited to sensitive, complex issues such as the withdrawal of life support technology.

However, different research projects and programs call for different disciplinary representation—not every perspective is relevant to every research question. Advances in our understanding of (not to mention improvement of) the care of patients at the end of life in the ICU will be best enhanced through transdisciplinary research. However, most investigative teams are not ideally represented by all potentially relevant disciplines. Clinicians who read literature on end-of-life care in the ICU, just like consumers of other published evidence, need to consider the influence (and absence) of different disciplinary perspectives on the results of the research they read. For example, what does the discipline of economics bring to the scrutiny of end of life decisions in the ICU? This discipline has traditionally been concerned with publicly visible, obviously expensive technologies such as ventilators, dialysis machines, and ICU beds,[7] yet it casts into bold relief not just the clinical but also the economic consequences of our end-of-life decisions.

The Potential Contribution of Qualitative Research

Clinicians are trained to think mechanically and to draw conclusions using pathophysiologic rationale and deductive reasoning. The biomedical literature reflects this orientation, and we are therefore most familiar with deductive, quantitative research. Quantitative studies (such as epidemiologic investigations and clinical trials) are designed to test well-specified hypotheses concerning a few predetermined variables. However, medicine is not only a mechanistic and quantitative science but also an interpretive art.

The goal of qualitative research is to develop theoretical insights that describe and explain social and emotional phenomena such as interactions, experiences, roles, and organizations. Examples include inquiry about the meaning and interpretation of illness to individuals and families, or the attitudes and behavior of patients and clinicians. Qualitative study is inductive, aiming to discover important variables and generate coherent theory.

In a recent qualitative study, we explored the purposes for which advanced life support technology is used in the care of critically ill, dying patients who are unable to make their own decisions.[8] We observed 25 ICU rounds and 11 family meetings in which withdrawal or withholding of advanced life support was addressed. We conducted semistructured interviews with intensivists, consultants, ICU nurses, the ICU nutritionist, the hospital ethicist, and pastoral services representatives, discussing patients about whom life support decisions were made, as well as life support practices in general. Interview transcripts and field notes were analyzed inductively to identify and corroborate emerging themes; data were coded following modified, grounded theory techniques.[9] Methods to ensure the validity of the work (i.e., triangulation) included corroboration among multiple sources of data, multidisciplinary team consensus, sharing results with participants, and theory triangulation.[10]

First we found that dialogue around withdrawal decisions barely resembled the popular imagery of pulling the plug. Withdrawal is not a decisive event, but an unfolding process. The orchestration of death was the most apt metaphor describing the process of determining which life support technologies come into play, to what ends, when, by whom, and for whom. Clinicians thus use technology to orchestrate the "best" death possible for critically ill patients under difficult circumstances. This goal is concerned less with health outcomes in the traditional sense than it is with the aesthetic, ethical, and social experiences of those involved in the patient's care (e.g., significant others, family members, and clinicians). In this context, technologies are considered analogous to orchestral instruments for expressing values and visions, as well as clinical instruments for producing health.

Second, the withholding or withdrawal of life support can be orchestrated to occur quickly or slowly, changing the tempo of the dying process. The pace at which life supports are withdrawn, and the sequential order of withdrawals, may be dominated by concerns such as the potential suffering experienced by the patient, vicarious suffering experienced by others, and the speed of the consequent death.

Third, life support creates an interlude during which people strive to harmonize their understandings, expectations, and plans for the patient. Family and clinicians work, and wait, for the synchronous acceptance of imminent death. The family may need time to overcome denial that the patient is dying, disbelief that treatment options have run out, or disagreements among themselves that death is ineluctable.

Fourth, at key points in life support decision making, family members and caregivers relate to life support technologies collectively as "technology" itself, rather than discretely as specific technological tools with specific therapeutic uses. Technology thus comes to represent a global approach to achieving the goals of care. Typically, this happens early in the ICU stay when there is a desire to "do everything," and when the objective is saving life.

Finally, the orchestration of life support often concerns the number of technologies in play at once, and whether to add new ones. Life support technologies initiated at an earlier time under a more optimistic prognosis or aggressive management plan may be continued, but additional interventions or life support measures may be withheld. At issue is the intensity of care overall, often more than the merits and demerits of specific interventions. A collective view of technology similarly appears toward the end of the ICU stay as an imperative to "stop doing everything." In this context, the use of technology seems morally offensive, degrading, or dehumanizing. The inherent goal of technology has thus shifted from life saving to death prolonging or pain inducing. In discussions, erstwhile useful instruments are transformed dismissively into "a whole bunch of machines" and a source of discord. A discrete technology (e.g., dialysis) can act as a synecdoche for the more general concept of life support technology and life support goals; by working through a decision about whether to use dialysis, for example, clinicians and family members can begin to address decisions regarding other life supports more generally.

In summary, when life support technology is viewed as a means to orchestrate a death in the ICU, this qualitative research highlights how it can perform functions not well appreciated by conventional frameworks for technology evaluation. Decision making at the end of life concerns not only whether to use life support technology but also how—the timing, intensity, and number of technologies. These decisions are negotiated and nuanced, and are individualized for each patient. Patient autonomy notwithstanding, the orchestration metaphor generated by our analysis alludes to "composers" and "conductors" who coordinate how technologies play out in the ICU.

Bias, Heuristics, and End of Life Decisions

Understanding the notion of bias has undeniably advanced clinicians' ability to critically appraise published research and has improved the design of new investigations. While bias may be characterized by systematic errors that result in deviation from the "truth," random errors "create noise" and may also obscure our understanding of the truth. The notion of bias has crept into several aspects of practice that bear on end-of-life care in the ICU. Bias is often associated with capricious decision making when the prognosis is futile and with whimsical allocation of life support resources including ICU beds.

There are several common clinical biases that form a typology of influences on end-of-life decisions. These include the propensity that clinicians might have to (1) minimize diagnostic uncertainty, (2) minimize prognostic uncertainty, (3) inflate treatment effectiveness, (4) deflate treatment effectiveness, (5) overvalue experience, (6) undervalue experience, (7) overemphasize supportive evidence, (8) underemphasize counterevidence, (9) confuse ignorance with uncertainty, and (10) personify excessive confidence (Table 6–1). Other chapters in this book (Chapters 5, 8, and 9) as well as original research and white papers in critical care literature[11-14] have addressed the foregoing biases (e.g., challenging to use of illness severity scoring systems to prognosticate, exposing misinterpretation or misapplication of the medical literature, and framing bias in talking to families).

A mirror image of these potential biases is embodied in the heuristics of practice.[15] Derived from common sense and experience rather than a set of systematic observations (published or unpublished), heuristics might be devalued by virtue of being potentially biased. Ironically, yet perhaps appropriately, heuristics are less encumbered by such negative connotations. Heuristics are necessary and valued determinants (but should not be the soul determinants) of practice. There are many situations in which clinicians rely heavily on experience and experiential shortcuts to manage information or make decisions.

Table 6–1. A typology of potential biases influencing end-of-life care

Potential bias	Potential consequence
Minimizing diagnostic uncertainty	Failing to extensively work up reversible etiologies of ARDS before approaching withdrawal of life support
Minimizing prognostic uncertainty	Undue reliance on illness severity scores as a predictor of very poor outcome
Inflating treatment effectiveness	Continuation of life support technology that is unlikely to provide sufficient interim support or to improve the underlying pathophysiology
Deflating treatment effectiveness	Withdrawing mechanical ventilation prior to a trial of aggressive lung-protective strategies in ARDS
Overvaluing experience	Focusing on the outcomes of similar prior patients without considering the unique features of each individual patient that might influence survivorship
Undervaluing experience	Failure to consider past experience (personal and global) with similar patients in formulating judgment about probability of mortality
Overemphasizing supportive evidence	Communicating to families about the likely benefit of rescue therapies without acknowledging the promising, albeit unproven, nature of the claim
Underemphasizing counter evidence	Dependence on one positive study favoring an intervention without considering the totality of the best available evidence that shows no treatment effect or harm
Confusing ignorance with uncertainty	Stating that an intervention is of uncertain benefit while remaining unaware of the literature supporting or refuting the statement
Personifying excessive confidence	Portraying, with conviction, that end-of-life decisions are either black and white or right and wrong

These potential biases may influence end-of-life care in the ICU, but they do not always create problematic consequences if patient, family, and caregiver goals are in synchrony.

ARDS, acute respiratory distress syndrome.

Heuristics give rise to helpful rules of thumb that guide us in daily practice. An age-old example is Occam's razor: "choose the simplest hypothesis that explains the observations."

Clinicians caring for patients at the end of life are seldom information-seeking, probabilistic decision makers. These evidence-based attributes are rarely in the forefront during decisions about withdrawal of life support when sound clinical reasoning is neither linear nor unidimensional. Many clinicians reason about individual patients on the basis of analogy, experience, heuristics,

and theory, and only sometimes on a foundation of research evidence[16] during
end-of-life decision making. The heuristics of end-of-life care are just beginning to be taught and studied in the ICU setting. Until recently, they have
been implicit rather than explicit in most training programs and research reports. An example might include the fundamental objective of focusing on the
goals of care. Like heuristics that guide practice in other fields, heuristics that
we use in caring for patients at the end of life in the ICU vary widely and
represent a largely unacknowledged and unmeasured set of influences on practice variation.

The Relation Between Confidence and Decisions

Studies of confidence in ICU decision making have focused on interpreting
results of diagnostic tests and estimating prognosis. In medical and nonmedical
studies, a poor correlation between the rates of "correct" decision making and
associated levels of confidence have been demonstrated. There is a tendency
for the level of confidence to increase as more information (whether relevant
or not) about a particular problem is supplied, as more time is spent on a given
problem, and as the experience of the decision maker with similar problems in
the past increases. Even taking these factors into account, the rate of "correct"
decision making is only modestly better when confidence is high than when it
is low.[17,18] To discuss examples of how confidence bears on end-of-life decisions
in the ICU, it is necessary to emphasize that "correct" decision making is an
untenable construct.

In a national survey of withdrawal of life support in different scenarios,[19] we
analyzed the association between the clinical scenario, the level of care chosen
by the respondents, confidence in the decisions, and the health care worker
group.[20] Responses for each scenario varied widely; the level of care chosen was
dependent on the scenario, the health care worker group, and the confidence
with which the decisions were made. Intensivists were less aggressive than the
ICU nurses, who were less aggressive than the housestaff, but the difference
was small. Overall, respondents were very confident about their decisions 34%
of the time. After adjustment for clinical scenario and chosen level of care,
intensivists were more confident than nurses, who were more confident than
house staff (40% of intensivists were very confident, vs. 29% of nurses, and
23% of house staff). In general, health care workers tended to be more confident when they chose extreme levels of care than when they chose intermediate levels of care. In summary, when given standard information, health care
workers made contradictory decisions yet were still very confident about the
level of care they would administer. Moreover, we found that while confidence
in decisions about withdrawal of life support increased with seniority and authority, consistency of decisions did not.

It is possible that clinicians are more confident at making extreme decisions, although the confidence is unwarranted. An alternative interpretation is

that an intermediate level of care may be chosen when clinicians are unsure of the correct course of action. Or, clinicians may report greater confidence when taking extreme measures, to reduce the cognitive dissonance between what they feel they must do and their uncertainty about the results of their actions.[21] These observations and interpretations indicate that clinicians can be very confident about opposite plans of care for the same patient. However, in reality, decisions about withdrawal of life support are rarely made by an individual, at least in North America; they are made by an ICU team of clinicians in consultation with patients and families. Moreover, a questionnaire is unlikely to capture all the complex information and cues that, in reality, guide clinical decisions. Nevertheless, the relation between confidence and decision making in the ICU requires further study.

Potential Insights From Cognitive Psychology

Several other clinical biases that can potentially influence end-of-life decision making have been studied empirically. The objective of one important study was to determine whether situations involving multiple options can paradoxically influence people to choose an option that would have been declined if fewer options were available.[22] In a mailed survey to family physicians, a case scenario of a 67-year-old male with severe osteoarthritis was described. In the first scenario, there was one nonsteroidal anti-inflammatory drug that he had not tried. In the second, there were two that he had not tried. The physicians were significantly more likely to say "refer to orthopedic surgery and do not start new medication" in response to the second scenario than the first scenario. This survey supports the finding that introduction of additional options can increase decision difficulty and the tendency to choose a distinctive option or maintain the status quo. Awareness of this bias may lead to offering few options in patient or family discussions, or to simplified decision-making processes in complex medical situations.

In a narrative review of selected psychology literature, Redelmeier and colleagues[23] described ways in which intuitive thought processes and feelings may lead patients to make "suboptimal" decisions. Two issues focused on perceptions of risk. The first issue relevant to end-of-life decisions is hindsight bias— the tendency to de-emphasize prior data that are contradictory or ambiguous, and to highlight prior data consistent with a specific outcome. This bias may make end-of-life decision making more comforting, by minimizing conflicting prior information incongruent with a decision to withdraw life support. The second phenomenon is about categorical safety and danger bias—the notion that the illusion of perfect safety is more appealing but less realistic than lowering the risk of an adverse effect. This phenomenon can inhibit a change in plans from the safety and certainty of full technologic support to plans that lower the risk of prolonging the dying process by means of technology.

Three additional themes cited in this review of the psychology literature are relevant to end-of-life care in the ICU. The first is a preference for maintaining the status quo, which we often see manifest as a reluctance to change current life support plans. This tendency is both common and psychologically adaptive for many families and clinicians. The second is loss aversion, or taking actual losses far more seriously than foregone gains. As most families grieve in the ICU setting, the temporal orientation is toward the present and the past. However, future losses experienced as foregone gains are also considered during the withdrawal process, and probably more intensely after the patient's death. It is possible that less emphasis on foregone gains may be psychologically protective in the ICU setting, lest families not be overwhelmed by concurrently experiencing loss across the time continuum of past, present, and future. Future research will be needed to determine whether an approach that de-emphasizes foregone gains allows clinicians to help families with difficult decisions about end-of-life care in the ICU. The third phenomenon that can affect end-of-life care in the ICU is poor prediction of future feelings and a failure to integrate knowledge of future health states with future feelings about future health states. As families grapple with the dying of their loved ones, we need to support them through their current experiences and feelings, and help them to consider (if they are not doing so) their projected future feelings about their loved ones' probable future quality of life. There are no empiric data to inform us how and to what extent decisions to withdraw life support follow the integration of emotional phenomena (e.g., feelings) and cognitive phenomena (e.g., knowledge).

Conclusions

The holistic, team-oriented approach to delivering compassionate critical care during difficult and emotionally loaded end of life decisions signifies the necessity for multifaceted research programs embracing both qualitative and quantitative methods informed by transdisciplinary perspectives. If we are open to evidence generated through such a process, then this empiric knowledge is sure to enlighten us, thereby helping to improve the care we give to dying patients in the ICU.

References

1. Ventres W, Nichter M, Reed R, Frankel R. Limitation of medical care: an ethnographic analysis. *J Clin Ethics* 1993;4:134–145.
2. Singer PA, Martin DK, Kelner M. Quality end-of-life care: patients' perspectives. *JAMA* 1999;281:163–168.
3. Zussman R. Intensive Care. Chicago: University of Chicago Press, 1992.
4. Chambliss DF. Death as an organizational act. In: Beyond Caring: Hospitals,

Nurses, and the Social Organization of Ethics. Chicago: University of Chicago Press, 1996.

5. Gjengedal E. The ethical impact of advanced biomedical technology: on means and ends in high-technology medicine. *Scand J Caring Sci* 1992;6:195–199.

6. Good MJ. Cultural studies of biomedicine: an agenda for research. *Soc Sci Med* 1995;41:461–473.

7. Cook DJ, Sibbald WJ. The progress, the promise and the paradox of technology assessment in the intensive care unit. *Can Med Assoc J* 1999;161:1118–1119.

8. Cook DJ, Giacomini M, Johnson N, Willms D, for the Canadian Critical Care Trials Group. Life support technology in the intensive care unit: a qualitative investigation of purposes. *Can Med Assoc J* 1999;161: 1109–1113.

9. Strauss A, Corbin J. Selective coding. In: Basics of Qualitative Research: Grounded Theory Procedures and Techniques. London: Sage Publishders, 1990, pp. 116–142.

10. Willms D, Best A, Taylor D. A systematic approach to qualitative methods in primary prevention research. *Med Anthropol Q* 1990;4:4(NS).

11. Luce JM. Physicians do not have a responsibility to provide futile or unreasonable care if a patient or family insists. *Crit Care Med* 1995;23:760–766.

12. Task Force on Ethics of the Society of Critical Care Medicine. Consensus report on the ethics of foregoing life-sustaining treatment in the critically ill. *Crit Care Med* 1990;18:1435–1439.

13. American Thoracic Society Bioethics Task Force. Withholding and withdrawing life sustaining therapy. *Am Rev Respir Dis* 1991;144:726–731.

14. Luce JM. Ethical principles in critical care. *JAMA* 1990;263:696–700.

15. McDonald CJ. Medical heuristics: the silent adjudicators of clinical practice. *Ann Intern Med* 1996;124:56–62.

16. Tanenbaum SJ. Sounding board: what physicians know. *N Engl J Med* 1993; 329:1269–1270.

17. Baumann AO, Deber RB, Thompson GG. Over-confidence among physicians and nurses: the "micro-certainty, macro-uncertainty" phenomenon. *Soc Sci Med* 1991; 32:167–174.

18. Paese PW. Influences on the appropriateness of confidence in judgement. Practice, effort, information and decision-making. *Organizat Behav Hum Decision Processes* 1991;48:100–130.

19. Cook DJ, Guyatt GH, Jaeschke R, Reeve J, Spanier A, King D, Molloy DW, Willan A, Streiner D, for the Canadian Critical Care Trials Group. Determinants in Canadian health care workers of the decision to withdraw life support from the critically ill. *JAMA* 1995;273:703–708.

20. Walter S, Cook DJ, Guyatt GH, Spanier A, Jaeschke R, Todd T, Streiner DL, for the Canadian Critical Care Trials Group. Confidence in life support decisions in the ICU: A survey of health care workers. *Crit Care Med* 1998;26:44–49.

21. Skrabanek P, McCormick J. Follies and Fallacies in Medicine. New York; Prometheus Press, 1989.

22. Redelmeier D, Shafir E. Medical decision-making in situations that offer multiple alternatives. *JAMA* 1995;273:302–305.

23. Redelmeier D, Rozin P, Kahneman D. Understanding patients' decisions: Cognitive and emotional perspectives. *JAMA* 1993;270:72–76.

Chapter 7

The Role of Quality of Life and Health Status in Making Decisions about Withdrawing Life-Sustaining Treatments in the ICU

J. RANDALL CURTIS

DONALD L. PATRICK

*T*here is growing concern that disproportionate amounts of health care budgets are spent for end-of-life medical care, and many authors have decried the high cost of dying in our society.[1–3] Part of the reason that this issue has received such attention is the aging of our population and the high proportion of deaths that occur in acute care hospitals.[4] Consequently, practioners and health economists have expressed increasing interest in finding ways to limit the aggressiveness and cost of care at the end of life. There is a widespread belief that older patients and patients with a reduced quality of life due to chronic disease do not want aggressive life-sustaining treatments at the end of life. In this chapter, we will examine empiric data to challenge this assumption and provide ICU clinicians an alternative way of viewing the role of quality of life in decisions about withdrawing life-sustaining therapy.

What is Quality of Life and How Is It Measured?

Quality of life is one of the commonly used "patient-assessed outcomes" that have increasingly been used in research about outcomes of ICU care.[5] If ICU clinicians are going to use data about of quality of life in their decision making in the ICU, it is important that they have a basic understanding of the terminology and methodologies used in this field. Patient-assessed health outcomes can be divided into four major categories: quality of life, health status, health state preferences, and satisfaction with care. In this chapter, we will focus on quality of life and health status measurement. Figure 7–1 shows the relationships between the terms used to describe health status and quality of life,

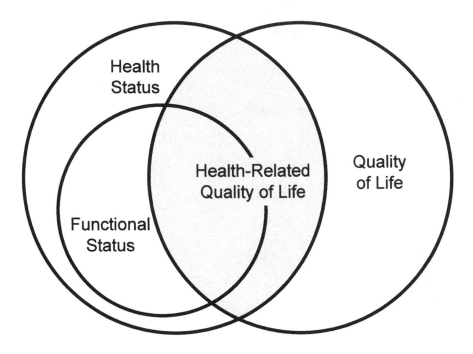

Figure 7–1. Diagram showing overlap of terms used to describe health status and quality of life.

although it is important to understand the distinctions and the overlap. This figure shows the overlap in the operational definitions of these terms; a useful conceptual model of the interactions between these terms and clinical variables has been constructed by Wilson and Cleary.[6] Quality of life and health status are important outcome measures in medicine, public health, and health policy.[7]

The term "quality of life" is widely used in clinical research and clinical care, but is sometimes used to mean different things by different authors. In its broadest definition, the quality of an individual's life is a holistic, self-determined evaluation of satisfaction with issues important to the individual. Quality of life is influenced by many factors, including financial status, housing, employment, spirituality, social support network, and health. Consequently, many medical investigators use the more restrictive term "health-related quality of life" (HRQOL) to mean quality of life as it is affected by health. The term "functional status" is used to describe an individual's ability to function in such diverse realms as physical, social, and emotional. These two terms, HRQOL and functional status, are often used interchangeably, but they represent different concepts. *Functional status* reflects the ability to perform the tasks of daily life, while *HRQOL* connotes the subjective experience of the impact of health status on the quality of life. Operationally, many of the instruments designed to measure HRQOL or functional status encompass both, which can make it difficult to distinguish these concepts in practical applications.

An increasing number of studies have tried to characterize the HRQOL of patients in the ICU.[8] Some studies assess HRQOL in the diverse population of critically ill patients[9] while others focus on individual diseases or syndromes. For example, there is a growing literature on the quality of life of survivors of the acute respiratory distress syndrome (ARDS).[10-14] McHugh and colleagues showed that the HRQOL of ARDS survivors improved during the first 6 months following hospital discharge, but then stabilized at a level significantly below normal.[10] Davidson and colleagues showed that patients with ARDS have a significantly lower HRQOL than critically ill patients with a similar severity of illness but without ARDS.[11] Similarly, other studies are uniform in their observation that survivors of acute lung injury and ARDS have significant reductions in HRQOL compared to population norms.[12-14] However, while HRQOL is an important outcome of critical care, measurement of HRQOL occurs infrequently in the critical care literature and the studies that do assess HRQOL frequently have important methodologic problems.[8]

How Does Quality of Life Affect Patients' Medical Decision Making?

Elderly individuals and patients with a burden of chronic diseases often suffer progressive decline in functional status and quality of life. It seems intuitive that as patients' quality of life decrease, so will their interests in undergoing aggressive life-sustaining medical treatments. If this is true, we should be able to use quality of life as one way to understand and communicate about patients' treatment preferences for life-sustaining care at the end of life.

There have been a number of studies that have examined patients' preferences for undergoing life-sustaining medical care as a function of their projected quality of life after such care. These studies have shown that most patients say that they would forego life-sustaining treatment if their quality of life after treatment is severely impaired.[15-18] This same finding is true for patients who know what it is like to receive intensive care because they have had a life-threatening illness treated in the ICU.[19] These studies convincingly show that most patients say they would not want aggressive medical care if the outcome of such care were a severely reduced quality of life such as persistent vegetative state or dependence on others for all of the activities of daily living.

However, these data should not be extrapolated to make the assumption that patients who currently have a low, but not severely reduced, quality of life prefer less aggressive medical care. The studies cited above use hypothetical future health states that involve a very poor quality of life, such as persistent vegetative state or severe stroke. In fact, many of these health states are so severely impaired that it is not possible to assess the patients' perspective of them. However, when studies measure patients' *current* quality of life, there is no or very little correlation between quality of life and patients' preferences for aggressive life-sustaining medical care.[15,20-23] This finding is also true for those patients who have received care in the ICU in the past and therefore know what this care entails.[20] In fact, in some studies, patients with decreased HRQOL and patients with depression actually prefer more aggressive medical treatment.[24]

Finally, it is important for clinicians to understand the role that the treatment itself may play in some patients' preference for life-sustaining therapy. In a study of patients' preferences for life-sustaining therapy in different health states, some patients reported that they would not want life-sustaining therapy even if the outcome were a health state that they considered to be preferable to death.[25] In these circumstances, patients seem to weigh the burdens of treatment itself into the decision to prefer to forego treatment. Nursing home residents and elderly outpatients are more likely to consider the burden of treatment than younger, healthy adults. Therefore, clinicians should consider the burden of treatment in discussions with patients and families about life-sustaining therapy.

How Does Quality of Life Affect Clinicians' Medical Decision Making?

There is evidence that physicians make the incorrect assumption that patients with lower current quality of life want less life-sustaining therapy. In a study of 258 elderly outpatients, there was no or very little significant correlation between patients' quality of life and their treatment preferences for CPR or mechanical ventilation.[21] However, when the patients' primary care physicians were asked whether the physician thought the patient would want CPR or mechanical ventilation, there was a significant correlation between physicians' impressions of patients' treatment preferences and patients' quality of life. These data suggest that physicians assume that patients with lower current quality of life want less life-sustaining therapy when in fact this is not the case. Since physician prediction of patients' treatment preferences may have an important effect on treatments received,[26] these findings imply that patients with poor, but measurable, quality of life may receive less life-sustaining medical care than they would otherwise choose. Therefore, physicians should be careful that they do not make incorrect assumptions about patients' treatment preferences based on the patient's quality of life.

Implications for Clinical Practice in the ICU

The belief that patients with lower quality of life prefer less aggressive medical care has made it into clinical practice and bedside decision making. Unfortunately, most clinicians are not aware of the weak connection between patients' current quality of life and their treatment preferences. Patients and doctors infrequently communicate about end-of-life care prior to life-threatening illness[27] and patients' family members and primary care physicians are frequently unable to predict patients' preferences for end-of-life care.[28-30] Therefore, current medical practice runs the risk of making inaccurate assumptions about patient treatment preferences based on physician or surrogate interpretation of patients' quality of life. Consequently, it is important that ICU clinicians not make assumptions about patient treatment preferences based on the patients' quality of life. Instead, clinicians should take the time to discuss treatment preferences and goals of therapy with patients and their families.

References

1. Bayer R, Callahan D, Fletcher J, Hodgson T., Jennings B, Monsees D, Sieverts S., Veatch R. The care of the terminally ill: mortality and economics. *N Engl J Med* 1983;309:1490–1494.

2. Schroeder SA, Showstack JA, Schwartz J. Survival of adult high-cost patients: report of a follow-up study from nine acute-care hospitals. *JAMA* 1981;245:1446–1449.

3. Turnbull AD, Carlon G, Baron R, Sichel W, Young C, Howland W. The inverse relationship between cost and survival in the critically ill cancer patient. *Crit Care Med* 1979;7:20–23.

4. Field MJ, Cassel CK, eds. Approaching Death: Improving Care at the End of Life. Institute of Medicine Report. Washington, DC: National Academy Press, 1997.

5. Curtis JR. The "patient-centered" outcomes of critical care: what are they and how should they be used? *New Horizons* 1998;6:26–32.

6. Wilson IB, Cleary PD. Linking clinical variables with health-related quality of life: a conceptual model of patient outcomes. *JAMA* 1995;273:59–65.

7. Patrick DL, Erickson P. Health Status and Health Policy: Quality of Life in Health Care Evaluation and Resource Allocation. New York: Oxford University Press, 1993.

8. Heyland DK, Guyatt G, Cook DJ, Meade M, Juniper E, Cronin L, Gafni A. Frequency and methodologic rigor of quality of life assessments in the critical care literature. *Crit Care Med* 1998;26:591–598.

9. Patrick DL, Danis ML, Southerland LI, Hong G. Qualtiy of life following intensive care. *J Gen Intern Med* 1988;3:218–223.

10. McHugh LG, Milberg JA, Whitcomb ME, Schoene RB, Maunder RJ, Hudson LD. Recovery of function in survivors of the acute respiratory distress syndrome. *Am J Respir Crit Care Med* 1994;150:90–94.

11. Davidson TA, Caldwell ES, Curtis JR, Hudson LD, Steinberg KP. Reduced quality of life in survivors of acute respiratory distress syndrome compared to critically ill controls. *JAMA* 1999;281:354–360.

12. Hopkins RO, Weaver LK, Pope D, Orme JF, Bigler ED, Larson-Lohr V. One year quality of life and neuropsychological outcome following adult respiratory distress syndrome (ARDS). *Chest* 1996;110:58S.

13. Schelling G, Stoll C, Hallar M, Briegel J, Manert W, Hummel T, Lenhart A, Heyduck M, Polasek J, Meier M, Preuss, U, Bullinger M, Schuffel W, Peter K.

Health-related quality of life and posttraumatic stress disorder in survivors of acute respiratory distress syndrome. *Crit Care Med* 1998;26:651–659.

14. Weinert CR, Gross CR, Kangas JR, Bury CL, Marinelli WA. Health-related quality of life after acute lung injury. *Am J Respir Crit Care Med* 1997;156:1120–1128.

15. Gerety MB, Chiodo LK, Kanten DB, Tuley MR, Cornell JE. Medical treatment preferences of nursing home residents: relationship to function and concordance with surrogate decision-makers. *J Am Geriatr Soc* 1993;1993:953–960.

16. Murphy DJ, Burrows D, Santilli S, Kemp AW, Tenners, Kreling B, Teno J. The influence of the probability of survival on patients' preferences regarding cardio-pulmonary resuscitation. *N Engl J Med* 1994;330:545–599.

17. Cohen-Mansfield J, Rabinovich BA, Lipson S, Fern A, Gerber B, Weissman S, Pawlson LG. The decision to execute a durable power of attorney for health care and preferences regarding the utilization of life-sustaining treatments in nursing home residents. *Arch Intern Med* 1991;151:289–294.

18. Schneiderman LJ, Pearlman RA, Kaplan RM, Anderson JP, Rosenberg EM. Relationship of general advance directive instructions to specific life-sustaining treatment preferences in patients with serious illness. *Arch Intern Med* 1992;152:2114–2122.

19. Elpern EH, Patterson PA, Gloskey D, Bone RC. Patients' preferences for intensive care. *Crit Care Med* 1992;20:43–47.

20. Danis ML, Patrick DL, Southerland LI, Green ML. Patients' and families' preferences for medical intensive care. *JAMA* 1988;260:797–802.

21. Uhlmann RF, Pearlman RA. Perceived quality of life and preferences for life-sustaining treatment in older adults. *Arch Intern Med* 1991;151:495–497.

22. Starr TJ, Pearlman RA, Uhlmann RF. Quality of life and resuscitation decisions in elderly patients. *J Gen Intern Med* 1986;1:373–379.

23. Tsevat J, Dawson NV, Wu AW, Lynn J, Soukup JR, Cook EF, Vidaillet H, Phillips RS. Health values of hospitalized patients 80 years or older. *JAMA* 1998;279:371–375.

24. Garrett J, Harris R, Norburn J, Patrick D. Life-sustaining treatments during terminal illness: who wants what? *J Gen Intern Med* 1993;1993:361–368.

25. Patrick DL, Pearlman RA, Starks HE, Cain KC, Cole WG, Uhlmann RF. Validation of preferences for life-sustaining treatment: Implications for advance care planning. *Ann Intern Med* 1997;127:509–517.

26. Orentlicher D. The illusion of patient choice in end-of-life decisions. *JAMA* 1992;267:2101–214.

27. The SUPPORT Principal Investigators. A controlled trial to improve care for seriously ill hospitalized patients: the Study to Understand Prognoses and Preferences for Outcomes and Risks of Treatments (SUPPORT). *JAMA* 1996;274:1591–1598.

28. Seckler AB, Meier DE, Mulvihill M, Cammer Paris BE. Substituted judgement: how accurate are proxy predictions? *Ann Intern Med* 1991;115:92–98.

29. Suhl J, Simons P, Reedy T, Garrick T. Myth of substituted judgement: Surrogate decision making regarding life support is unreliable. *Arch Intern Med* 1994;154:90–96.

30. Uhlmann RF, Pearlman RA, Cain KC. Physicians' and spouses' predictions of elderly patients' resuscitation preferences. *J Gerontol* 1988;43:M115–M121.

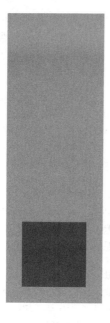

Chapter 8

Advance Care Planning in the Outpatient and ICU Setting

JOAN M. TENO

*A 70-year-old man with acute respiratory distress syndrome from a viral pneumonia is in the ICU, intubated and requiring PEEP to maintain oxygenation. The attending physician speaks with his second wife and his children from his first marriage. Doris, his wife, notes that he has a living will that states that he does not want life-sustaining treatment if incurably ill. She notes, "John does not want to be kept alive on machines if there is no hope of recovery. I want to honor those wishes. What I don't know is when to stop? When is there no hope?"**

*K*nowing when to stop," or when to implement treatment wishes in an advance directive, is an important and difficult decision that health care providers are faced with on a daily basis in caring for seriously ill patients in an ICU. These are rightfully difficult and thought-provoking decisions. In the past three decades, Americans have successfully grappled with the morality of withdrawal or foregoing of life-sustaining treatment. Through court cases[2,3] and guidelines from the Presidential Commission on Biomedical Ethics,[4] a broad-based consensus has developed that it is ethical to withhold or withdraw life-sustaining treatment. Indeed, the legal and ethical guidance on the withholding and withdrawal of life-sustaining treatment has been an important success of the advance directive movement. This movement has focused on providing guidance for these paradigmatic court cases through the use of legal documents (called advance directives) that allow competent persons to state their wishes for medical treatment or name a surrogate in advance of a period of diminished mental capacity. While this focus on the legality and morality of these paradigmatic cases was an important step forward, this effort did not address the more difficult and challenging decision that we are faced with on a daily basis: knowing when to stop.

*This case is based on a narrative case from the Study to Understand Prognosis and Preferences for Outcomes and Risks of Treatments (SUPPORT).[1]

Key to knowing when to stop is the patient's disease trajectory, outcomes with and without available medical treatments, and information about the patients' values and treatment preferences. Many patients are cognitively impaired at the time treatment is stopped or foregone. Thus, we must rely on a process of communication and negotiation with the patient and/or the appropriate surrogate decision maker to arrive at treatment goals. An important component of this process of communication and negotiation is *advance care planning* (ACP)[5,6] which should start at the time of the patient's diagnosis and is best if it occurs in the outpatient setting. Communication and negotiation with patients comprise the first step of ACP. The second key step is the formulation of contingency plans, which ensure that the patient's preferences are honored, if possible.[6] In this chapter, I will outline ACP in the outpatient setting. It is important that critical care clinicians understand this process to facilitate high quality end-of-life care in the ICU. In addition, this same process that might be useful in the most difficult of circumstances—with seriously ill patients in an ICU. This chapter will provide a conceptual framework for communication during ACP as well as suggested "icebreakers" for health care providers to begin a dialogue with either a seriously ill patient or the appropriate surrogate decision maker. Communication skills in ACP are as important to the intensivist as the proper placement of a Swan-Ganz catheter. Chapter 9 contains additional information about communicating with patients and families about end-of-life care in the ICU.

Advance care planning in the outpatient setting has many of the same features as communication with patients and families in the ICU. This communication is at its most difficult and time pressured for the seriously ill ICU patient. Unlike with a seriously ill person in the outpatient setting, in the ICU the health care provider is faced with a medical crisis that may require a decision in the next several minutes. The patient's diminished acuity due to illness and the urgency of the situation make communication of ACP an important challenge for health care providers. Despite the urgency of the patient's situation, this communication still remains a process—one which the patient and/or loved ones° must be willing and ready to undertake. In the ICU, ACP starts when clinicians first meet the patient and the family. Often health care providers are faced with breaking bad news—telling patients and their loved ones that they are in a crisis that necessitates ICU level of medical care. In order to build a trusting and collaborative relationship, bad news must be told in a sensitive manner (see Table 8–1). Buckman has outlined a six-step protocol for breaking bad news in palliative care.[7] Each of these steps is important to ACP with a competent patient. First and foremost, one must choose the proper setting (step 1), come to understand how the patient and/or loved ones understand the patient's disease and prognosis (step 2), and listen to how much information they want to know (step 3).

°The use of the term "loved one" acknowledges that many patients make medical decision in conjunction with a family member or other persons who are important in their life.

Table 8–1. Use of Buckman's six steps to breaking bad news in advance care planning in the ICU

Step no.	Buckman's six steps	Applying six steps to advance care planning in an ICU setting
Step 1	Use the right physical context	Getting the context right may be difficult in the setting of urgent decision making. Introduce yourself and your role in the medical care of their loved one and sit down in a quiet setting, if at all possible.
Step 2	Find out how much information the patient and/or family knows	It is important to listen to the patient and the family to determine what they know about the illness, especially with regard to how they frame the patient's prognosis.
Step 3	Find out how much information the patient and/or family wants to know	Even if the patient and/or family do not want information on the patient's prognosis, you should still discuss treatment plans with them.
Step 4	Share information (educating)	Through actively listening to the patient, you should be able to tailor the presentation of information to the "mental model" of the patient and their family. For example, a family that speaks of probability based on medical information on the Internet should have the information tailored to their need for probabilistic information based on the scientific evidence. When there is uncertainty, openly discuss it with the patient and/or surrogate. Educating and clarifying misperceptions are often an important part of sharing information.
Step 5	Respond to the patient's and/or family's feelings	Being empathetic is key to advance care planning. One must be cognizant of how far one can push a patient or family in decision making if they have fully come to terms with their response to their situation.
Step 6	Plan and follow through	Key to closure is summarizing the situation, stating the plan, and setting a time for the next meeting.

One must listen carefully to what the patient's "mental model" is regarding what is going on, as well as to whether or how the patient uses probability in talking about his or her medical condition. Although many persons are not educated about probability, increasingly, consumers are beginning to understand the use of probability as applied to medical decisions. Consumers are educating themselves through Internet sites and other sources on the probability of survival with and without various treatment modalities. It may not be unusual to encounter a person with precise information from a Medline search, now available free of cost on the Internet. Nonetheless, some of their understanding of medical information may be wrong because of they used the wrong sources or misunderstood medical information. Health care providers must educate the patient and/or the family (step 4) after coming to understand what their framework is for understanding the patient's illness and prognosis.

Decisions regarding transition in the goals of care are life-defining and emotionally difficult decisions. Health care providers must be empathetic to the patient and/or family (step 5). One must weigh the urgency of decisions with how far one can "push" patients and/or their families to deal with their circumstances on an emotional level, assimilate that information, and make a decision. This is a process that under ideal circumstances needs to occur over time. In some urgent situations in which a decision must be made, one outcome of the conversation is that no decision is made. The failure to make a decision to withhold life-sustaining treatment is by default making the decision that those treatments will be utilized in life-threatening situation. Finally, ACP in the context of breaking bad news should end with the clinician summarizing the conversation and the plan of care, and when the clinician's next contact with the patient will be (step 6).

Ideally, ACP occurs in the outpatient setting with the patient's primary health care provider. It should be a process that progresses in content and specificity over the course of the patient's disease. For healthy persons, the focus during ACP should be on naming a proxy and stating unusual preferences (e.g., a patient is a Jehovah's Witness and would never want to receive a blood transfusion). For the person diagnosed with a serious illness, the focus of ACP is to educate the patient about the projected course of their illness and the likely outcomes that they may encounter. Values history forms or scenario-based advance directives such as the medical directive may serve as communication aides. Once the patient has reached the point in their care when they have a life-threatening illness or by virtue of old age, death is expected shortly, the ACP should be focused on achieving the patient's desired specificity and a plan of care should be developed that would achieve those goals and values. The primary care provider should discuss with the patient their hopes and expectations for this final phase of life. Once the patient's preferences are clarified, the clinician should develop a plan that will ensure that the patient's preferences will be honored. For example, noting in the chart that the patient does not want to be intubated is not enough in the patient with severe chronic obstructive pulmonary disease (COPD). Most of these patients will have terminal dyspnea. Without the proper plans for palliation of dyspnea, the patient will either die with severe dyspnea or end up in the emergency room.

Under ideal circumstances, the ICU clinician would speak with patients about their preferences and formulate a plan of care prior to a period of diminished mental capacity. Too often, this does not occur. Research among seriously ill adults has shown that only one in five persons has completed a written advance directive prior to a serious illness and that physicians are rarely involved in counseling patients about that directive.[8] In addition, nearly one-half of persons with a written advance directive and a preference to forego resuscitation do not have a do-not-resuscitate (DNR) order written.[8] Even when seriously ill patients complete an advance directive, the vast majority of these directives do not provide information that would guide decision making in the seriously ill beyond the naming of a proxy.[9] This and other research have clearly shown that advance directives, as they currently are used, do not impact the cost of care in the ICU[10,11] and do not change end-of-life decision making in the ICU.[8]

Sadly, many patients have not discussed their preferences with a physician and the intensive care clinicians are faced with making decisions for a patient with diminished decision-making capacity. In this case, the goal is to gather from available sources valid information with convincing evidence of the patient's informed preferences. A clear statement written in an appropriately completed advance directive (i.e., a competent patient who is informed of his or her treatment options) is considered to be the best source of information for the mentally incompetent patient. From there, one can assess information sources on the basis of how close they are is to the patient's own statements about his or her values and goals of care. A direct conversation between a health care provider and the patient would be an excellent source of information. Other sources of information are one more step removed from the patient. Usually, one must turn to a surrogate to "speak for the patient." In some situations, surrogates either report direct conversations they had with the patient or they infer the patient's preferences from conversations with the patient's loved one(s). When there is no evidence based on a direct conversation with the patient and surrogate, the surrogate should be asked to provide the clinician with information on the patient's goals on the basis of the surrogate's knowledge of that person. It is important to note here that surrogates are not being asked to "pull the plug" or make the decision. Rather, their task is to help the clinician make decisions based on knowledge of their loved one and what that person would want.

Written advance directives are viewed from a legal standpoint as a preferred source of evidence of the patient's wishes. However, the current implementation of formulating advance directives remains problematic, as previously discussed. The main difficulty is that most advance directives are *not* formulated with health care providers playing an active role in counseling and they often contain vague statements that need additional interpretation. Without appropriate counseling, even the most explicit statements could reflect inadequate counseling and not the patient's valid preferences for medical care. For example, the statement "no CPR, no Vents, no G-tubes" seems to be an explicit and clear wording of patient preferences. Indeed, this was inserted in a living will of a person enrolled in the Study to Understand Prognoses and Preferences for Outcomes and Risks of Treatments (SUPPORT)[9] However, the patient changed his preferences after speaking with a physician. This case emphasizes the importance of physician–patient communication in the completion of written advance directives. Knowledge that a patient has an advance directive provides the physician with an important opportunity to clarify the patient's goals and values. For example, a physician might ask, "Mr. _____, I see that you have a living will . . . tell me about what concerns led you to sign one."

Over emphasis has been placed on resuscitation, or getting the DNR order, as the focus of ACP in the hospital. Instead, the conversation should focus on understanding where the patient is in his or her disease trajectory—for example, "Mrs. _____, tell me about how your dad has been doing at home." Is the patient at the point in the disease trajectory when the quality of life is greatly diminished? Or does the patient want to focus on aggressive treatment? Understanding where the persons are in their disease trajectory and how it has impacted their quality of life is an important first step in guiding these conversations. For the patient who has reached a critical turning point when the disease has resulted in a drastically diminished quality of life and death is preferred over continued existence, the physician's role is to acknowledge that and formulate a plan that focuses on the patient's comfort and quality of life. The following sequence is an example of how a physician might state this: "Mrs. _____, it seems that you have reached a point in your illness where you want the medical care to focus on your comfort. Given those preferences, I would recommend that we do not use a breathing machine. Instead, we are going to focus on your comfort by using morphine to keep you as free of pain and discomfort as possible."

For patients who desire continued aggressive care, physicians must inform them of the treatment outcomes, including the burdens of that treatment choice. Patients have the authority to request continued aggressive care up to society-imposed constraints on resources or to medical futility. The decision to pursue aggressive care may increase the patient's suffering. While every attempt should be made to keep the patient as free of pain as possible, many of the procedures utilized in the ICU can cause significant suffering. The patient should be informed that clinicians will discuss with the patient on a daily basis, his or her treatment options, and that the patient always has the option of changing his or her mind.

In the case of family members asking for continued aggressive care, one must be sure that they are acting in good faith. Are they acting in concert with the patient's wishes, if these are known? Would one reasonably infer that the patient would want this treatment course, given prior knowledge of the patient? In some cases, families may choose aggressive care that seems contrary to the patients' wishes. As a first step in such cases, the ICU clinicians should organize a multidisciplinary team meeting including the patient's primary care doctors. In this meeting, it is important to acknowledge the difficult decision that the family and the health care team are faced with—e.g., "Today, we are here to discuss a tough decision in John's medical care." Yet, the clinician must remind the family of the task of honoring the patient's wishes if they are known. To continue with the above example, "John's advance directive stated that he didn't want to be on a ventilator if he didn't wake up from a coma in a week. This is a difficult decision, but a final gift of love is for us to honor and respect his wishes." In the case where the family member persists despite attempts to resolve the conflict through involvement of an ethics committee, the clinician must consider court involvement to ensure that the patient's informed wishes are respected. This should be a exceedingly rare event.

Advance care planning is a fundamental skill that practitioners working in an ICU should understand. With increasing patient longevity, decisions about withholding and withdrawal of life-sustaining treatment involves weighing tradeoffs of quality of life, longevity, and potentially, quality of dying. Patient preferences are important given that a reasonable person may disagree with each of these tradeoffs. Advance care planning is a process of communication and planning that develops patient goals and a set of contingency plans that will allow these preferences to be honored. Often, breaking bad news is part of ACP. An approach has been outlined here that applies Buckman's six steps to ACP. It is important to remember that this is a process that ideally should have started in the outpatient setting. Often, ICU clinicians are faced with the failure of ACP in the outpatient setting. In this instance, the clinicians must assess the degree to which they can compact this process and how much progress the patient or family can make toward arriving at treatment goals and accepting their potential loss. Skillful communication, with focus on the patient's goals and the patient's understanding of treatment during the course of illness, can lead to decisions that honor the patient's autonomy.

References

1. Teno JM, Stevens M, Spernak S, Lynn J. Role of written advance directives in decision making: insights from qualitative and quantitative data. *J Gen Intern Med.* 1998;13:439–46.
2. In re Quinlan 7NJ13A26cd4US9. 1976.
3. Cruzan v. Dirctor, Missouri Department of Health, 110 S. Ct. 284.2855.
4. President's Commission for the Study of Ethical Problems in Medicine and Biomedical and Behavioral Research; *Deciding to Forego Life-Sustaining Treatment.* Washington, DC: Government Printing Office; 1983.
5. Teno JM, Nelson HL, Lynn J. Advance care planning. Priorities for ethical and empirical research. *Hastings Cent Rep* 1994;24:S32–S36.
6. Teno JM, Lynn J. Putting advance-care planning into action. *J Clin Ethics* 1996; 7:205–213.
7. Buckman, R. Communication in Palliative Care: A Practical Guide. Dereck Doyle GWCHNM. *Oxford Textbook of Palliative Medicine.* Second ed. Oxford, England: Oxford University Press; 1998:141–158.
8. Teno J, Lynn J, Wenger N, et al. Advance directives for seriously ill hospitalized patients: effectiveness with the patient self-determination act and the SUPPORT intervention. SUPPORT Investigators. Study to Understand Prognoses and Preferences for Outcomes and Risks of Treatment [see comments]. *J Am Geriatr Soc* 1997;45:500–570.

 9. Teno JM, Licks S, Lynn J, et al. Do advance directives provide instructions that direct care? SUPPORT Investigators. Study to Understand Prognoses and Preferences for Outcomes and Risks of Treatment [see comments]. *J Am Geriatr Soc* 1997;45:508–512.

10. Schneiderman LJ, Kronick R, Kaplan RM, Anderson JP, Langer RD. Effects of offering advance directives on medical treatments and costs [see comments]. *Ann Intern Med* 1992;117:599–606.

11. Teno J, Lynn J, Connors AF Jr, et al. The illusion of end-of-life resource savings with advance directives. SUPPORT Investigators. Study to Understand Prognoses and Preferences for Outcomes and Risks of Treatment [see comments]. *J Am Geriatr Soc* 1997;45:513–518.

12. Tulsky JA, Fischer GS, Rose MR, Arnold RM. Opening the black box: how do physicians communicate about advance directives? *Ann Intern Med* 1998;129:441–449.

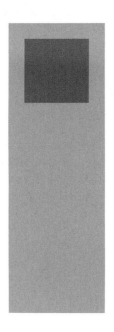

Part III

Practical Skills Needed to Manage Death in the ICU

Chapter 9

How to Discuss Dying and Death in the ICU

J. RANDALL CURTIS

DONALD L. PATRICK

*B*ecause of the severity of illness of the patients, the ICU is a setting where death is common. Of patients who die in the hospital, approximately half are cared for in an ICU within 3 days of their death and one-third spend at least 10 days in the ICU during their final hospitalization.[1] A recent study showed that 90% of deaths in the ICU in 1992 and 1993 involved withholding or withdrawing at least one life-supporting intervention, a dramatic increase when compared to 5 years previously.[2] Similarly, many other investigators have shown that most deaths in the ICU involve withholding or withdrawing multiple life-sustaining therapies.[3-11] Thus, the ICU represents a setting where decisions about managing the dying and death of patients are made on a frequent basis. These decisions are difficult not only because discussions about dying evoke fear and anxiety but also because the dominant culture of the ICU is oriented toward saving lives.[12,13] Because of the "rule of rescue,"[14] effective communication about end-of-life care is especially difficult. Clinicians in the ICU need to learn effective communication skills to provide quality end-of-life care to patients and their families.

Several studies have shown that family members with loved ones in the ICU rate communication with health care providers as one of the most important skills for these providers.[15,16] In fact, most families rate clinicians' communication skills as equally or more important than clinical skills.[16,17] A study of family satisfaction after a loved one died in the ICU has shown that satisfaction of family members was associated with having a single ICU attending physician and the same nurse caring for the patient on consecutive days.[18] This finding suggests that continuity of care and sustained communications with these clinicians are important to family members. Similarly, in one qualitative study, family members reported that communication with physicians and nurses was the most important part of their experiences of having a loved one die in the ICU.[15]

What Is Different About Discussing Dying and Death in the ICU?

A number of review articles and books provide clinicians with advice on how to communicate with patients and families when delivering bad news[19–22] and discussing palliative medicine.[23] While these reviews provide valuable insights, they focus on communication with patients in outpatient settings. In the ICU, these conversations usually concern patients incapable of participating in these discussions because of the severity of their illness, and often clinicians and the family do not have a prior relationship.[2–4] The ICU setting frequently involves complicated, confusing, and even discordant data that can be overwhelming to family members and make the family more dependent on the health care team for assistance with decision making.[24] For example, a critically ill patient may have improvement in one organ system while showing deterioration in several others. There are also more likely to be discordant views about the appropriate treatment among ICU team members, consultants, and primary care physicians as well as different family members.[24] Each of these features have the potential for making communication about dying more difficult in the ICU setting. Because the ICU is unique in these ways and is the location in which decisions about withholding and withdrawing life-sustaining therapy are commonly made,[2] ICU clinicians should make special efforts to improve their skills in this area.

Why Doesn't Advance Care Planning with Outpatients Take Care of this Problem?

In the 1980s, many prominent investigators believed that advance directives would allow patients to inform their physicians of what kind of care they would want if they became too sick to speak for themselves.[25–27] A logical extension of this argument is that advance directives could diminish the need for critical care clinicians to discuss end-of-life care with patients and families. However, numerous studies have suggested that advance directives do not significantly affect the aggressiveness or costs of ICU care[28–30] and do not change end-of-life decision making in the ICU.[31–33] These studies have led many to lose faith in advance directives.[34–36] Advance care planning, defined as an ongoing discussion among patients, family members, and providers, may be more effective than advanced directives at allowing patients' wishes to be followed if they become too ill to speak for themselves. However, to date there are no data to support or refute this view.

Understanding advance care planning occurring prior to hospitalization should remain an important component of end-of-life communication in the ICU (see Chapter 8). Advance directives or advance care planning, however, will not obviate the need to discuss with families the withholding and withdrawal of life support in the ICU. Furthermore, as our population continues to age and as we develop new technology and treatments for chronic and life-threatening diseases, therapeutic trials of intensive care may become more common.[37] When these therapeutic trials do not result in success, ICU clinicians will be in the position to discuss withholding and withdrawing life-sustaining therapy with patients and their families.

Whom Do We Talk with About End-of-Life Care in the ICU?

Prior studies have suggested that less than 5% of patients are able to communicate with clinicians at the time that decisions are made about withholding or withdrawing life-sustaining therapies in the ICU.[2] When ICU clinicians discuss these issues, most often the discussions are with patients' families and loved ones. Nonetheless, ICU clinicians should not assume that the patient can't participate just because the patient is in the ICU. There are circumstances where patients can, and therefore should, participate in these discussions despite being in the ICU or even on mechanical ventilation.

If patients can no longer communicate their wishes for medical care, the legal surrogate decision maker is usually identified in a hierarchical fashion. First priority usually goes to an individual named in a Durable Power of Attorney for Health Care and then to family members. In most states and countries, the family members primarily responsible for decision making are, in order, legal spouse, parent, adult children, and siblings. If there is more than one individual at a given level in the hierarchy, such as occurs in a family with several adult children, many states require that the decision be based on group consensus (see Chapter 18 for more details.) Although the law may specify a legal decision maker, in most cases the actual decision-making process occurs in a series of family conferences with all individuals who have strong ties to the patient.[38] Decision making is usually facilitated if all interested individuals are involved as early and as completely as possible.

How Well Do We Discuss End-of-Life Care in the ICU?

There has been no prior research on the quality of clinician–family communication in the ICU, although one study used audiotapes of family meetings in the ICU to describe methods for seeking consensus in decisions about withdrawing or withholding life support.[39] These researchers found that decision making to withhold or withdraw life support therapy involved "complex, difficult processes" that were fertile ground for further study.

Previous researchers have assessed the quality of patient–clinician communication with hospitalized patients about do not resuscitate orders.[40] These studies found substantial shortcomings in the communication skills of physicians, noting that typically physicians spent 75% of the time talking and missed important opportunities to allow patients to discuss their personal values and goals of therapy. These investigators also showed that most of these physicians felt that they did a good job discussing DNR orders, but that they had very little training about how to hold these types of discussions with patients.[41] In a more recent study, these same investigators examined communication between physicians and outpatients about advance directives.[42,43] In this study, investigators again found that physicians rarely elicited information about patient goals and values, avoided discussing uncertainty, and rarely asked patients to explain why they had specific treatment preferences or what was important to them about their quality of life after treatment. In summary, these data suggest that the quality of patient–physician communication about end-of-life care is poor and is unlikely to improve under our current system of health care delivery and medical education. These studies challenge us to develop better ways to teach end-of-life communication skills to ICU clinicians in training and in practice.[24]

What Is the Role of the ICU Team in Communication with Patients and Families?

The ICU team is made up of a number of health care professionals including physicians, nurses, social workers, respiratory therapists, and others. Different team members may play varying roles in different ICUs. It is important that all team members who are directly involved in communication with patients and families be involved as much as possible in the process of end-of-life care in the ICU. Consensus within the ICU team is a vital step in the process of making decisions about withholding or withdrawing life-sustaining therapy. Of the few legal cases that have been brought against physicians for end-of-life decisions, most have been initiated by disgruntled colleagues. In addition, it is important that all members be informed about the medical situation and plan of therapy so that patients and families do not receive different messages from different staff members.

Critical care nurses play a pivotal role in clinician–family communication in the ICU.[44-46] Prior research with family members after the death of a loved one in the ICU suggests that families' communication with nurses occur mostly during informal conversations at the bedside.[15] In addition, families rate the nurses' skill at this communication as one of the most important clinical skills of ICU clinicians.[16,17,47,48] In a meta-analysis of studies assessing the needs of family members who have a loved one in the ICU, 8 of the 10 needs identified relate to communication with clinicians, and most of these communication needs are primarily addressed by nurses.[16] There are, however, data to suggest that nurses are not better at communication about end-of-life care than physicians[49] and, consequently, could also benefit from efforts to improve the quality of this communication.

Social workers often play an important role in ICUs in identifying and contacting family members, coordinating and scheduling family conferences, and keeping in contact with family members during the ICU stay. This is a very important role in providing sensitive care in the ICU and in communicating with patients' families. The person filling this role must be aware of the medical prognosis and treatment plans and be an active part of the ICU team.

One method of improving communication within the ICU team is to have the entire team make ICU morning rounds. This is a relatively simple solution that can have a profound effect on team communication, but it may require reorganization of morning rounds to allow all team members to be present. Another important foundation for team communication is that the culture of the ICU be one of a team approach where every team member's views are heard and valued.

When Should We Talk About End-of-Life Care in the ICU?

It is impossible to be prescriptive about the "right" time to discuss end-of-life care in the ICU, except to say that we should talk about it earlier than we usually do. Often, ICU clinicians, particularly physicians, wait until they have decided that life-sustaining treatments are no longer indicated before they initiate communication about end-of-life care with patients or families. Families may be just beginning to think about withdrawing life support while clinicians are feeling increasingly frustrated at providing the care they believe is no longer indicated. Alternatively, sometimes the family is considering withdrawal of life-sustaining treatments well before the medical team. The ICU team itself may also vary in the timing with which they believe that life-sustaining therapy should be withdrawn. Often, nurses come to this conclusion earlier than physicians, which can be an area of extreme frustration for some critical care nurses[50,51] and a source of interdisciplinary conflict for physicians and nurses.[52]

A potential solution to this difficulty is to begin discussions among the ICU team, patients, and families earlier in the course of the ICU stay. Early in the ICU stay, however, these discussions are likely to have a different focus. Rather than discussing withdrawal of life-sustaining therapy, clinicians may focus discussion on prognosis, goals of therapy, and the patients' values and attitudes toward medical therapy. These discussions may foreshadow or set the stage for subsequent discussions about withdrawing or withholding life-sustaining treatments and can be a very helpful way to avoid situations where ICU team

members and family members have very different views of the utility of ongoing intensive care.

How Should We Talk About End-of-Life Care in the ICU?

Because discussing end-of-life care with patients and families is an important
part of providing high-quality intensive care, we should approach these discussions with the same care and planning as that with which we approach other
important ICU procedures. For example, we should (1) put time and thought
into the preparations we need to make prior to holding this discussion, (2) plan
where this discussion should take place, (3) talk with the family about who
should be present and what will be covered during the discussion, and (4)
anticipate what is likely to happen after the discussion. These issues address
the processes that ideally should occur prior to the discussion, during the discussion, and after the discussion. Table 9–1 outlines some of the steps that may
facilitate good communication about end-of-life care in the ICU. These are
described in more detail below.

Making preparations prior to a discussion

A common mistake that some ICU clinicians make is to embark on a discussion
about end-of-life care with a patient or family without having made the necessary preparations for the discussion. Clinicians should review what is known
about the patient's disease process including the diagnoses, prognosis, treatment options, and likely outcomes with different treatments. Clinicians should
identify gaps in their knowledge by systematically reviewing this information
and seeking out the information they need before they find themselves in a
discussion with patients or their families.

It is also important for clinicians to review what they know about the patient and the family, including their relationships with one another, their attitudes toward illness, treatment, and death, and their prior reactions to information about illness and death. If, for example, there are family members who
have had strong emotional reactions to bad news, it may be helpful to mobilize
the aid of a family member or staff member, such as a social worker or chaplain, who can support them through and after the discussion with the clinician.

It is also useful for clinicians to consider their own feelings of grief, anxiety,
or guilt prior to holding a discussion about end-of-life care with patients or
families. This may be especially important in cases when the clinician has
known the patient or family for a long time, when the clinician and patient or
family have been through a lot together, or when the clinician has some feelings of inadequacy about the patient's condition or treatment. Self-awareness of
these feelings can help clinicians avoid projecting their own feelings or biases
onto the patient or family. In addition, the clinician's own feelings of guilt

Table 9–1. Components of a discussion about end-of-life care in the ICU

Making preparations prior to a discussion about end-of-life care in the ICU

Review previous knowledge of the patient and/or family
Review previous knowledge of the patient's attitudes and reactions
Review your knowledge of the disease—prognosis, treatment options
Examine your own personal feelings, attitudes, biases, and grief
Plan the specifics of location and setting: a quiet, private place
Have advance discussion with the patient or family about who will be present

Holding a discussion about end-of-life care in the ICU

Introduce everyone present
If appropriate, set the tone in a nonthreatening way: "This is a conversation I have with all my
    patients . . ."
Find out what the patient or family understands
Find out how much the patient or family wants to know
Be aware that some patients do not want to discuss end-of-life care
Discuss prognosis frankly in a way that is meaningful to the patient
Do not discourage all hope
Avoid temptation to give too much medical detail
Make it clear that withholding life-sustaining treatment is *not* withholding caring
Use repetition to show that you understand what the patient or family is saying
Acknowledge strong emotions and use reflection to encourage patients or families to talk about
    these emotions
Tolerate silence

Finishing a discussion of end-of-life care in the ICU

Achieve common understanding of the disease and treatment issues
Make a recommendation about treatment
Ask if there are any questions
Ensure basic follow-up plan and make sure the patient and/or family knows how to reach you for
    questions

or inadequacy can lead the clinician to avoid the family or to avoid talking with the family about death. Reviewing these feelings by oneself or with another clinician can be the first step to becoming more comfortable with discussing dying and death with a patient or family. For more information about the clinician's own feelings toward dying and death, see Chapter 14.

An additional step in preparing for an end-of-life discussion in the ICU is to plan where the discussion will take place and who will be there. Ideally, these discussions should take place in a quiet and private room where there is some assurance that people, phones, or pagers will not interrupt the discussion. It should be a room that is comfortable for all the participants without a lot of medical machinery or other distractions such as medical diagrams. All parties should be sitting at the same level and it should be around a table or chairs in a circle. It is best to avoid having a clinician sitting behind a desk with the family in front of a desk. If the patient can participate in the discussion but is too ill to leave their ICU bed, efforts should be made to make the ICU room comfortable for everyone present.

The clinician, patient, and family should discuss, prior to the scheduled discussion about end-of-life care, who should be present for the discussion. In addition, the clinician should make certain that all appropriate members of the staff are consulted about whether they should be present, including the medical staff, nursing staff, chaplains, and trainees that have been involved with the patient or family. Ideally, someone should take responsibility for scheduling the conference at a time when as many participants as possible can be present. It may be helpful for some families to be told that they can write down any questions they have prior to the scheduled conference to ensure that their questions will be answered.

Holding a discussion about dying and death in the ICU

The first step of a discussion about dying and death is to be sure that everyone participating in the discussion has met everyone else present. Some staff members present for the discussion may not have met all family members. Take the time to go around the room to be sure that everyone has met everyone else and knows their role either on the staff or in the family.

Introducing the issue of dying and death or end-of-life care can be an important and difficult part of these discussions. Often, by the time these discussions occur in the ICU, everyone in the room knows that the discussion will focus on how to help the patient die in comfort and with dignity. But sometimes patients or families may not be aware that this is part of the clinician's agenda. In those situations, the clinician should make the patient or family as comfortable as possible talking about dying and death. In these latter situations, it may be helpful to frame the discussion by saying that these are discussions that the clinician has with all patients or families in this situation.

Not everyone present will have the same level of understanding of the patient's condition, thus it is often helpful to first find out what the patient or family understands of the patient's situation. This can be a useful way for the clinician to determine how much information can be given, the level of detail that will be understood, and the amount of technical language that can be used. It can also be useful in some settings to ask the patient or family how much they want to hear on this day as a way to gauge how much information and detail to give. Clinicians should be careful to avoid unnecessary amounts of technical jargon and be cautious about using technical jargon to avoid saying words like "dying" or "death". It is important for clinicians to avoid the temptation to give too much technical detail about physiology or pathophysiology as a way of dealing with their own discomfort, but they should be aware that some patients or families may want to hear this type of detail. Clinicians should also be cautious about using physiologic detail to cover an uncomfortable message about the patient's prognosis. For example, it is not unusual for clinicians to say things like "the patient's blood pressure has stabilized on dopamine and levophed" in settings where a stable blood pressure on pressor agents is of little or no relevance to the overall prognosis. In this way, the clinician can get the positive rewards of giving some good news, but may be misleading the family.

During these discussions, it is important to discuss prognosis in an honest way that is meaningful to patients and their families. For example, the term "median survival" is not very useful to most family members. In discussing prognosis, clinicians should also be honest about the degree of uncertainty in the prognosis. Finally, it is also important to provide honest information about the prognosis without completely discouraging hope from those patients or families that would like to maintain their hope. This can be a tricky balancing act for clinicians, but it is a part of the art of holding these discussions. There are several specific ways that clinicians can allow patients or families to maintain their hope in the face of a poor prognosis. First, the clinician can allow the patient or family some time to get used to a poor prognosis. Sometimes this can take days, but it can be very helpful to patients or families if they are allowed to make this transition at their own pace. Second, the clinician can help the patient or family redirect their hope and move from a hope for recovery to hope for some quality time together or for a comfortable death without pain or dyspnea and with as much dignity and meaning as possible.

An important goal of end-of-life discussions in the ICU is to align the clinicians' and the patient's or families' views of what is happening. The discussions about end-of-life care that are most difficult are those in which the families' views and the clinicians' views are dramatically different. Making the effort to discover these differences and working to minimize them can be time consuming, but it is usually time well spent, as it can greatly facilitate decisions about end-of-life care.

It is extremely important in discussions about end-of-life care in the ICU that the patient and/or family understand that if the decision is made to withhold or withdraw a particular treatment, the clinicians themselves are not withdrawing from caring for the patient. While this may seem obvious to some clinicians, it should be stated explicitly to patients and families to avoid any misunderstanding. In some ICU settings, withholding or withdrawing life-sustaining therapy may mean that the patient will be transferred out of the ICU and to another set of clinicians. If this is the case, clinicians should discuss this with patients and family members and ensure that the transfer does not mean or give the appearance that the patient will no longer receive aggressive, timely, and appropriate treatment, even if that treatment is palliative.

After discussing prognosis and treatment options at the patient's or family's level of understanding, it is important to spend some time exploring the patient's and/or family's reactions to what was discussed. Clinicians should under-

stand that patients and families will react to their perception of what was said
and they may not react in the way the clinician expects. There are several
useful techniques that clinicians can use to explore patients' or families' reactions. First, it can be helpful to repeat what patients or families have said as a
way to show that the clinician has heard them. This can be particularly useful
when the clinician and the patient or family have different views of what is
happening or what should happen. Second, it is important to acknowledge
strong emotions that come up in these discussions. Whether the strong emotion is anger, anxiety, or sadness, it is useful for the clinician to acknowledge
the emotion in a way that allows the person with the emotion to talk about why
they feel that way. In acknowledging such emotions, it can be useful for the
clinician to use reflection to show empathy and to encourage discussion about
the emotion. For example, a clinician can say, "it seems to me that you are very
angry about the care that your father has received, can you tell me why that
is?" as a way to show some empathy for a family member and allow that family
member to talk about their feelings. Finally, another technique clinicians can
use in discussions with a patient or family is to tolerate silences. Sometimes it
is after what seems like a long silence that patients or family members will ask
a particularly difficult question or express a difficult emotion.

How should we finish a discussion about end-of-life care in the ICU?

Prior to finishing a discussion about end-of-life care, there are several steps
that clinicians should take. First, it is important that clinicians make recommendations during the discussion. With the increasing emphasis on patient
autonomy and surrogate decision making, there may be a tendency for some
clinicians to describe treatment options to a patient or family, but to then feel
they shouldn't make a recommendation.[53] On the contrary, it is important that
clinicians offer their expertise to patients and their families. Part of offering
their expertise is making a recommendation. This is especially important in
discussions with family members about withholding or withdrawing life support. It is a disservice to leave family members feeling like they made the
decision to "pull the plug" on a loved one in situations in which ongoing life
support therapy is unlikely to provide significant benefit.

Prior to finishing a discussion about end-of-life care, clinicians should summarize the major points and ask patients or family members if there are any
questions. This is a good time to tolerate silence, as it may take a while for the
uncomfortable questions to surface.

Finally, before completing a discussion about end-of-life care, clinicians
should ensure that there is an adequate follow-up plan. This often means a
plan for when the clinician will meet with the patient or family again, and a

way for the patient or family to reach the clinician if questions arise before the next meeting.

How Can We Help Families With the Decision to Withhold or Withdraw Life Support?

When families are faced with making the decision of whether to withdraw life support for a loved one, there are several ways clinicians can help (for a summary, see Table 9–2). First, it is crucial that families understand the basic principle of surrogate decision making. Family members are being asked what they think the patient would want if the patient were able to speak for him- or herself. The reason the family members are being asked this question is that they generally are the ones in the best position to determine what the patient would want. Clinicians should make it clear to family members that they are not being asked to decide what they (the family members) want for the patient or even what they would want if they were in the patient's situation. Making this clear to families can be extremely useful for family members who feel torn between deciding to continue life-sustaining therapy because they do not want their loved one to die, and deciding to stop life-sustaining therapy because they feel the loved one would not want this treatment in this circumstance.

Sometimes clinicians may arrive at the decision that withdrawing life-sustaining therapy is in the patient's best interest before the family does. These situations can be very contentious and can be a source of conflict between ICU clinicians and the family. In these situations, often the family needs time to accept and understand the patient's prognosis and to come to terms with the loss of a loved one. Allowing families the time to make these adjustments can be an important use of ICU resources. Furthermore, pushing families to make

Table 9–2. Helping families make decisions about withdrawing life support in the ICU

Focus the family on what the patient would want, not what the family wants

If life-sustaining therapy is to be withdrawn, emphasize that
 Life-sustaining therapy cannot reverse the underlying disease process
 Withdrawal of life-sustaining therapy allows the natural course of the disease to occur
 Aggressive palliative therapy will be used to ensure that the patient is comfortable

Some families need time to adjust to withdrawing life-sustaining therapy; such time can be an important use of ICU resources

Educate the family about what will likely happen after life-sustaining therapy is withdrawn
 Discuss the likely time to death as well as the variability and uncertainty
 Discuss agonal respirations and myoclonus

Elicit family preferences about extubation

Mention organ donation, but leave discussion to the organ procurement team the decision to withdraw life-sustaining therapy before they are ready can set up an antagonistic relationship between clinicians and families and can erode the confidence that families have in the clinicians. Once this confidence is eroded, it is often difficult to regain.

Frequently, part of the decision for a family member is whether the patient would want to be resuscitated in the event of cardiac arrest. It is our opinion that in helping families make this decision, it is important that advanced cardiac life support (ACLS) not be broken down into components, but instead be presented as a package. Dividing ACLS into components (chest compressions, anti-arrhythmic drugs, pressor agents, intubation) makes these decisions unnecessarily complex and can lead to an absurd resuscitation status such as compressions and all drugs, but no intubation. There are circumstances in which patients are already intubated or receiving pressors and the decision is made to withhold resuscitation, but in general, ACLS should be viewed as a single package that will be used to the extent indicated or will be withheld.

There are several reasons why discussing withholding ACLS and cardiopulmonary resuscitation (CPR) is different from discussing other treatments. First, many families have unrealistic expectations about the efficacy of CPR and assign this treatment enormous symbolic significance.[54] Second, discussion about situations in which ACLS is not indicated or desired can open the door to a discussion of withholding other ICU treatments. Finally, it is important that all members of the team understand that withholding CPR does not necessarily mean that other ICU treatments are not indicated.[55]

If the decision is made to withdraw life-sustaining therapy, clinicians should emphasize to family members that life-sustaining therapy was not able to reverse the underlying disease and the removal of life-sustaining therapy is allowing the disease to take its natural course. In addition, clinicians should reassert that aggressive therapy in the form of palliative care will be provided to ensure the patient's comfort.

If families decide to withdraw life-sustaining therapy, it is important that clinicians teach them about this process. This should include discussing the likely period of time from life support withdrawal to death and the variability and uncertainty in determining this time. Families are often worried about the patient's suffering. Clinicians should discuss the treatments available to prevent pain and suffering during the withdrawal of life-sustaining therapy. Clinicians should also discuss the possibility of agonal respirations and myoclonus so family members are prepared. For patients who are intubated, clinicians should elicit family preferences about extubation and discuss the advantages and disadvantages of extubation (for more details on this decision, see Chapter 11). Finally, clinicians should mention the option of organ donation, if that is appropriate. If available, organ procurement teams should have this discussion with families rather than the clinicians, as organ donation is more likely to occur if an organ procurement team has this discussion with the family than if the clinician has the discussion.[56]

How Does Medical Futility Fit in?

It can be helpful for clinicians to have a framework to think through the indications for initiating or continuing life-sustaining therapy before approaching the patient or family. The principle of medical futility can be useful in this framework provided that it is used in a precise and accurate way. The principle of medical futility states that a therapy is futile if there is no or a very low likelihood that the therapy will result in a successful outcome.[57,58] There is considerable controversy about the role of this principle in making unilateral decisions,[59] but in our experience, this principle can be useful in a framework for discussing the use of specific treatments. One approach to such a framework is outlined in Figure 9–1. First, the clinician should elicit from the patient or family the patient's wishes for therapy and outcome. These wishes should be formulated into reasonable therapeutic goals. Often this goal is discharge from the hospital alive or discharge to home, but for some patients a goal might include surviving until the arrival of a family member or the birth of a child. Once the goals have been elicited, the clinician should use published literature and clinical experience to determine whether the treatment in question can achieve one of the goals. If the treatment can achieve one of the goals, then the patient or family should be asked if the patient would want the treatment. If, however, treatment cannot achieve one of the goals, the treatment is medically futile and, in general, should not be offered. Once this determination is made, the clinician should review the basis for this determination to be sure that there are adequate data or clinical experience to support it. Prior research has shown that some physicians make a determination of medical futility in settings where it does not apply.[60] If the determination of medical futility stands up to this scrutiny, this therapy should not be offered to patients or families, but the determination of futility should be discussed with them. In most cases, patients or families will agree with this determination and will appreciate not being asked to choose to forego a treatment that is not indicated.[61] However, in some circumstances, patients and families will not agree with foregoing a futile treatment. In these situations, a process should be initiated to reconcile these differences, as described in a paper from the American Medical Association,[62] and treatment should be offered until differences can be reconciled.

Understanding Our Own Discomfort with Discussing Death

Discomfort with discussing death is universal. This is not a problem unique to physicians, nurses, or other health care providers, but has its roots in our society's denial of dying and death. Medical schools and nursing schools have only recently begun to teach students how to help patients and families through the dying process and still do so in a limited way.[63] Major medical textbooks have

1. Elicit patient wishes about therapy and outcomes.

2. Formulate these wishes into appropriate therapeutic goals (such as discharge to home with independent living or survive until granddaughter is born).

   Treatment Decision:

3. Determine whether treatment can acheive at least one reasonable therapeutic goal

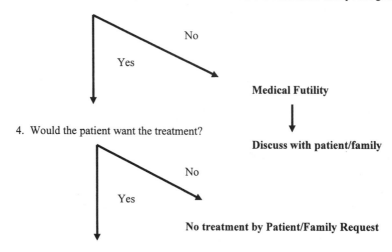

Provide treatment and periodically reassess goals and indications

Figure 9–1. A framework for discussing specific interventions and a view of where medical futility fits.

had very little information about end-of-life care.[64] For all these reasons, it is not surprising that many clinicians have difficulty talking with their patients and families about end-of-life care. Furthermore, the ICU culture is one of using technology to save lives. For many clinicians, discussing dying and death is even more difficult in this technologic, aggressive care setting. To compound this difficulty, clinicians in the ICU can also feel that a patient's death reflects poorly on their skills as an ICU clinician and represents a failure on their part to save the patient's life.

It is important for ICU clinicians to recognize the difficulty they have discussing dying and death. If clinicians acknowledge this difficulty, they can work to minimize some of the common effects that such discomfort can take (see Chapter 14). For example, discomfort discussing death may cause clinicians to give mixed messages about a patient's prognosis or to use euphemisms for dying and death. This discomfort discussing dying and death can even cause clinicians to avoid speaking with a patient or a family. Recognizing this discomfort and being willing to confront it is the first step in overcoming these barriers to effective communication about dying and death with patients and their families.

Summary

Discussing dying and death with patients and their families is an extremely important part of providing good quality care in the ICU. While there is very little empiric research to guide ICU clinicians in choosing the right time or the most effective way to have these conversations, there is developing experience with and increasing emphasis on making this an important part of the care clinicians provide and an important part of training for medical and nursing students. Much like other ICU procedures or skills, providing sensitive and effective communication about end-of-life care requires training and practice as well as planning and preparation. We have reviewed some of the fundamental components of discussing end-of-life care in the ICU that should be part of the care of most patients with life-threatening illnesses in the ICU.

References

1. The SUPPORT Principal Investigators. A controlled trial to improve care for seriously ill hospitalized patients: the Study to Understand Prognoses and Preferences for Outcomes and Risks of Treatments (SUPPORT). *JAMA* 1996;274:1591–1598.
2. Pendergast TJ, Luce JM. Increasing incidence of withholding and withdrawal of life support from the critically ill. *Am J Respir Crit Care Med* 1997;155:15–20.
3. Faber-Langendoen K. A multi-institutional study of care given to patients dying in hospitals. Ethical practices and implications. *Arch Intern Med* 1996;156:2130–2136.
4. Smedira NG, Evans BH, Grais LS, Cohen NH, Lo B, Cooke M, Schecter WP, Fink C, Epstein JG, May G. Withholding and withdrawal of life support from the critically ill. *N Engl J Med* 1990;322:309–315.
5. Vincent JL, Parquier JN, Preiser JC, Brimioulle S, Kahn RJ. Terminal events in the intensive care unit: review of 258 fatal cases in one year. *Crit Care Med* 1989; 17:530–533.
6. Eidelman LA, Jakobson DJ, Pizov R, Geber D, Leibovitz L, Sprung CL. Foregoing life-sustaining treatment in an Israeli ICU. *Intensive Care Med* 1998;24:162–166.
7. Keenan SP, Busche KD, Chen LM, McCarthy L, Inman KJ, Sibbald WJ. A retrospective review of a large cohort of patients undergoing the process of withholding or withdrawal of life support. *Crit Care Med* 1997;22:1020–1025.
8. Koch K. Changing patterns of terminal care mangement in an intensive care unit. *Crit Care Med* 1994;22:233–243.
9. Vernon DD, Dean JM, Timmons OD, Banner W, Allan-Webb EM. A. Modes of death in the pediatric intensive care unit: Withdrawal and limitation of supportive care. *Crit Care Med* 1993;21:1798–1802.
10. Youngner SJ, Lewandowski W, McClish DK, Juknialis BW, Coulton C, Bartlett ET.

Do not resuscitate orders: incidence and implications in a medical intensive care unit. *JAMA* 1985;253:54–57.

11. Bedell SE, Pelle D, Maher PL, Cleary PD. Do not resuscitate orders for critically ill patients in the hospital: how are they used and what is their impact? *JAMA* 1986;256:233–237.

12. Caswell D, Omrey A. The dying patient in the intensive care unit: making the critical difference. *Clin Issues Crit Care Nurs* 1990;1:178–186.

13. Nelson JE. Saving lives and saving deaths. *Ann Intern Med* 1999;130:776–777.

14. Jonsen AR. Bentham in a box: technology assessment and health care allocation. *Law Med Health Care* 1986;14:172–174.

15. Shannon SE. Families' experiences with proxy decision making for critically ill patients. Presented at Summer Seminar in Ethics, Copper Mountain, Colorado, 1996.

16. Hickey M. What are the needs of families of critically ill patients? A review of the literature since 1976. *Heart Lung* 1990;19:401–415.

17. Molter NC. Needs of relatives of critically ill patients: a descriptive study. *Heart Lung* 1979;8:332–339.

18. Johnson D, Wilson M, Cavanaugh B, Bryden C, Gudmundson D, Moodley O. Measuring the ability to meet family needs in an intensive care unit. *Crit Care Med* 1998;26:266–271.

19. Campbell ML. Breaking bad news to patients. *JAMA* 1994;271:1052.

20. Buckman R. Breaking bad news: why is it still so difficult? *BMJ* 1984;288:1697–1599.

21. Buckman R. How to Break Bad News. Baltimore: Johns Hopkins University Press, 1992.

22. Quill TE, Townsend P. Bad news: delivery, dialogue, and dilemmas. *Arch Intern Med* 1991;151:463–468.

23. Lo B, Quill T, Tulsky JA, for the ACP-ASIM End-of-Life Care Consensus Panel. Discussing palliative care with patients. *Ann Intern Med* 1999;130:744–749.

24. Danis M, Federman D, Fins JJ, Fox E, Kastenbaum R, Lanken PN, Long K, Lowenstein E, Lynn J, Rouse F, Tulsky J. Incorporating palliative care into critical care education: Principles, challenges, and opportunities. *Crit Care Med* 1999;27:2005–2013.

25. Singer PA, Siegler M. Advancing the cause of advance directives. *Arch Intern Med* 1992;152:22–24.

26. Emanuel LL, Emanuel EJ. The medical directive. *JAMA* 1989;261:3288–3293.

27. Emanuel LL, Barry MJ, Stoeckle JD, Ettelson LM, Emanuel EJ. Advance directives for medical care—a case for greater use. *N Engl J Med* 1991;324:889–895.

28. Schneiderman LJ, Kronick R, Kaplan RM, Anderson JP, Langer RD. Effects of offering advance directives on medical treatment and costs. *Ann Intern Med* 1992;117:599–606.

29. Danis M, Mutran E, Garrett JM. A prospective study of the impact of patient preferences on life-sustaining treatment and hospital cost. *Crit Care Med* 1996;24:1811–1817.

30. Danis M, Southerland LI, Garrett JM, Smith JL, Hielma F, Pickard CG, Egner DM, Patrick DL. A prospective study of advance directives for life-sustaining care. *N Engl J Med* 1991;324:882–888.

31. Teno J, Lynn J, Connors AF, Wegner N, Phillips RS, Alzola C, Murphy DP, Desbiens N, Knaus WA. The illusion of end-of-life savings with advance directives. *J Am Geriatr Soc* 1997;45:513–518.

32. Teno JM, Lynn J, Wegner N, Phillips RS, Murphy DP, Connors AF Jr, Desbiens N, Fulkerson W, Bellamy P, Knaus WA. Advance directives for seriously ill hospitalized patients: Effectiveness with the Patient Self-Determination Act and the SUPPORT intervention. *J Am Geriatr Soc* 1997;45:500–507.

33. Teno JM, Licks S, Lynn J, Wegner N, Connors AF Jr, Phillips RS, OConnor MA, Murphy DP Fulkerson WJ, Desbiens N, Knaus WA. Do advance directives provide instructions that direct care. *J Am Geriatr Soc* 1997;45:508–512.

34. Block JA. Living wills are overrated. *Chest* 1993;104:1645–1646.

35. Dresser R. Confronting the "near irrelevance" of advance directives. *J Clin Ethics* 1994;5:55–56.

36. Tonelli MR. Pulling the plug on living wills—a critical analysis of advance directives. *Chest* 1996;110:816–822.

37. Danis M. Outcomes research and end of life issues. *New Horizons* 1998;6:110–118.

38. Swigart V, Lidz C, Butterworth V, Arnold R. Letting go: family willingness to forgo life support. *Heart Lung* 1996;25:483–494.

39. Miller DK, Coe RM, Hyers TM. Achieving consensus on withdrawing or withholding care for critically ill patients. *J Gen Intern Med* 1992;7:475–480.

40. Tulsky JA, Chesney MA, Lo B. How do medical residents discuss resuscitation with patients? *J Gen Intern Med* 1995;10:436–442.

41. Tulsky JA, Chesney MA, Lo B. See one, do one, teach one? House staff experience discussing do-not-resuscitate orders. *Arch Intern Med* 1996;156:1285–9.

42. Tulsky JA, Fischer GS, Rose MR, Arnold RM. Opening the black box: how do physicians communicate about advance directives? *Ann Intern Med* 1998;129:441–449.

43. Fischer GS, Tulsky JA, Rose MR, Siminoff LA, Arnold RM. Patient knowledge and physician predictions of treatment preferences after discussion of advance directives. *J Gen Intern Med* 1998;7:447–454.

44. Jamerson PA, Scheibmeir M, Bott MJ, Crighton F, Hinton RH, Cobb AK. The experiences of families with a relative in the intensive care unit. *Heart Lung* 1996;25:467–474.

45. McClement SE, Desgner LF. Expert nursing behaviors in care of the dying adult in the intensive care unit. *Heart Lung* 1995;24:408–419.

46. Hampe SO. Needs of the grieving spouse in a hospital setting. *Nurs Res* 1975;24:113–120.

47. Daley L. The perceived immediate needs of families with relatives in the intensive care setting. *Heart Lung* 1984;13:231–237.

48. Rodgers CD. Needs of relatives of cardiac surgery patients during the critical care phase. *Focus Crit Care* 1983;10:50–55.

49. Maguire PA, Faulkner A. Helping cancer patients disclose their concerns. *Eur J Cancer* 1996;32A:78–81.

50. Asch DA. The role of critical care nurses in euthanasia and assisted suicide. *N Engl J Med* 1996;334:1374–1379.

51. Asch DA, Shea JA, Jedrziewski MK, Bosk CL. The limits of suffering: critical care nurses' views of hospital care at the end of life. *Soc Sci Med* 1997;45:1661–1668.

52. Shannon SE. The roots of interdisciplinary conflict around ethical issues. *Crit Care Nurs Clin North Am* 1997;9:13–28.

53. Quill TE, Brody H. Physician recommendations and patient autonomy: finding a balance between physician power and patient choice. *Ann Intern Med* 1996;25:763–769.

54. Diem SJ, Lantos JD, Tulsky JA. Cardiopulmonary resuscitation on television: miracles and misinformation. *N Engl J Med* 1996;21:235–242.
55. Tittle MB, Moody L, Becker MP. Nursing care requirements of patients with DNR orders in intensive care units. *Heart Lung* 1992;21:235–242.
56. Gortmaker SL, Beasley CL, Sheehy E, Lucas BA, Brigham LE, Grenvik A, Patterson RH, Garrison RN, McNamara P, Evanisko MJ, Improving the request process to increase family conset for organ donation. *J Transplan Coordination* 1998;8:210–217.
57. Schneiderman LJ, Jecker NS, Jonsen AR. Medical futility: its meaning and ethical implications. *Ann Intern Med* 1990;112:949–954.
58. Schneiderman LJ, Jecker NS. Futility in practice. *Arch Intern Med* 1993;153:437–441.
59. Lantos JD, Singer PA, Walker RM, Gramelspacher GP, Shapiro GR, Sanchez-Gonzalez MA, Stocking CB, Miles SH, Siegler M. The illusion of futility in clinical practice. *Am J Med* 1989;87:81–84.
60. Curtis JR, Park DR, Krone MR, Pearlman RA. Use of the medical futility rationale in do-not-attempt-resuscitation orders. *JAMA* 1995;273:124–128.
61. Curtis JR, Patrick DL, Caldwell E, Collier AC. The attitudes of patients with advanced AIDS towards use of the medical futility rationale in decisions to forego mechanical ventilation. *Arch Int Med* 2000;160:1597–1601.
62. Council on Ethical and Judicial Affairs AMA. Medical futility in end-of-life care. *JAMA* 1999;281:937–941.
63. Billings JA, Block S. Palliative care in undergraduate medical education: status report and future directions. *JAMA* 1997;278:733–738.
64. Rabow MW, McPhee SJ, Fair JM, Hardie GE. A failing grade for end-of-life content in textbooks: what is to be done? *J Palliat Med* 1999;2:153–155.

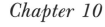

Chapter 10

Pain and Symptom Control in the Dying ICU Patient

KATHLEEN M. FOLEY

$\mathcal{T}$he care of the critically ill dying patient requires the knowledge, skills, compassion, and resources of a multidisciplinary team. To manage the common symptoms in this patient population, assessment and treatment strategies must be integrated with the needs of the individual patient. The goal of symptom management varies with the specific goals of care for each individual patient. For the dying patient, the goals of care are to provide adequate control of major physical and psychological symptoms to allow the patient to die in comfort and to enhance their quality of living during their last days of life. Some patients may remain conscious during the dying process; others may be obtunded or comatose secondary to central nervous system disease or dysfunction or from pharmacologic agents administered for symptom control.[1] Balancing the adequate control of symptoms with an acceptable level of cognitive function is difficult in the critically ill patient. Health care professionals need to be familiar with the theoretical and practical aspects of pain and symptom control in this patient population. Pharmacologic therapy is the mainstay of treatment to manage the multiple symptoms in providing humane, compassionate care.

Scope of the Problem

Detailed studies of the epidemiology of pain and other symptoms in ICUs are not available. It is well recognized, however, that multiple symptoms have an impact on the quality of life of patients in ICUs, and the assessment and management of pain, anxiety, and agitation in this patient population have received increased attention in the critical care literature.[2-13] There are many reasons for patients experiencing pain in ICUs, all of which are related to tissue injury–from prolonged immobilization, repeated exposure to a wide variety of procedures, continuous instrumentation of sensitive tissues, and preexisting or new pain syndromes associated with surgery, trauma, burns, or other medical illnesses such as cancer.[4,8,14–17]

Surveys of patients recently discharged from ICUs report that anxiety and pain are the most commonly remembered experiences, with lack of rest, placement of the endotracheal tubes, and application of face masks being events associated with pain and anxiety.[12,17–20] In one study of pain in ICU patients, the patients reported that they used eye signals, facial expressions, and hand and leg motions to alert ICU staff that they were in pain.[17] Patients treated with only paralyzing agents such as succinylcholine without coadministration of opioids or anxiolytics reported experiencing profound anxiety following recovery.[13]

Most of these limited data on approaches to symptom control come indirectly from surveys of patterns of use of opioid and sedative drugs to manage pain, provide sedation, or control agitation.[13,19–22] These studies have also identified that pain and anxiety are often undertreated in this patient population because they are difficult to assess.[10,23] The authors of the Study to Understand Prognoses and Preferences for Outcomes and Risks of Treatment (SUPPORT) reported that pain was a common symptom in patients with serious life-threatening illness, with patients or their surrogates reporting moderate to severe pain in up to 50% of patients in the last 3 days of life.[14] Few data are available on the exact prevalence of anxiety, agitation, delirium, nausea and vomiting, fatigue, constipation, etc., but studies of patients with advanced cancer as well as studies of patients with AIDS and elderly patients in the last weeks of life all suggest a list of common symptoms occurring in seriously ill patients that clearly interfere with patients' quality of life.[24] For purposes of this chapter, I will focus on the assessment and treatment of the common symptoms of pain, anxiety, nausea and vomiting, dyspnea, and agitation.

Symptom assessment

Researchers have developed symptom assessment tools to provide accurate information about patients' experiences.[25] These assessment tools have been combined with algorithms to improve the quality of symptom management in ICU patients.[12,22,26,27] Much of the research to date has focused on the assessment and management of the symptom pain in critical care patients, because their inability to communicate and the nature of the procedures employed, cause this patient population to be at risk for unrelieved pain. Comprehensive assessment methods that combine both verbal and nonverbal tools with systematic behavioral and physiological indicators of pain are now those most commonly used.[4,14,20,28] The routinization of such measurements can provide data on the effectiveness of various symptom management interventions,[29] a wide variety of tools are currently available to rapidly assess symptoms in patients. For valid assessment of pain, for instance, a visual analog scale combined with word scores was used in the Memorial Pain Assessment Card, or a 0–10 pain scale was used as a "fifth vital sign" to be recorded regularly along with the patient's blood pressure and temperature on the vital signs sheet.[30] These two approaches are commonly used as part of institutional programs of continuous quality improvement in pain management.[27,29] For those patients who are cognitively impaired, behavioral signs such as grimacing, withdrawing, and moaning are used on the basis of pediatric models of assessment. Tools for assessing patients who are obtunded or unconscious help to provide physicians and nurses with useful criteria for the dosing of analgesics. A wide variety of both individual symptom assessment scales as well as more generalized approaches, including the Memorial Symptom Assessment Scale and the Edmonton Symptom Assessment Scale,[25,31,32] and individual tools to measure cognitive function, anxiety and depression, dyspnea, and nausea and vomiting are also available for routine clinical use. A more detailed discussion of some of these assessment tools can be found in Chapter 12. Such tools should be employed to measure the quality of care of dying ICU patients. Specific toolkits for measurement are currently in development.[33]

Management of Pain and Other Symptoms

Effective analgesia is not only a humanitarian requisite of good ICU care but also has important physiological consequences that can both decrease complications and improve patient outcome. In a recent review of the literature, techniques of effective pain control were shown to have measurable effects on the recovery of patients who suffer from major trauma or critical illness. Neuroendocrine distress, cardiovascular dysfunction, and pulmonary function improve following adequate management of pain in critically ill patients.[13]

The American Pain Society, The Agency for Health Care Policy and Research, The World Health Organization, and a variety of other organizations have published specific guidelines for pain management.[26,28,34-36] All agreed that analgesic drug therapy is the mainstay of treatment. Such therapy includes the combination of nonopioid, opioid, and adjuvant analgesic drugs used alone or in combination, individualized to the needs of the patient and titrated to provide effective analgesia. Drug therapy is only one part of a multimodal approach for enhancing the quality of living. The delivery of optimal therapy depends on an understanding of the clinical pharmacology of the analgesic drugs and a comprehensive assessment of the pain, the patient's medical condition, and the psychosocial status of the patient.

In describing the use of analgesic drug therapy in the dying ICU patient, these guidelines are sufficiently general to cover the spectrum of patients who may be cognitively intact and who wish to remain alert for as long as possible while concurrently receiving adequate analgesia. These same guidelines apply to the patient who is sedated but in whom behavioral responses to painful stimuli need to be assessed to determine adequate analgesia. In our experience, all attempts should be made to maintain patients cognitive function for as long as possible to allow them to interact with their families and have the opportunity to come to closure as they are dying.

The World Health Organization's three-step analgesic ladder is a useful tool for framing the discussion of analgesic drug therapy.[35,36] This approach emphasizes the intensity of pain rather than a specific etiology or mechanism as the prime consideration in analgesic selection. Step 1 is for patients with mild to moderate pain; here a nonopioid alone or in combination with an adjuvant drug is used. Aspirin, acetaminophen and nonsteroidal anti-inflammatory drugs (NSAIDs) make up the nonopioid regimen. Step 2 is for patients who are relatively nontolerant and who have failed a trial with a nonopioid analgesic or are not able to tolerate aspirin or NSAIDs. Weak opioids such as codeine, oxycodone, and tramadol alone or in combination with a nonopioid and adjuvant analgesic are used.[37] This three-step approach is important in the ICU, especially for patients who would like to achieve pain control while remaining as alert as possible. However, frequently the ICU clinician must go directly to step 3 because of the intensity of the pain encountered in this setting.

Nonopioid Analgesics

These drugs are most commonly used for the management of patients with mild to moderate pain. This class includes aspirin and other NSAIDs as well as acetaminophen. In contrast to opioid analgesic drugs, they have a "ceiling" effect for analgesia, and increasing the dosage above a set range will not provide additive analgesia. Neither tolerance nor physical dependence develops as a result of these agents, but their serious adverse effects, including bleeding disorders, ulcer diathesis, and impaired renal function, significantly alter their use. Drug selection and the use of peptic cytoprotective agents can modify the risk of gastrointestinal bleeding. The nonacetylated salicylates such as choline magnesium trisalicylate and salicylate have less effect on platelet aggregation and no effect on bleeding time at usual clinical dosages. Misoprostol is the preferred agent for the prevention of NSAID-related peptic ulcers in patients because it decreases the risk of duodenal and gastric ulcers, unlike H_2 antagonists, which do not prevent gastric ulceration.[38]

Acetaminophen has fewer adverse effects than the NSAIDs, and hepatic toxicity is rare when the ceiling dosage of 4000 mg/day is observed. At the current time, the only NSAID available by parenteral or intravenous use in the United States is kelorolac.[39,40] This drug may have particular value in critically ill patients as it can provide analgesia comparable to 10 mg of intramuscular/ intravenous morphine. Because of its gastrointestinal toxicity, its use is limited to no more than 5 days at a time. The advantages of ketorolac over an opioid include its ability to provide analgesia without an effect on ventilatory responses to CO_2. It has no effect on gastric emptying. Cox-2 inhibitors, which are safer nonsteroidal anti-inflammatory drugs, have become recently available. At the present time, none of these drugs are available for intramuscular or intravenous administration, thus limiting their use in the critically ill patient to oral administration alone.

These nonopioid drugs represent the first-line approach; the choice and use of each can be individualized. If these are appropriate for the intensity of pain, the patient should be given an adequate trial of one nonopioid analgesic before switching to an alternative one. The trial should include administration of the drug to maximum levels at regular intervals. If pain relief is not obtained, adding an opioid to a nonopioid provides additional analgesia.

Opioid Analgesics

Opioid analgesics, of which morphine is the prototypic drug, vary in their potency, efficacy, and adverse effects. These drugs produce their analgesic effects by binding to discrete opioid receptors in the peripheral and central nervous system. In contrast to nonopioid analgesics, opioid analgesics do not appear to have a ceiling effect, that is, as the dose is escalated on a log scale, the increment in analgesia is linear to the point of a loss of consciousness. Effective use of opioid drugs requires the balancing of the most desirable effects of pain relief with the undesirable effects of nausea, vomiting, mental clouding, sedation, respiratory depression, constipation, tolerance, and physical and psychological dependence. In the critically ill patient, judicious use of opioids can both provide analgesia, anxiolysis, and sedation and secondarily stabilize neuroendocrine, cardiovascular, and pulmonary function.

Before considering the general principles that guide their clinical use, it is important to distinguish the use of opioids for analgesia from their use for sedation and anxiolysis. In the ICU, opioids are commonly used to achieve all three effects, most commonly in the mechanically ventilated patient. In the patient not receiving ventilatory support, excessive sedation is commonly associated with a higher risk of respiratory depression. In such cases, the use of nonopioids or specific anesthetic agents, such as ketamine, or the phenothiazine analgesic, methotrimeprazine, may be more appropriate.[41,42] Alternatively, the use of epidural local anesthetics to treat chest wall pain or pain in the lower extremities might be considered.

Choosing specific analgesic therapy

The use of opioids in the ICU is directed by the first guideline principle: *choose a specific analgesic therapy on the basis of individual patient charac-*

teristics. These include *the type of pain*—somatic, neuropathic, or visceral; *the intensity of pain*—opioids for severe pain, nonopioids, and adjuvants for mild pain or neuropathic pain; *the site and cause of pain*—e.g., epidural local anesthetics for hip fracture; *patient-specific factors*—i.e., the patient's history of drug allergy and side effects from other opioid drugs; and the *patient's prior opioid exposure.* Increased opioid requirements will be necessary for patients chronically taking opioids for pain or for the treatment of drug addiction prior to admission to the ICU.

Numerous studies have demonstrated that there is a marked degree of variable responsiveness of different types of pain to opioid analgesics.[43] The concept of a continuum of opioid responsiveness rather than an all or nonquantal phenomenon has been clearly observed. *Opioid responsiveness* is defined as the degree of analgesia achieved during dose escalation to either intolerable side effects or adequate analgesia. Patient-characteristic, pain-related factors and drug-selective effects influence this variable response. The practical application of this concept is that patients require dose titration to limiting side effects before one is able to determine whether they will achieve adequate analgesia with the specific choice of drug.

In choosing a specific opioid analgesic, the clinician has available a wide variety of opioid analgesics. These include morphine and its congeners— codeine, oxycodone, hydromorphone, oxymorphone, and levorphanol. Morphine is considered the standard analgesic against which all other agents are compared. Morphine is available in a wide variety of oral, parenteral, and epidural preparations for various routes of administration. It has a half-life of 3–4 hours and an active metabolite, morphine-6-glucoronide (M-6-G), which is twice as potent as morphine as an analgesic and accumulates in renal dysfunction.[21] Various factors may influence the levels of both M-6-G and morphine and M-3-G, including route (increased M-6-G following oral administration), male sex (decreased morphine and M-6-G plasma concentrations), use of ranitidine (increased morphine) and of rifampin (decreased morphine) and renal dysfunction. Studies of morphine in ICU patients revealed that patients experienced periods of prolonged sedation, which was attributed to persistently elevated levels of M-6-G. This metabolite has been demonstrated to readily cross the blood-brain barrier to produce central nervous system (CNS) effects. In contrast to morphine, it has a long half-life of 12 hours and accumulates in renal dysfunction.[21,44,45]

The other alternative morphine congeners that are commonly used include hydromorphone, oxycodone, oxymorphone, and levorphanol. All of these drugs are available by both the oral and parenteral route except for oxycodone, which is only available orally, and oxymorphone, which is only available parenterally. Hydromorphone has poor oral availability; it has a short half-life of 2–3 hours, is highly soluble, and is available in a high-potency parenteral form of 10 mg/ml. Because of its short half-life, it is commonly used in elderly patients.

Oxycodone, which is not available by the parenteral route, is available in both immediate-release and slow-release preparations. Its half-life is approximately 3–4 hours. Oxymorphone is currently available only by the intravenous and rectal routes and serves as an alternative to morphine. It has less of a histamine effect and may be of use in those patients who complain of headache or itch following opioid administration.[46] Levorphanol has a high bioavailability but a prolonged plasma half-life of approximately 12–16 hours. It can accumulate with repeated administration but may have special advantages in patients who are unable to tolerate morphine, hydromorphone, or oxymorphone. It is available in oral and parenteral forms.

Fentanyl is a synthetic opioid analgesic, which is commonly used for acute postoperative pain as well as chronic pain associated with serious medical illness. It has a relatively short half-life of 1–2 hours and is currently available in transmucosal, transdermal, intravenous, and epidural preparations.[47–49] The availability of transdermal fentanyl is of special advantage to patients unable to take drugs by mouth by providing them with continuous opioid analgesia through the transdermal approach. Patches are currently available in 25–100 μg/hr doses. Following patch placement, full analgesia is not achieved until 12–16 hours, requiring that either intravenous or oral analgesia be available to patients in the titration phase. Rescue medications should also be available by either the oral, intravenous or transmucosal route. The oral transmucosal formulation of fentanyl has been demonstrated to be effective in "breakthrough pain." This formulation may be useful in the conscious ICU patient for rapid pain relief. Fentanyl is administered intravenously by continuous infusion via a patient-controlled analgesia (PCA) pump.

Methadone is also an effective opioid analgesic commonly used to manage patients with chronic pain and is available in oral and parenteral preparations. The bioavailability of methadone is higher than that of morphine—85% vs. 35%. Its analgesic potency also differs, with a parenteral to oral ratio of 1:2, in contrast with 1:6 with morphine.

The plasma half-life of methadone is 17–24 hours, with reports of up to 50 hours in some patients, but with duration of analgesia of only 4–8 hours. The discrepancy between analgesic duration and plasma half-life of methadone has made it a drug that requires particularly careful titration. Methadone has been commonly recommended as a second-line agent in patients who are experiencing inadequate pain control on high doses of morphine, hydromorphone, or fentanyl.[45,50–52] In such patients, switching to methadone can often provide adequate analgesia. When switching to methadone from other opioid analgesics, specifically morphine and hydromorphone, the starting dose of methadone needs to be significantly reduced to 25% of the equianalgesic dose calculated.[45] Several authors have developed protocols for switching patients from morphine and hydromorphone to methadone based on the patient's prior opioid exposure. Care should be taken to make these opioid dose adjustments. For example, for patients on a dosage of morphine <80 mg/24 hr, the ratio of methadone to morphine is 1:4; a dosage of >100–200 mg/24 hr, has a ratio of 1:6, and for >200 mg/24 hr the ratio is 1:8.[52]

Meperidine is not used chronically in the management of patients with pain. It has a poor parenteral-to-oral ratio and is currently only available by the oral and intramuscular routes. Repetitive intramuscular administration is associated with local tissue fibrosis and sterile abscess. Repetitive dosing of meperidine can lead to normeperidine accumulation; subtle mood effects, followed by tremors, multifocal myoclonus, and occasional seizures, are characterized by hyperirritability. The accumulation of normeperidine occurs most commonly in patients with renal dysfunction, but it can also occur following repeated administration to patients with normal renal function.[53]

The role of mixed agonist antagonists such as pentazocine, butorphanol, and nalbuphine is particularly limited in the management of pain in patients who are critically ill, and these drugs do not appear to offer any special advantages in this patient population. Moreover, in patients chronically receiving opioids, the introduction of mixed agonist antagonists such as pentazocine can precipitate withdrawal, markedly exacerbating the pain in the individual patient.

Equianalgesic dosage

The second important principle of opioid drug therapy is to *know the equianalgesic dosage of the drug and its route of administration* (see Table 10–1.). Knowing the proper equianalgesic dosages can ensure more appropriate drug use; lack of attention to these differences in drug dosage is the most common cause of undermedication or overdosage of pain patients. Table 10–2 lists the most commonly used equianalgesic dosages, which have been derived from the assessment of the relative analgesic potency of the drug. Relative potency is the ratio of the dosages of two analgesics required to produce the same effect. Estimates of relative potency provide the basis for selecting the appropriate dosage when switching dosage or route of administration of the same drug. The equianalgesic dosage is the recommended starting dosage, with the optimal dosage for each patient being determined by dosage adjustment.

Increasing attention has been focused on the role of opioid rotation in providing patients with ongoing analgesia. In a study of 100 consecutive patients evaluated by investigators at the Memorial Sloan-Kettering Cancer Center Pain and Palliative Care Service, most of the patients required at least one change in opioid to maximize analgesia and minimize side effects.[51] Up to 40% of patients required two changes. This study points out the need for clinicians to know how to use multiple opioids and to switch drugs in patients to minimize side effects and maximize analgesia. Empiric data suggest that opioid tolerance is incomplete.[24] It is suggested that one-third to one-half of the equianalgesic dose should be used as a starting dosage when switching patients

Table 10–1. Equianalgesic opioid dosage

Drug	IM	PO	Half-life (hr)
Morphine	10	20–30 60[b]	2–3.5
Codeine	130	200	2–3
Oxycodone	15	30	3–4
Hydromorphone	1.5	7.5	2–3
Methadone	10	20	15–120
Meperidine	75	300	2–3
Oxymorphone	1	10	2–3
Levorphanol	2	4	12–16
Fentanyl	0.1[a]	—	1–2[c]
Tramadol	100	120	3–4

IM, intramuscular; PO, by mouth.

[a]Empirically, transdermal fentanyl at 100 μg/hr = 2–4 mg/hr intravenous morphine.

[b]Derived from single-dose studies.

[c]Single-dose data. Continual infusion produces lipid accumulation and prolonged terminal excretion.

from one opioid to another. Specific recommendations have been previously described when switching to methadone.[52]

Route of administration

The third principle of opioid drug therapy is *choose the route of administration appropriate to the patients' needs.* There are numerous methods of drug delivery that can be used to maximize pharmacologic effects and minimize side effects. Patients commonly require multiple routes of drug administration in the course of their pain management.[45,51] The oral route is preferable and easy, and a wide variety of slow-release preparations of morphine, hydromorphone, and oxycodone are now available for convenient dosing in patients on an 8-, 12-, and 24-hour basis. Morphine, oxymorphone, hydromorphone, and methadone are also available in a suppository form, and both slow-release oxycodone and morphine preparations have been demonstrated to be effective rectally.[54] In the ICU patient, nasogastric or rectal administration of slow-release preparations is feasible, but these drugs should not be cut or pulverized. The recent introduction of transmucosal fentanyl has provided a novel route of administration for patients with breakthrough pain; this requires an alert patient and an intact oral cavity.

In the critically ill patient, subcutaneous and intravenous routes of administration are most commonly used. Intermittent and continuous intravenous infusions delivered through patient controlled pumps [PCA] designed to infuse a drug continuously but with options for bolus administration are now

Table 10–2. Guidelines for analgesic drug therapy

1. Choose a specific analgesic therapy individualized to patients' needs
   Type of pain (somatic, neuropathic, visceral)
   Intensity of pain (mild, moderate, severe)
   Site and cause of pain (focal versus diffuse, acute versus chronic)
   Patient-specific factors (drug allergies, side effects)
   Prior opioid exposure (degree of tolerance to adjust equianalgesic dosage)

2. Know the equianalgesic dosage of drug for the route of administration

3. Choose the route of administration appropriate to the patient's needs
   Oral
   Buccal
   Rectal
   Transmucosal
   Transdermal
   Subcutaneous
   Intravenous
   Epidural
   Intrathecal
   Intraventricular

4. Develop a dose titration protocol
   Schedule dosage intervals for baseline pain
   Give rescue doses for breakthrough pain
   Switch opioids to maximize analgesia and minimize side effects
   Use 25% of equianalgesic dose when switching to methadone in patients on high doses of morphine or hydromorphone

5. Use a combination of drugs to increase analgesic efficacy or treat side effects

6. Choose an adjuvant analgesia for the specific type of pain

7. Understand the phenomena of tolerance, physical dependence, and psychological dependence
   Use tapering opioid schedule to prevent acute withdrawal

the most common approaches for managing pain.[55,56] Such continuous intravenous approaches are preferred for patients who require the rapid onset of analgesia, for rapid changes in dose requirements, and to circumvent impaired swallowing or gastrointestinal obstruction. The value of continuous infusion is that it limits problems associated with bolus effects by providing the patient with a continuous minimal effective concentration of drug. It also allows staff to provide a rapid change in drug administration for pain by the PCA method. Often these are nurse- rather than patient-administered boluses. For patients taking drugs orally, patients should be given an around-the-clock dosing schedule to prevent pain from recurring and provide continuous pain relief.

Dose titration protocols

The fourth principle of opiod drug therapy is *develop a dose titration protocol*. Rescue medication should be provided to treat breakthrough pain.[32] The integration of scheduled dosing with rescue doses provides a method for a safe and rational dosage escalation and is applicable to all routes of opioid administration. The rescue dosage is generally identical to that administered on a continuous basis. Clinical experience suggests that the size of the rescue dose should be equivalent to approximately 5%–15% of the 24-hour baseline dose. The frequency with which rescue doses can be administered depends on the time to peak effect for the drug and the route of administration. Oral rescue doses can be offered up to every 60 minutes and parenteral rescue doses through a PCA device can be offered up to every 15 minutes. In selecting an initial dosage, a patient with severe pain who is relatively non-tolerant of pain should begin with one of the opioid agonists at a dosage equivalent to 10 mg of intramuscular morphine every 4 hours. If a switch from one opioid drug to another is required because of unacceptable side effects, the equianalgesic dosage table can be used as a guide to the starting dosage of the new drug. In those patients with adequate pain control, the starting dosage of the new drug should be reduced to one-third to one-half the equianalgesic dosage to account for incomplete cross-tolerance. If the patient has had inadequate pain control on a previous opioid, a small reduction in dosage is used and the starting dosage of the new drug can usually be 75%–100% of the equianalgesic dosage. As previously mentioned, additional caution should be exercised when the change is to methadone. Inadequate pain relief should be addressed through a gradual escalation of the opioid dosage until acceptable analgesia is reported or intolerable side effects occur.

For patients who are chronically receiving opioid analgesics, it is important to remember that the analgesic response to opioids increases linearly with the log of the dosage and therefore dosage escalations of <30%–50% are not likely to significantly improve analgesia. Large-dose increments may be necessary for a meaningful change in effect. The severity of the pain should determine the ratio of dose titration. In those patients with severe pain who need rapid relief, repeated parenteral dosing every 15–30 minutes until the pain is partially relieved is an appropriate method. After intravenous loading with a short half-life opioid, such as morphine, an approximate hourly maintenance dosage can be calculated by dividing the total loading dose by twice the elimination half-life of the drug. Rapid-dose titration is most commonly used in those patients with an acute pain crisis.

For dying patients with pain, continuous opioid infusions are delivered preferably through PCA pumps to facilitate the delivery of prompt-rescue medications, which are particularly important for patients with acute exacerbations of breakthrough pain. The use of continuous infusions instead of boluses has practical consequences. They are easier for the nursing staff to administer; they reduce the bolus effect, which is associated with increased sedation or respiratory compromise; and they protect nurses and physicians from feeling guilty that they may be hastening the patient's death if the patient dies shortly after a bolus dose. Open discussions about the use of opioid analgesics in this setting, the dose titration, and the indications for and intent of their use are critical to developing an approach to provide comfort for dying patients.

Use of combinations of drugs

The fifth principle of opiod drug therapy is *use a combination of drugs to increase analgesic efficacy without escalating the opioid dosage and to treat side effects.* Combinations of an opioid and other anti-inflammatory nonsteroidal drugs provide additive analgesia, as do combinations of opioids with 100 mg of hydroxyzine.[45] A wide range of adjuvant agents are commonly used to treat side effects or enhance analgesia. The side effects of opioid analgesics, the most common ones being respiratory depression, sedation, nausea, vomiting, constipation, and multifocal myoclonus and seizures, can compromise or limit their use.

Respiratory depression can be associated with opioid use, but the rapid development of tolerance to this side effect commonly protects patients who are chronically receiving opioids. This is not an issue in the mechanically ventilated ICU patient. In the nonventilated patient, the risk of respiratory depression is accepted, so that comfort might be provided to the dying patient. Alternative analgesics, such as methotrimeprazine and ketamine, can be used instead.[42,45]

In the care of the dying patient, sedation and drowsiness, which may vary with the drug and dosage, can be addressed by reducing the individual drug dose and prescribing the drug at more frequent intervals or switching to an analgesic with a shorter plasma half-life. Amphetamine, methylphenidate, pemoline, and caffeine can be used to counteract these sedative effects.[57-59] It is important to discontinue all other drugs, including a wide variety of medications such as cimetidine, barbiturates, and other anxiolytic medications, that might exacerbate the sedative effects of the opioid analgesic. Patients and their families often request that patients be as awake as possible to allow time for them to say good-bye. In this case, pharmacologic adjustments are required to maximize pain relief and reduce side effects.

The use of antiemetics, including the use of sequential trials of compazine, haloperidol, metaclopromide, and ondasteron, is important for reducing opioid-induced nausea and vomiting. Opioid rotation, by switching to a different drug and/or a different route, has been shown to be effective in reducing these side effects.[48,50,51,60] Constipation can be prevented by using a prophylactic bowel regimen with senna derivatives and stool softeners as the first line of therapy.

Multifocal myoclonus can commonly occur in patients on chronic doses of morphine and its congeners. Switching to another opioid such as methadone may allow for a reduction in the amount of opioid used and markedly reduce this complication. Alternatively, the use of clonazepam is appropriate to suppress myoclonus if switching opioids is not a practical alternative and the patient is dying imminently.[61]

Seizures from opioid analgesics alone rarely occur, except with meperidine, and most commonly they are dose related, occurring with very high doses.

Again, switching a patient to another analgesic at a lower dosage and using intravenous benzodiazepines are alternative approaches to prevent seizures in the dying patient.

Adjuvant drugs are used not only to enhance analgesia and treat side effects but also to provide pain relief in certain pain states, e.g., neuropathic pain.[42-44,62-68] Table 10–3 lists the commonly used types of adjuvant drugs. Because of the lack of data from controlled studies and lack of well-defined guidelines, these drugs require sequential trials with dose titration to determine their clinical efficacy. For patients with neuropathic pain, several adjuvant drugs may provide analgesia. Some antidepressant drugs, including amitryptyline, desipramine and paroxetine, have selective analgesic efficacy.[62,63] They are only available orally, thus their role in the ICU patient population is limited. Phenytoin, which is available by the pareteral route, has been reported to provide analgesia in patients with lancinating pain. In contrast, both carbamazepine and gabapentin, which are only available orally, have been shown in controlled trails to be effective in treating trigeminal neuralgia (carbamazepine), post-herpetic neuralgia, and diabetic neuropathy (gabapentin).[62,64] For patients with cutaneous neuropathic pain, local applications of an eutectic mixture of local anesthetics (EMLA) cream provides substantial relief. This is applied topically and can reduce pain from various procedures such as intravenous placement and

Table 10–3. Adjuvant drugs for pain and symptom control

1. Adjuvants to increase analgesia

Acetaminophen
Nonsteroidal anti-inflammatory drugs
Cox-2 inhibitors
Hydroxyzine

2. Adjuvants to treat side effects

Nausea and vomiting: antiemetics (compazine, metaclopromide, ondansetron)
Sedation: psychostimulants (caffeine, methylphenidate, dextroamphetamine, pemoline)
Constipation: laxatives (senna)
Anxiety: benzodiazepines (alprazolam, lorazepam, clonazepam)
Delirium: neuroleptics (haloperidol, chlorpromazine)

3. Adjuvants to treat neuropathic pain

Antidepressants (amitriptyline, desipramine, paroxetine)
Anticonvulsants (phenytoin, carbamazepine, gabapentin,baclofen)
Oral and IV local anesthetics (mexiletine, lidocaine)
Corticosteroids (dexamethasone, prednisone)
Benzodiazepines (lorazepam, clonazepam)
Neuroleptics (methotrimeprazine, haloperidol, chlorpromazine)
NMDA antagonists (dextromethorphan, ketamine)
Alpha$_2$ adrenergic agonists (clonidine)

arterial blood draws.[45,62] Intravenous lidocaine has been reported in numerous case reports to provide analgesia in patients with nerve injury pain.[66]

The corticosteroids have been demonstrated to reduce pain in cancer patients with epidural cord compression and in patients with inflammatory rheumatic disorders.[45] The benzodiazepines have been reported anecdotally to reduce neuropathic pain, but the data are limited.[62] Methotrimeprazine, a phenothiazine analgesic with antiemetic and anxiolytic properties, is commonly used for patients who require these three effects for the quality of their dying.[45,68] Methotrimeprazine is commonly used to manage escalating pain for patients who have failed to respond to increasing opioids and who develop intolerable side effects. Doses start at 5 mg. and should be titrated to analgesia. The major side effects are postural hypotension and at high doses, extrapyramidal effects.

Ketamine given at subanesthetic doses has been shown to provide analgesia for patients with neuropathic pain.[42,62] It is currently used to treat patients who have not had adequate analgesia with opioids. From clinical experience, the drugs most commonly used in a dying patient with neuropathic pain are corticosteriods, local anesthetics, methotrimeprazine, and ketamine.[6,45,61] In most cases, these drugs are added to existing opioid regimens in an attempt to enhance analgesia through the selective role these drugs play in neuropathic pain.

Tolerance and physical dependence

The sixth principle of opioid drug therapy is *understand the phenomena of tolerance and physical dependence.* Tolerance is characterized by the need to use escalating opioid dosages to maintain the same analgesic effect. Experience with the use of opioids in patients with chronic pain due to cancer has shown that there is no limit to tolerance.[24] Patients can continue to obtain analgesia over a wide range of opioid doses. In fact, most patients require an escalation in dosages to manage increasing pain from demonstrable progression of disease. For a patient who is tolerant and experiencing inadequate analgesia, it is critical to remember that a 50%–75% increase in drug dosage may be necessary to provide analgesia, because opioid response increases linearly with the log of the dosage. For example, for a patient on 100 mg of intravenous morphine/hr who complains of severe, persistent pain, 150–175 mg of intravenous morphine/hr may be necessary to provide additive analagesia. In cancer patients, the range in opioid doseag for dying patients varies 20-fold from 15–30 mg/24 hr to 300–500mg/hr.

Physical dependence also occurs with chronic opioid administration, and abrupt withdrawal of opioid analgesics is contraindicated, as it will lead to the development of a full-blown withdrawal syndrome. For patients whose opioid analgesic dosage is to be discontinued or who become comatose because of CNS or metastatic disease, a tapering schedule should be instituted. Data suggest that using 25% of the total opioid dose can prevent signs of withdrawal, thus the opioid should be slowly tapered at 25% intervals daily. Naloxone should be used cautiously in dying patients, if at all.[69,70] When administered to a patient chronically receiving opioids, it should be diluted 10-fold and administered slowly to prevent the development of a withdrawal syndrome.[45]

Assessment and Management of Other Symptoms

Anxiety

Anxiety is one of the more common symptoms experienced by critically ill patients in the ICU. The management of such distress can dramatically improve the quality of life for the patient. Patients with a history of prior anxiety states, including phobias, panic attacks, and major anxiety disorders, are at high risk for these symptoms. Specific anti-anxiety agents should be used in such patients and, in general, anxiolytics should be the drug of choice for these symptoms. Benzodiazepines are the most commonly used drugs for sedation in the ICU.[2,3,5,9,13,22,71-75] They work through the inhibitory neurotransmitter gamma-amino buytyric acid (GABA) at the level of the limbic system. They have no intrinsic analgesic properties and concurrent administration of opioids may help those patients who require treatment of anxiety and pain relief. These drugs impair memory acquisition and cause anterograde amnesia, making them useful in limiting patients' memories of stressful experiences.

Diazepam, lorazepam, and midazolam are also commonly used drugs for anxiety.[2,3,5,9,71-75] Diazepam, because of its long half-life and active metabolite, is less frequently used than midazolam, which is the most commonly used agent in ICUs and for patients in palliative care and hospice units. Midazolam has a rapid onset of action and a short half-life. Because of its short half-life, it requires administration by continuous infusion. Various drug interactions, e.g., with heparin (increases the free fraction) and cimetidine (increases plasma levels), can alter its pharmacokinetic profile. Patients in renal failure have increased free drug, thus a lower dosage than is standard is required. Lorazepam has a half-life of 4–12 hours and can be administered by continuous and intermittent infusions. Lorazepam is metabolized by a glucuronyl transferase and not the p-450 system. Therefore, drugs such as anticonvulsants, rifampin, and cimetidine do not affect its pharmacokinetics. Lorazepam is less expensive than midazolam. Both drugs are commonly used by the intravenous or subcutaneous route, but because of their akaline nature they cannot be easily coadministered with other drugs and often require a separate intravenous line for administration. Standard dosages of these drugs exist, but both the initial dose and dose titration must be individualized.

Clonazepam and alprazolam are commonly used by the oral route. Both drugs are significantly less sedating than lorazepam or midazolam. Clonazepam has a long half-life, allowing it to be administered every 12 hours. Alprazolam has a short half-life, thus repeated administration every 3 to 4 hours is required, for example, to manage panic attacks.

With continuous infusions, tolerance develops rapidly after several days and an increase in dosage is required to maintain symptom control. Similarly, withdrawal symptoms can occur following discontinuation of such infusions and slow tapering of the drug is suggested for those patients on infusions for a prolonged period of time (1 week or longer).[2,71,72]

Barbiturates are also commonly used with pentobarbital and phenobarbital. These are commonly administered intravenously but phenobarbitol suppositories have been described anecdotally in the hospice literature as being useful for sedation in the home-based palliative care patient.[73,74]

Delirium

Agitated delirium is commonly observed in the critically ill patient. Aggressive management of delirium is required to calm these patients, to prevent them from injuring themselves, and to comfort the families, who become profoundly distressed when seeing family members having major symptoms and acting out of control. There is a wide differential diagnosis for delirium in such patients and the goals of care need to be defined early on to facilitate both the assessment and treatment. Haloperidol is the drug of choice for agitated delirium and has been demonstrated in controlled studies to be more effective than lorazepam and chlorpromazine in the management of delirium in critically ill patients.[75] Haloperidol should be started at a dosage of 0.5 to 1 mg and be rapidly titrated up to 5 mg every 4 hours or higher if symptoms are not readily brought under control. In some instances, switching to a different opioid, and titrating the dose of a benzodiazepine concurrently with that of haloperidol are required to obtain the appropriate effect. Methotrimeprazine, a phenothiazine with analgesic and sedative properties, can be useful for those patients in whom the opioid used for analgesia may be causing the delirium. Intramuscular administration of 15 mg of methotrimeprazine is equivalent to 10 mg of intramuscular morphine and can be used to improve analgesia, reduce the respiratory depressant effects, and provide sedation.[41,45] Although available in only a parenteral formulation, it can be given orally, subcutaneous, or intravenously. As previously stated, all attempts to maintain the patient's consciousness and cognitive function should be the first consideration, but such approaches are often not possible. Patients who have developed uremic encephalopathy or hepatic encephalopathy or who have multiple brain metastases or underlying CNS disease need to have their delerium managed to prevent harm to themselves.

Dyspnea

Dyspnea, an uncomfortable awareness of breathing, seriously affects the quality of life of patients and is associated with patients' significant fear of suffocation. Appropriate management of dyspnea in ICU patients requires knowledge of the multidimensional nature of the symptom, of the clinical syndromes that cause dyspnea, and the indications and limitations of the available therapeutic approaches.[76] A wide variety of specific therapies can address the treatment of dyspnea related to specific causes. There are also many treatments that have been suggested for the management of dyspnea, e.g., placing the patient in an upright position so that the patient is leaning forward, with the upper extremities supported on a table. Oxygen therapy has been reported to alleviate dyspnea in hypoxemic patients, but its role in nonhypoxemic patients is not well defined. Low-dose intravenous morphine has been demonstrated to be useful for controlling dyspnea in patients with chronic obstructive pulmonary disease, and data suggest that early use with intravenous opioids, specifically morphine, is effective in reducing physical and psychological distress and exhaustion in patients.[77] The data on nebulized morphine are controversial. Several centers have demonstrated some improvement in exercise endurance, but further studies are necessary before this route can be suggested as an alternative approach.

Sedatives and anxiolytic drugs, including chlopromazine and lorazepam, have also been tried for managing dyspnea, with some providing a slight improvement in the patient's condition. Further studies are necessary to clearly define specific agents that are most effective. Low doses of intravenous morphine—1–2 mg in a nontolerant patient, or titrated to higher doses in a tolerant patient—have been associated with symptomatic relief and should therefore be considered a first-line therapy.

Nausea and vomiting

Nausea and vomiting are also common symptoms in dying patients. It is beyond the scope of this chapter to discuss the potential mechanisms of nausea and vomiting in such patients, but the first line of management should be to reverse the causes of nausea and vomiting if they can be appropriately diagnosed. Intestinal obstruction is one of the more common causes. Dramatic benefit can be achieved by using a protocol for the medical management of intestinal obstruction: the patient is maintained on intravenous or subcutaneous fluids, a draining percutaneous gastrostomy is placed to prevent continuous vomiting, and antiemetics, in combination with antispasmotics and octreotide, is administered to decrease gastrointestinal secretions. For those patients in whom nausea and vomiting are drug induced, the antiemetics of choice include compazine, corticosteroids, haloperidol, metoclopramide, and ondansteron. No direct, comparative data exist to assess the efficacy of any one of these agents in patients experiencing nausea and vomiting, but each drug has been shown to be effective as an antiemetic and sequential trials may be necessary to provide adequate control of nausea and vomiting.

The Role of Sedation

Dying patients commonly have diminished consciousness. In a randomized study of cancer deaths, the proportion of patients who were able to interact at 24 hours,

12 hours, and 1 hour prior to death fell from one-third to one-fifth to one-tenth. Ventafridda and colleagues reported that approximately 50% of patients followed in an Italian home-based palliative care program required sedation to control intractable symptoms.[78] Recent controversy has arisen over the role of sedation in the care of the dying, with some authors suggesting that it is a form of "slow euthanasia."[79] A 1997 Supreme Court decision on physician-assisted suicide strongly endorsed sedation in the imminently dying as appropriate palliative care, and distinguished it from physician-assisted suicide and euthanasia.[80]

Numerous surveys of physicians, nurses, and specialty physician groups suggest that clinicians are confused about the application of ethical principles in the care of the dying.[81] For example, in a recent survey of neurologists, 40% reported that administering intravenous morphine to a dyspneic amyotrophic lateral sclerosis (ALS) patient could be considered a form of euthanasia.[82]

Intensive care units need to develop guidelines for the use of sedative agents in the management of pain and other symptoms in dying patients. Such guidelines must include the parameters for the choice of drug and dosage, and a titration method correlated to symptom assessment and individualized to the major symptom complex. Dose titration without clear indications should not occur merely to protect the professional and moral integrity of all involved. Continuous infusions rather than bolus injections are preferable to prevent the acute exacerbation of pain, dyspnea, or delirium in the patient.[83] Family members may press staff to hurry the process of dying along, and staff should address these requests directly through a family conference to define the goals of care and the role of sedation in providing comfort, not hastening death. Some patients may linger following withdrawal of life support; increased attention must then be focused on supporting the family and the staff through a slow dying process. Families need to be assured that the patient is not suffering and staff need to clearly define how they are assessing the quality of care. For more details on the withdrawal of life support, see Chapter 11.

Careful charting of the drugs administered and of the rationale for dose increases, and open discussions about the plan of end-of-life care can clarify the distinction between aggressive palliative care and euthanasia.

Recent data on patients requiring sedation have shown that patients who received morphine during withdrawal of ventilatory support lived longer than those patients who did not, suggesting that morphine protected patients from the acute stressors of critical illness.[22] Similarly, in a comparison of patients sedated for symptom control versus those who were not, in both hospital and home-based palliative care units, there was no significant difference in the patients' time to death.[5] In a study of opioid dosages in patients cared for in an inpatient palliative care unit, there was no correlation between the opioid dosage and the timing of patients' deaths.[84] The opioid dosages commonly used to sedate critically ill patients are significantly lower than those used to treat pain in postoperative patients. Therefore, there is no empiric evidence that a higher dosage of palliative mediation hastens death.

In short, sedation in the imminently dying patient occurs in the setting of a complicated and rapidly changing clinical situation. Such situations are more uncomfortable for clinicians who lack knowledge about the use of analgesics and sedative agents in such patients and who may confuse their lack of knowledge and experience with their ambivalence about their role in such patient care. Open discussion, clear documentation, and the acknowledgment of ambivalence, ignorance, and lack of competency can provide the environment in which to provide quality care of patients.[85,86]

In summary, the management of physical and psychological symptoms in the dying patient in the ICU should focus on patient comfort and should be guided by the use of an assessment tool, protocols, and careful documentation of goals and plans of care. Aggressive symptom management for the dying is complex, often requiring rapid dosage escalations or drug changes to maintain effective control of symptoms. The application of existing guidelines focused on the special needs of the patient will encourage a more coherent plan of care and create a environment in which new therapies can be tested and existing ones shown to be evidence based.[16] The development of scientifically based guidelines that are tailored to the needs of the individual patient to provide comfort in dying is the current challenge to clinicians who care for the dying.

References

1. Bernat JL, Goldstein ML, Viste KM Jr. The neurologist and the dying patient. *Neurology* 1996;46:598–599.
2. Berger I, Waldhorn RE. Analgesia, sedation and paralysis in the intensive care unit. *Am Fam Physician* 1995;51:166–172.
3. Burns AM, Shelly MP, Park GR. The use of sedative agents in critically ill patients. *Drugs* 1992;43:507–515.
4. Caswell DR, Williams JP, Vallejo M, et al. Improving pain management in critical care. *J Comm J Qual Improv* 1996;22:702–712.
5. Chaters S, Viola R, Paterson J, Jarvis V. Sedation for intractable distress in the dying- a survey of experts. *Palliat Med* 1998;12:255–269.
6. Cherny NI, Coyle N, Foley KM. Guidelines in the care of the dying cancer patient. In: Hematology/Oncology Clinics of North America: Pain and Palliative Care (Cherny NI, Foley KM, eds.). Philadelphia: W.B. Saunders, 1996, pp. 235–259.
7. Cherny NI, Coyle N, Foley KM. Suffering in the advanced cancer pain: a definition and taxonomy. *J Palliat Care* 1994;10:57–70.
8. Christoph SB. Pain assessment. The problem of pain in the critically ill patient. *Crit Care* 1991;3:11–16.
9. Dasta JF, Fuhrman TM, McCandles C. Use of sedatives and analgesics in a surgical intensive care unit: a follow-up and commentary. *Heart Lung* 1995;24:76–78.
10. Lasch K, Carr DB. Pain assessment in seriously ill patients: its importance and need for technical improvement. *Crit Care Med* 1996;24:1943–1944.
11. Mayer SA, Kossoff SB. Withdrawal of life support in the neurological intensive care unit. *Neurology* 1999;52:1602–1609.

12. Tittle M, McMillan SC. Pain and pain-related side effects in an ICU and on a surgical unit: nurses' management. *Am J Crit Care* 1994;3:25–30.

13. Veselis RA. Sedation and pain management for the critically ill. *Crit Care* 1988; 4:167–181.

14. Desbiens NA, Mueller-Rizner N, Connors AF Jr, Wenger NS, Lynn J. The symptom burden of seriously ill hospitalized patients. *J Pain Symptom Manag* 1999;17:248–255.

15. Morrison RS, Ahronheim JC, Morrison GR, Darling E, Baskin SA, Morris J, Choi C, Meier DE. Pain and discomfort associated with common hospital procedures and experiences. *J Pain Symptom Manag* 1998;15:91–101.

16. Prendergast TJ, Claessens MT, Luce JM. A National Survey of End-of-Life Care for Critically Ill Patients. *Am J Respir Crit Care Med* 1998;158:1163–1167.

17. Puntillo KA. Pain experiences of intensive care unit patients. *Heart Lung* 1990; 19:526–533.

18. Gujol MC. A survey of pain assessment and management practices among critical care nurses. *Am J Crit Care* 1994;3:123–128.

19. Puntillo KA. Stitch, stitch . . . creating an effective pain management program for critically ill patients. *Am J Crit Care* 1997;6:259–260.

20. Puntillo KA, Miaskowski C, Kehrle K, Stannard D, Gleeson S, Nye P. Relationship between behavioral and physiological indicators of pain, critical care patients' self-reports of pain, and opioid administration. *Crit Care Med* 1997;25:1159–1166.

21. Tiseo P, Thaler HT, Lapin J, Inturrisi CE, Portenoy RK, Foley KM. Morphine-6-glucurinide concentrations and opioid related side effects-a survey in cancer patients. *Pain* 1995;61:47–54.

22. Wilson WD, Smedira NG, Fink C, McDowell JA, Lance JM. Ordering and administration of sedatives and analgesics during the withholding and withdrawal of life support from critically ill patients. *JAMA* 1992;267:949–953.

23. Wild L. Pain management. *Crit Care* 1990;2:537–547.

24. Foley KM. Clinical tolerance to opioids. In: Towards a New Pharmacotherapy of Pain: Dahlem Konfrenzen (The Dahlem Conference) (Basbaum AL, Besson JM, eds.). Chichester, UK: John Wiley & Sons, 1991, pp. 181–204.

25. Ingham JM, Portenoy RK. Symptom assessment. In: Hematology/Oncology Clinics of North America: Pain and Palliative Care (Cherny NI, Foley KM, eds.). Philadelphia: W.B. Saunders, 1996, pp. 21–40.

26. American Pain Society. Principles of Analgesic Use in the Treatment of Acute Pain and Cancer Pain, 4th ed. IL: American Pain Society.

27. Bookbinder M, Coyle N, Kiss M, Goldstein ML, Holritz K, Thaler H, Gianella A, Derby S, Brown M, Racolin A, Ho MN, Portenoy RK. Implementing national standards for cancer pain management. *J Pain Symptom Manag* 1996;12:334–347.

28. Carr DB, Jacox AK, Chapman CR, et al. Acute Pain Management, No. 1. A HCPR Publication No. 95-0034. Rockville, MD: U.S. Department of Health and Human Serivces, Public Health Service, Agency for Health Care Policy and Research, 1995.

29. American Pain Society, Quality of Care Committee. Quality improvement guidelines for the treatment of acute pain and cancer pain. *JAMA* 1995;274:1874–1880.

30. Fishman B, Pasternak S, Wallerstein SL, et al. A valid instrument for the evaluation of cancer pain. *Cancer* 1987;60:1151–1158.

31. Bruera E, MacDonald S. Audit methods: Edmonton Symptom Assessment System. In: Clinical Audit in Palliative Care (Higginson I, ed.) Oxford: Radcliffe Medical Press, 1993, pp. 61–77.

32. Portenoy RK, Hagen NA. Breakthrough pain: definition, prevalence and characteristics. *Pain* 1990;41:273.
33. Fowler FJ, Coppola KM, Teno JM. Methodological challenges for measuring quality of care at the end of life. *J Pain Symptom Manag* 1999;17:114–119.
34. Jacox AK, Carr DB, Payne R, et al. Management of Cancer Pain, Clinical Practice Guidelines, No. 9. AHCPR Publication No. 94-0592. Rockville, MD: U.S. Department of Health and Human Services, Public Health Service, Agency for Health Care Policy and Research, 1994.
35. World Health Organization Cancer Pain Relief and Palliative Care. Geneva: World Health Organization, 1996.
36. World Health Organization. Cancer Pain Relief, 2nd ed. With a Guide to Opioid availability, Cancer Pain Relief and Palliative Care: Report of the WHO Expert Committee. *World Health Organ Tech Rep Ser* 1996;804.
37. Aronson MD. Nonsteriodal anti-inflammatory drugs, traditional opioids and tramadol: contrasting therapies for the treatment of chronic pain. *Clin Ther* 1997; 19:420–432.
38. Henry D, Lim LL-Y, Rodriguez LAG, et al. Variability in risk of gastrointestinal complications with individual nonsteriodal anti-inflammatory drugs: results of a collaborative meta-analysis. *BMJ* 1996;312:1563–1566.
39. Brandon-Bravo L, Mattie H, Spierdijk J, et al. The effects on ventilation of ketorolac in comparison with morphine. *Eur J Clin Pharmacol* 1988;35:491–494.
40. Litvak KM, McEvoy GK. Ketorolac, and injectable nonnarcotic analgesic. *Drug Rev* 1990;9:921–935.
41. Lasagna L, DeKornfeld TJ. Methotrimeprazine: a new phenothiazine derivative with analgesic properties. *JAMA* 1961;178:887–890.
42. Portenoy RK. Adjuvant analgesics in palliative care. In: Textbook of Palliative Medicine. Oxford: Oxford University Press, 1998, pp. 361–390.
43. Portenoy RK, Foley KM, Inturrisi CE. The nature of opioid responsiveness and its implications for neuropathic pain. *Pain* 1990;43:273.
44. Cherny NI, Thaler HT, Friedlander-Klar H, Lapin J, Foley KM, Houde RW, Portenoy RK. Opioid responsiveness of cancer pain syndromes causes by neuropathic or nociceptive mechanisms: a combined analysis of controlled, single-dosed studies. *Neurology* 1994;44:857–861.
45. Foley KM. Management of cancer pain. In: Cancer Principles and Practice of Oncology, 3rd ed. (DeVita VT, Hellman S, Rosenberg SA, eds.) Philadelphia: J.B. Lippincott, 1997, pp. 2807–2841.
46. Rogers AG. Considering histamine release in prescribing opioid analgesics. *J Pain Symptom Manag* 1991;6:44–45.
47. Biddle C, Gilliland C. Transdermal and transmucosal administration of pain-relieving and anxiolytic drugs: a primer for the critical care practitioner. *Heart Lung* 1992;21:115–124.
48. Cherny NI, Chang V, Frager G, Ingham JM, Tiseo PJ, Popp B, Portenoy RK, Foley KM. Opioid pharmacology in the management of cancer pain. *Cancer* 1995; 76:1283–1293.
49. Farrar JT, Cleary J, Rauck R, Busch M, Nordbrook E. Oral transmucosal fentanyl citrate: randomized, double-blinded, placebo-controlled trial for treatment breakthrough pain in cancer patients. *J Nat Cancer Inst* 1998;90:611–616.
50. Bruera E, Pereira J, Watanabe S, et al. Opioid rotation in patients with cancer pain:

a retrospective comparison of dose ratios between methadone, hydromorphone and morphine. *Cancer* 1996;78:852–857.

51. Mercadante S, Casuccio A, Agnello A, Barresi L. Methadone response in advanced cancer patients with pain followed at home. *J Pain Symptom Manag* 1998;18:188–192.

52. Ripamonti C, Groff L, Brunelli C, Polastri D, Stravrakis A, De Conno F. Switching from morphine to oral methadone in treating cancer pain: what is the equianalgesic dose ratio? *J Clin Oncol* 1998;16:3216–3221.

53. Kaiko RF, Foley KM, Grabinski PY, Heidrich G, Rogers AG, Inturrisi CE, Reidenberg MM. Central nervous system excitatory effects of meperidine in cancer patients. *Ann Neurol* 1983;13:180–185.

54. De Conno F, Ripamonti C, Saita L, et al. Role of rectal route in treating cancer pain: a randomized crossover clinical trial of oral versus rectal morphine administration in opioid-naive cancer patients with pain. *J Clin Oncol* 1995;13:1004–1008.

55. Stanik JA. Use of patient-controlled analgesia with critically ill patients: a risk-benefit analysis. *Crit Care Nurse* 1991;2:741–747.

56. Bedder MD, Soifer BE, Mulhall JJ. A comparison of patient-controlled analgesia and bolus prn intravenous morphine in the intensive care environment. *Pain* 1991;7:205–208.

57. Bruera E, Chadwick S, Brenneis C, Hanson J, MacDonald RN. Methylphenidate associated with narcotics for the treatment of cancer pain. *Cancer Treat Rep* 1987;71:67–70.

58. Forrest WH, Brown BW, Brown CR, et al. Dextroamphetamine with morphine for treatment of postoperative pain. *N Engl J Med* 1977;296:712–715.

59. Laska EM, Sunshine A, Mueller F, et al. Caffeine as an analgesic adjuvant. *JAMA* 1984;251:1711–1718.

60. Ashby MA, Martin P, Jackson KA. Opioid substitution to reduce adverse efects in cancer pain management. *Med J Aust* 1999;170:68–71.

61. Cherny NI, Portenoy RK. Sedation in the management of refractory symptoms: guidelines for evaluation and treatment. *J Palliat Care* 1994;10:31–39.

62. Hewitt DJ, Portenoy RK. Adjuvant drugs for neuropathic cancer pain. In: *Topics in Palliative Care, Vol. 2.* (Bruera E, Portenoy RK, eds.) New York: Oxford University Press, 1998, pp. 41–62.

63. Max MB, Lynch SA, Muir J, Shoaf SE, Smoller B, Dubner R. Effects of desipramine, amitriptyline, and fluoxetine on pain in diabetic neuropathy. *N Engl J Med* 1992;326:1250–1256.

64. Rosenberg JM, Harrell C, Ristic H, Werner RA, de Rosayro AM. The effect of gabapentin on neuropathic pain. *Clin J Pain* 1997;13:251–255.

65. Ettinger AB, Portenoy RK. The use of corticosteriods in the treatment of symptoms associated with cancer. *J Pain Symptom Manage* 1988;3:99–103.

66. Brose WG, Cousins MJ. Subcutaneous lidocaine for treatment of neuropathic cancer pain. *Pain* 1991;45:145–148.

67. Backonja M, Arndt G, Gombar KA, Check B, Zimmerman M. Response of chronic neuropathic pain syndromes to ketamine: a preliminary study. *Pain* 1994;56:51–57.

68. Foley KM. The relationship of pain and symptom management to patient requests for physician-assisted suicide. *J Pain Symptom Manage* 1991;6:289–297.

69. Fins JJ. Acts of omission and commission in pain management: the ethics of naloxone use. *J Pain Symptom Manage* 1991;17:120–124.

70. Manfredi PL, Ribeiro S, Chandler SW, Payne R. Inappropriate use of naloxone in cancer patients with pain. *J Pain Symptom Manage* 1996;11:131–134.
71. Bergman I, Steves M, Burckart G, Thompson A. Reversible neurologic abnormalities associated with prolonged intravenous midazolam and fentanyl administration. *J Pediatr* 1991;119:644–649.
72. Reves JG, Fragen RJ, Vinik HR, Greenblatt DJ. Midazolam: pharmacology and uses. *Anesthesiology* 1985;62:310–324.
73. Green WR, Davis WH. Titrated intravenous barbiturates in the control of symptoms in patients with terminal cancer. *South Med J* 1991;84:332–338.
74. Troug RD, Berde CB, Mitchell C, Greir HE. Barbiturates in the care of the terminally ill. *N Engl J Med* 1992;327:1678.
75. Brietbart W, Marotta R, Platt MM, Weisman H, Derevenco M, Grau C, Corbera K, Raymond S, Lund S, Jacobsen P. A double-blind trial of haloperidol, chlorpromazine, and lorazepam in the treatment of delirium in hospitalized AIDS patients. *Am J Psychiatry* 1996;153:231–237.
76. Dudgeon DJ, Rosenthal S. Management of dyspnea and cough in patients with cancer. In: Hematology/Oncology Clinics of North America: Pain and Palliative Care (Cherny NI, Foley KM, eds.) Philadelphia: W.B. Saunders, 1996, pp. 157–171.
77. Allard P, Lamontagne C, Bernard P, Tremblay C. How effective are supplementary doses of opioids for dyspnea in terminally ill cancer patients? A randomized continuous sequential clinical trial. *J Pain Symptom Manag* 1999;17:256–265.
78. Ventafridda V, Ripamonti C, De Conno F, Tamburini M, Cassileth BR. Symptom prevalence and control during cancer patients' last days of life. *J Palliat Care* 1990;6:7–11.
79. Billings JA, Block SD. Slow euthanasia. *J Palliat Care* 1996;12:21–30.
80. Burt RA. The Supreme Court speaks: not assisted suicide but a constitutional right to palliative care. *N Engl J Med* 1997;337:1234–1236.
81. Solomon M, O'Donnell L, Jenning B, et al. Decisions near the end of life: professional views of life-sustaining treatments. *Am J Public Health* 1993;83:14–21.
82. Carver AC, Vickrey BG, Bernat JL, et al. End of life care: a survey of US neurologists' attitudes, behavior and knowledge. *Neurology* 1999;53:284–293.
83. Fainsinger RL, Landman W, Hoskings M, Bruera E. Sedation for uncontrolled symptoms in a South African hospice. *J Pain Symptom Manag* 1998;16:145–152.
84. Brescia F, Portenoy R, Ryan M, Drasnoff L, Gray G. Pain, opioid use and survival in hospitalized patients with advanced cancer. *J Clin Oncol* 1992;10:149–155.
85. Mount B. Morphine drips, terminal sedation, and slow euthanasia: definitions and facts, not anecdotes. *J Palliat Care* 1996;12:31–37.
86. Portenoy RK. Morphine infusions at the end of life: the pitfalls in reasoning from anecdote. *J Palliat Care* 1996;12:44–46.

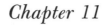

Chapter 11

Principles and Practice of Withdrawing Life-Sustaining Treatment in the ICU

GORDON D. RUBENFELD
STEPHEN W. CRAWFORD

Most deaths in intensive care units occur after decisions to limit or withdraw life support.[1-4] Despite extensive literature on whether to withdraw life support, little attention has been given to how to withdraw it.[5-12] For example, a recent edition of a critical care textbook covers the ethical and legal aspects of life-support withdrawal, but provides no recommendations for carrying it out.[13] Only recently, in the wake of growing data that problems may exist in providing palliative care in the ICU, has attention been directed to the practical aspects of withdrawing life support.[14] Many practical questions about withdrawal of life support are perplexing and controversial.[15] Should the endotracheal tube be left in place? Should interventions be weaned slowly or quickly? When should sedation be increased? How can concerns about relieving suffering be reconciled with fears of killing the patient? Should neuromuscular blockade be discontinued? These questions are important because clinicians face them frequently and yet are still confused by the goals and process of withdrawing life support, and because patients who die after withdrawal of life support may receive inadequate pain relief.[16,17]

Principles of Withdrawing Life-Sustaining Treatments

In this era of evidence-based medicine, there are inadequate data to direct clinicians in the optimal management of the dying, critically ill patient. Despite the lack of data on optimal management of some aspects of withdrawing life-sustaining treatment, a general consensus exists on the ethical and clinical principles that should guide this care. These six principles are listed in Table 11–1.

Understanding that the goal of withdrawing life-sustaining treatments is to

Table 11–1. Principles of withdrawing life support

1. The goal of withdrawing life-sustaining treatments is to remove treatments that are no longer desired or do not provide comfort to the patient.

2. The withholding of life-sustaining treatments is morally and legally equivalent to their withdrawal.

3. Actions with the sole goal of hastening death are morally and legally problematic.

4. Any treatment can be withheld or withdrawn.

5. Withdrawal of life-sustaining treatment is a medical procedure.

6. Corollary to 1 and 2: when circumstances justify withholding an indicated life-sustaining treatment, strong consideration should be given to withdrawing current life-sustaining treatments.

remove unwanted treatments rather than to hasten death is essential in clarifying the distinction between active euthanasia (providing drugs or toxins that hasten death) and death that accompanies the withdrawal of life support in the ICU. There is no doubt that withdrawing unwanted life-sustaining treatments will hasten death more than if they were continued; however, ethicists draw a line between withdrawing life-sustaining treatments when the expected but unintended effect is to hasten death and providing a treatment with the sole intent of hastening death. Despite the well-established principle that "withholding and withdrawing are equivalent," some clinicians find it difficult to stop treatments that are currently being provided and choose to withhold future treatments while continuing current levels of support. Frequently, clinicians are faced with multiple decisions about a variety of current or potential life-sustaining treatments. When a decision is made to withhold or withdraw one life-sustaining treatment—for example, if dialysis is withheld from a patient with worsening acidosis and anuria—clinicians should strongly consider whether continuing other life-sustaining treatments makes sense. When clinicians discuss options with families, they may put life-sustaining treatments into different categories such as "heroic measures" or "ordinary treatment"; however, these terms do not have a defined clinical meaning or ethical value. There is no distinction from an ethical or medical standpoint between mechanical ventilation, antibiotics, blood products, intravenous fluids, or nutrition. All medical treatments, even nutrition and fluids, can be legally, ethically, and compassionately stopped in the appropriate setting.

The recommendations in this chapter are based on the premise that the withdrawal of life-sustaining treatments is a clinical procedure, and, as such, merits the same meticulous preparation and expectation of quality that clinicians provide when they perform other procedures to initiate life support. Therefore, the steps clinicians take when they withdraw life-support should parallel the steps they take when they perform a thoracentesis, lumbar puncture, or appendectomy (Table 11–2). By providing a familiar framework to

Table 11–2. Routine steps in performing a procedure

The decision is made to perform the procedure.

Informed consent is obtained.

An explicit plan for performing the procedure and handling complications is formed.

The patient is moved to an appropriate setting.

Adequate sedation and analgesia are begun.

The plan is carried out.

The process is documented in the medical record.

The outcomes are evaluated in an attempt to improve the procedure.

guide clinical practice and by proposing a protocol for the procedure, we hope to improve the quality of care to patients at the end of life.

The Decision to Withdraw Life-Sustaining Treatments

Ethical and legal guidelines for decisions to withdraw life-sustaining treatments are well established and have been presented elsewhere (see Chapters 2 and 8).[18–21] Competent, informed patients may refuse any life-sustaining treatment. For incompetent patients, appropriate surrogates may refuse life-sustaining treatments on the basis of written advance directives or, in almost all U.S. states, the patient's previously stated wishes, values, or best interests . In some circumstances, it is ethically appropriate for physicians to limit treatment in the absence of a surrogate or advance directive.[22]

There should be a consensus among the health care team about the decision to withdraw life support. Frequently, members of the critical care team will reach the conclusion to limit life-sustaining treatment at different times. While the attending physician must take ultimate responsibility for the decision, it would be imprudent to insist on a plan in the face of persistent, thoughtful disagreement by members of the health care team. Withdrawing life support is seldom an emergency decision and time should be taken to resolve disagreements among the staff and with family members. Strategies to improve consensus include allaying fears of legal liability, encouraging face-to-face discussions between health care professionals who disagree on the prognosis, eliciting the views of clinicians providing bedside care, and consulting with a senior clinician or ethics committee. When engaging in these discussions, clinicians should temper the certainty of their convictions about the utility of life-sustaining treatment with the knowledge that a large body of data shows that clinicians apply personal values and biases rather than ethical principles and outcome data when making clinical decisions.[23–25] All team members, particularly those in direct patient care roles, should feel that they have had meaningful input into the final plan.

Informed Consent

Like other medical procedures, withdrawal of life support should be accompanied by informed consent and documentation of this consent in the medical record. Detailed recommendations about communication with family and staff about end-of-life decisions are presented in Chapter 9. Competent patients or the surrogates of incompetent patients should understand and agree with the decision to withdraw life support. In many cases, patients or families will initiate the request that life support be withdrawn. In rare cases, patients or surrogates may insist on interventions that the health care team regards as futile. While there is no ethical obligation to provide futile care, there is considerable controversy over which interventions are futile and can be withdrawn over the objections of the patient or surrogate.[26] Fortunately, almost all patients or surrogates eventually agree with physicians' recommendations to withdraw or withhold interventions.[4] Helpful strategies for reaching agreement include instituting open and honest communications with family members from the time of admission, identifying and correcting any misunderstandings, paying special attention to emotional needs, attempting time-limited therapeutic trials, and obtaining assistance from the hospital ethics committee.[27] In exceptional cases, even with the use of these techniques, agreement cannot be negotiated and clinicians may choose to withhold or withdraw futile interventions despite family requests. In these extraordinary cases, the ethical principles of truth-telling and respect for persons dictate that either families be informed of the decision or clinicians determine that the decision makers do not wish to be informed.[22] Although these discussions can be uncomfortable for clinicians and family members, this does not justify covert clinical activity such as "slow codes" or replacing vasopressor drips with normal saline.[28]

Physicians must provide clear recommendations while respecting the right of patients or their surrogates to make decisions about the process. It is important to explain to the family members how interventions will be withdrawn, to solicit their feedback, and to respect strong preferences regarding how interventions will be withdrawn. Some patients or their families may assign particular symbolic significance to certain aspects of care. For example, there may be strong wishes to remove the endotracheal tube while mechanical ventilation is being withdrawn or to continue feeding and hydration when dialysis and vasopressors are stopped. These wishes should be respected as long as they do not interfere with the primary goal of enhancing patient comfort and removing technology that does not fulfill the shared goals. Although it is important for patients and families to have some control over the dying process, it is confusing and inhumane to ask family members to give specific consent for each step of the withdrawal process. Clinicians should specifically avoid providing patients with an entire menu of life-sustaining treatment options to choose from. Families who are not medically sophisticated may have unrealistic expectations and understanding of life-sustaining technology.[29] Generally, once families set the goals of care—for example, to maximize comfort and forego attempts to prolong survival—it is up to clinicians to decide how to meet these goals.

Appropriate Setting and Monitoring

Transforming the ICU into a suitable place to fulfill the new goals of terminal care is not a simple task. The ICU and its staff are poised to respond to minor physiologic changes. Comfort, dignity, family access, and quiet may not always receive the highest priority. Particularly when family members and friends will be in attendance, the goal should be to have the patient lying comfortably, cleanly, and privately in a quiet room devoid of technology and alarms. The following are suggestions for creating a humane and private environment for the dying patient and family or surrogate:

- Separate the patient from the commotion of the ICU by moving the patient to a separate area or an isolated room. In open units, curtains should be closed.
- Turn off monitors and, if possible, remove them from the room. Remove electrocardiographic leads, pulse oximeter, and hemodynamic monitoring catheters. There is no point in monitoring physiologic parameters when the data generated will not alter care. Families attending the dying patient can become preoccupied with irrelevant numbers and waveforms instead of focusing their attention on the patient. Removing monitors also eliminates the alarms that will sound as patients die. Intensive nursing care supplemented by physical examination of the patient for blood pressure, pulse, and respiratory rate is sufficient to identify manifestations of suffering and to determine when death occurs. We feel that removing patients from electronic monitoring is an essential step in the transition from curative to comfort care. Unfortunately, it is extremely difficult for clinicians to give up this technologic tether precisely because this step symbolizes the break from the physiologic monitoring that identifies the ICU.
- Remove all tubes, lines, and drains if this can be done without significant discomfort. Catheter removal that would lead to painful obstruction, for example, of Foley catheters or biliary drains, may be left in place. Intravenous access should be maintained to administer analgesic medication. Remove unused intravenous pumps, resuscitation carts, and other mobile technology from the room.

- Liberalize visitation to the extent that it does not interfere with the delivery of care to other patients. Children should be allowed to visit if their parents approve.[30]
- Do not obtain further laboratory or imaging studies.

Sedation and Analgesia

Prior to performing uncomfortable procedures, clinicians provide patients with adequate medication to prevent anxiety and suffering. Critically ill, hemodynamically unstable patients may not receive optimal sedation when drug-related hypotension or respiratory suppression compromises the goals of maintaining life or liberation from mechanical ventilation. However, when the goal of care is changed to assuring patient comfort, any dosage of medication that is required to meet this goal is justified, even if it hastens death. The sole purpose of administering sedatives to dying patients is to relieve symptoms associated with this process. Although rare in the modern ICU, patients capable of communicating their wishes during the withdrawal of life-sustaining treatments should determine how much sedation they receive. Before patients are removed from life support, they should be completely comfortable as judged by the cessation of tachypnea, grimacing, agitated behavior, and autonomic hyperactivity. This is accomplished by titrating medication until objective signs of discomfort have been eliminated. In many cases this will require medication sufficient to induce unconsciousness. Doses should not be increased in the absence of demonstrable signs of discomfort or for behavior that cannot plausibly be interpreted as distress. For example, increased sedation may be indicated for coughing or tachypnea, but not for eye movements. When these goals are achieved, further increases in sedation are unnecessary and ethically problematic.

Although variations in clinical practice are expected, some regimens are unacceptable. Large boluses of medication similar to those used for the induction of general anesthesia are excessive unless smaller doses have failed to provide adequate sedation. There is an important ethical difference between escalating sedative doses to achieve rapid relief of symptoms and administering a large initial bolus intended to induce apnea or hypotension. There is no role for paralytic agents in the withdrawal of life-sustaining treatments. In fact, these drugs are contraindicated because they will hide manifestations of discomfort such as grimacing and tachypnea.

Given the variability in individual responses and drug tolerance, it is impossible to outline a single pharmacologic regimen to apply in every case. Current guidelines on the management of pain and anxiety in critical care recommend a combination of morphine or similar narcotic with a benzodiazepine.[31] These medications, dosed appropriately, will provide adequate analgesia and sedation in virtually all cases when life support is withdrawn. The individual clinician's experience or the failure of the opiate/benzodiazepine combination may justify the use of barbiturates, haloperidol, or propofol.[32]

We suggest the following guidelines for therapy:

- Specific doses of medication are less important goals than titration to achieve the desired effect. In patients with painful surgical wounds, high ventilatory drives, or prior exposure to narcotics, morphine doses of over 70 mg/hr may be necessary to achieve comfort. Perhaps the most important concept is that no ceiling should be placed on dosage if the goal of relieving patient distress has not been achieved. There is no substitute for close bedside evaluation in assessing the efficacy of the sedative medication.

- Because of its flexibility and reliability, continuous infusion is the route of choice for drug delivery. Increases in dosage should be preceded by a bolus so that steady-state levels are achieved rapidly.

- Critical care nurses, who have extensive experience in evaluating suffering in patients who cannot communicate, should be afforded wide latitude in drug dosing, with clear indications for changing the dose. For example, the order might read: "Titrate morphine drip to keep respiratory rate <30 and heart rate <100, and eliminate grimacing and agitation." Clinical events that necessitate increases in medication and the response to the new dose must be documented in the medical record.

A Plan for Withdrawal

Before physicians perform procedures like intubation or central venous catheterization, they have a clear plan of action as well as contingency plans for complications. A similar plan should be developed for withdrawing life support. Physicians need to consider which life-support measures will be discontinued, in what order, and by whom.

Once a decision has been made to orient the patient's care to comfort, the only criterion for judging whether a treatment should be initiated, withheld, or withdrawn is whether it contributes to the patient's comfort. All treatments can be withdrawn, including vasopressors, drugs, antibiotics, blood transfusions, and nutritional support. We recognize that clinicians and, occasionally, some families are uncomfortable discontinuing certain interventions they view as basic care. For example, some clinicians may feel that intravenous fluids, nutrition, and even antibiotics are basic enough to be included as comfort care.[33] There is little evidence that these treatments contribute to the comfort of dying patients.[34] Some families may choose to continue nutrition and hydration because of the symbolic nature of these treatments even after their lack of contribution to palliative care has been explained. These requests should be respected. When discussing these treatments, clinicians should avoid the use of emotionally charged terms like "starvation" and "dehydration," which probably do not apply to terminally ill patients whose symptoms have been appropriately palliated.

Many health care workers feel more comfortable withholding treatments rather than withdrawing them after they have been initiated.[35] Unfortunately, this leads many clinicians to a strategy that withdraws life support in a series of steps over several days.[33] In this "stuttering withdrawal" process, clinicians adopt a combination of withholding increases in vasopressor medication or ventilator pressures while continuing other treatments such as antibiotics and transfusions. Rarely, such measures are indicated as negotiating techniques with family members or to fulfill specific goals such as trying to sustain life until a relative can arrive while still minimizing burdensome treatments. Clinicians may engage in this stepped withdrawal because a gradual series of steps minimizes the psychological linkage between their actions and the patient's death.[36] Although potentially psychologically reassuring, a gradual approach to withdrawing life-sustaining treatments over several days is not ethically or legally necessary.[19,37] Generally, circumstances that justify withholding one indicated life-sustaining treatment also justify the withdrawal of current life-sustaining treatments.[19,38] For example, if clinicians and the family decide to withhold dialysis in a patient with cirrhosis, sepsis, and progressive hyperkalemia with acidosis, strong consideration should be given to withdrawing ventilatory support and other life-sustaining treatments. When partial treatment strategies are entertained, clinicians should be clear about the goals of care and the rationale for their decision and to ensure that this rationale is based on a specific family request rather than on their own discomfort with withdrawal of a particular life-sustaining treatment.

The time course over which a life-sustaining treatment should be withdrawn is determined by the potential for discomfort as the life-sustaining treatment is stopped. The only rationale for weaning or slowly tapering a life-sustaining treatment is to allow time to meet the patient's needs for pain relief. Mechanical ventilation is one of the few life-support devices whose abrupt termination is likely to lead to profound discomfort due to dyspnea and therefore deserves specific attention to the time course of its withdrawal. There is little justification for "weaning" other interventions. After adequate sedation has been achieved, vasopressors, pacemakers, intraaortic balloon pumps, and other therapy not oriented toward meeting the comfort goals of care should be turned off. Tapering these treatments serves no role other than delaying death. Since the withdrawal of mechanical ventilation poses the greatest problems with ensuring comfort, all other life-support devices should be withdrawn before the ventilator. Patients requiring high levels of hemodynamic support may sustain a rapid cardiac death just from withdrawal of hemodynamic support before any attention can be devoted to the ventilator. Physically turning off these devices can be an emotional task, and the attending physician should be prepared to perform this task or be present when it occurs. Physicians-in-training do not perform other medical procedures independently prior to demonstrating their competence in a supervised setting, and the same rules should apply to the withdrawal of life support.

Withdrawing mechanical ventilation

Unless the patient specifically requests otherwise, sedation and analgesia sufficient to prevent grimacing or response to painful stimuli should be provided before withdrawal of mechanical ventilatory support (Table 11–3). After adequate sedation is achieved, we reduce the inspired oxygen concentration to 0.21, remove positive end expiratory pressure, and set the ventilator at an intermittent mandatory ventilation (IMV) rate equal to the patient's spontaneous respiratory rate or to a level of pressure support (PS) sufficient to fully meet the patient's ventilatory requirements. These ventilator settings give the patient a fully supported ventilator breath with every inspiratory attempt and allow clinicians time to modify the sedation before completely removing ventilator assistance. Air hunger, as manifested by tachypnea or agitation, should be treated with a bolus of the chosen sedative followed by an increase in the continuous infusion. After the patient is comfortable, ventilatory support is weaned rapidly in either IMV or PS mode until the patient is comfortable with an IMV rate of zero or a PS of 5 cm H_2O, at which point the patient can be placed on a T-piece with humidified air. Unless extraordinary levels of dyspnea are encountered or in the unusual case in which clinicians are trying to withdraw ventilatory support from an awake patient and maintain some level of consciousness in the patients there is no reason for the transition from full ventilatory support to T-piece or extubation to take more than 15 to 30 minutes. Families may wish to be present for this process or not—if they choose to attend, they should be prepared for the possibility of some transient increases in agitation or respiratory rate as sedation is being titrated. It is extremely important to disable ventilator alarms during this period as patients' terminal hypoventilation may trigger them. Some ventilator alarms cannot be disabled

Table 11–3. Procedure for removing a patient from mechanical ventilation

Task	Approximate time (minutes)
Ensure adequate sedation	5–10
Reduce inspired oxygen to 21% (air) Remove positive end expiratory pressure (PEEP)	1–5
Set ventilator to IMV or PS level to fully meet patient's ventilatory needs	1–5
Observe and modify sedative medication while gradually reducing IMV rate or PS level to 5	5–20
Extubate or leave on humidified air by T-piece	

and this should direct clinicians to use a T-piece or to extubate rather than to leave the patient attached to the ventilator. An experienced physician should attend this early phase of withdrawal from the bedside to reassure the patient and family and observe for complications such as intractable discomfort that would require immediate intervention.

Our practice is to leave the endotracheal tube in place when mechanical ventilation is withdrawn. This prevents gasping and airway occlusion that may be uncomfortable for the patient and observers. It also facilitates suctioning in patients who are uncomfortable because of profuse secretions. Nevertheless, it may be appropriate to extubate the patient, particularly when the patient may be able to communicate or prolonged survival off of life support is expected. Some families or providers may feel strongly that the endotracheal tube be removed. Although these wishes should be respected, specific plans should be formulated to anticipate secretion problems and agonal airway obstruction when the endotracheal tube is removed. There are few data to determine the best practice in this area; however, if other aspects of the withdrawal of life-sustaining treatments are managed well, including communication with the family and adequate sedation, the management of the endotracheal tube is not of paramount importance.

The time course leading to death will vary according to the clinical situation and cannot be predicted accurately in every case. However, caregivers should inform the patient and family of the probable course of events once life support is withdrawn. The critically ill patient on several vasopressor agents who is pacemaker dependent will survive for only a few minutes when these are discontinued. A neurologically devastated teenager with a closed head injury whose only life support is an endotracheal tube, antibiotics, and enteral nutrition will have a more prolonged course. Plans should be made for alternative care sites if death is delayed. When patients are transferred out of the ICU, the ICU team should communicate the goals and plan to the new team and introduce the new team to the patient and family so that continuity of care is maintained.

Pastoral, Nursing, and Emotional Support

Before interventions are withdrawn, the family should be asked if a priest, pastor, rabbi, or other religious advisor should be called. Caring for patients after life-sustaining technology is withdrawn can require the same level of vigilance and time that aggressive life support requires. Nursing attention should be directed to hygiene, skin care, interacting with family members, and maintaining a quiet environment within the busy ICU. Treatments that may alleviate or prevent uncomfortable complications should be instituted or continued. For example, cooling blankets, antipyretics, and anticonvulsants fulfill the goals of patient comfort and should usually be continued. Suggestions and feedback from the family members should be regularly solicited. Members of the health care team should ask the family in an open-ended manner how they feel things are going and whether they have any questions about or suggestions for supportive care. Our approach is to invite the family to play an active role in the care, without making them feel responsible for how interventions are withdrawn.

Just as potential medical complications should be anticipated, the health care team needs to plan how to respond to the family's emotional reactions and needs. Family members, as well as some members of the health care team, often believe that they are causing the patient's death by withdrawing interventions. The physician should address these issues directly: "Many family members ask themselves whether they are causing the patient's death by agreeing to withdraw the ventilator. Do you feel that way?" Generally, people feel more comfortable with withdrawing interventions after these feelings are acknowledged, legitimized as common reactions, and discussed openly. Until these issues are addressed on an emotional level, it is unproductive to discuss the lack of philosophical and legal distinctions between withdrawing and withholding interventions.

If the patient survives longer than expected, family members and health care workers may feel impatient, frustrated, or angry. Again, the best course is to address the issue directly. A simple comment may broach the topic: "It's hard to have to wait like this, isn't it?" Our approach emphasizes that the exact time of death is out of the hands of the physicians and nurses. Some health care workers may feel comfortable saying, "It is now in God's hands." Death is traditionally marked by ceremonies and rituals that extend support and sympathy to the survivors. Health care workers can ask open-ended questions such as "Tell me about his life as a young man." After the patient dies, the attending physician can observe a moment of silence, say a few words of remembrance, and console the family. Empathetic comments such as "It must be hard to accept" or "This must be very painful for you," and questions such as "How can I be of help" are better received than identification with the family, such as "I know how you feel," or reassurance, such as "Time makes it easier" or "God had a purpose."[39] Physicians and nurses need not hide their tears. Physical acts of sympathy, from a handshake to a hug, are appropriate; but these will vary with the cultural and personal backgrounds of the health care workers and families.

Documentation

Progress notes in the medical record should document the meetings leading up to the decision to withdraw support, the specific plans for withdrawal, and the pharmacologic plan for sedation. This is particularly important because nurses or covering physicians who implement the plan may not have been involved in the original decision or discussions. Although meetings with surrogates need not address specific decisions regarding every piece of life-support technology, communication with other health care providers must be detailed. This is particularly important when clinicians choose to withhold some life-sustaining treatments while continuing others. In these cases, the rationale, proscribed treatments, and plan should be clearly documented in the progress notes and orders.

Specific orders for withdrawing interventions and for sedation should be written in the medical record. Orders that simply say "no heroic measures" or "comfort care only" can be confusing to a covering physician who must make decisions about antibiotics or blood transfusions. Institutions should develop guidelines, pathways, preprinted orders, and nursing and respiratory care documentation standards for the withdrawal of life support, as they currently do for other common clinical situations. See Figure 11–1 for an example of preprinted orders and principles.

Evaluation

Quality improvement procedures are important for evaluating the withdrawal of life support and the process of dying, just as they are for other hospital procedures. Members of the hospital critical care committee should review the circumstances of these deaths to evaluate the care. Those involved in the withdrawal of care, including family members, should have the opportunity to evaluate the quality of dying and suggest improvements for the future. These suggestions should be incorporated into the processes in this document and made a part of the local ICU guidelines.

Special Cases

Withdrawal of mechanical ventilation with potential survival

Some patients and families, particularly in cases of severe pulmonary or neuromuscular disease, request that ventilatory support be withdrawn when survival off the ventilator is unlikely but possible. Such requests pose a dilemma for clinicians because the goals of care are mixed. It is difficult to provide sedation to minimize distress *and* simultaneously treat the patient to maximize respiratory function to provide the best chance at survival without a ventilator. In these cases the latter goal is favored and sedation should be held to a minimum; respiratory function should be optimized with bronchodilator therapy, antibiotics, diuresis, and pulmonary toilet; and the patient should be extubated to supplemental oxygen. If it is consistent with the patient's goals, noninvasive

DATE	TIME	ADMITTING SERVICE/ATTENDING

Complete the following:
- ❏ Do Not Attempt Resuscitation (DNAR) order written
- ❏ Note written in chart that documents rationale for comfort care, discussions with attending and discussions with family (or attempts to contact family)

1) Discontinue all previous orders including routine vital signs, medication, enteral feeding, intravenous drips, radiographs, laboratory tests. See below for new orders.
2) Remove devices not necessary for comfort including monitors, blood pressure cuffs, and leg compression sleeves. See below for orders related to the ventilator.
3) Remove all devices (cardiac output computer, transfusers, defibrillator, intra-aortic balloon pump, ventricular assist device, temporary pacemaker) from ICU room.
4) Liberalize visitation.

SEDATION AND ANALGESIA:
5) Select one:
   - ❏ Morphine drip at current rate (assuming patient comfortable at that dose) or 10 mg/hr or _____ mg/hr
     For signs of discomfort, up to Q 15 min, give additional morphine equal to current hourly drip rate and increase drip by 25%
   - ❏ Fentanyl drip at current rate (assuming patient comfortable at that dose) or 100 ug/hr or _____ ug/hr
     For signs of discomfort, up to Q 15 min, give additional fentanyl equal to current hourly drip rate and increase drip by 25%
   - ❏ Other narcotic: _____

6) Select one:
   - ❏ Lorazepam drip at current rate (assuming patient comfortable at that dose) or 5 mg/hr or _____ mg/hr
     For signs of discomfort, up to Q 15 min, give additional lorazepam equal to current hourly drip rate and increase drip by 25%
   - ❏ Midazolam drip at current rate (assuming patient comfortable at that dose) or 10 mg/hr or _____ mg/hr
     For signs of discomfort, up to Q 15 min, give additional midazolam equal to current hourly drip rate and increase drip by 25%
   - ❏ Other benzodiazepine, barbiturate, or propofol: _____

VENTILATOR:
7) Initial ventilator setting: IMV rate _____, PS level _____, (Choose IMV or PS not a combination), F_iO_2 _____, PEEP _____.
8) Reduce apnea, heater, and other ventilator alarms to minimum setting.
9) Reduce F_iO_2 to room air and PEEP to zero over about 5 minutes and titrate sedation as indicated for discomfort.
10) As indicated by level of discomfort, wean IMV to 4 or PS to 5 over 5 to 20 minutes and titrate sedation as indicated for discomfort.
11) When patient is comfortable on IMV rate 4 or PS of 5, select one:
   - ❏ Extubate patient to air
   - ❏ T-piece with air (not CPAP on ventilator)

PHYSICIAN SIGNATURE		DATE:	TIME:	RN's SIGNATURE		DATE	TIME
	M.D.				R.N.		

PT.NO.

NAME

D.O.B

COMFORT CARE ORDERS FOR THE WITHDRAWAL OF LIFE SUPPORT IN ADULTS IN THE ICU

Page 1 of 2

Figure 11–1. Example protocol orders for withdrawing life sustaining treatment in the ICU.

ventilatory support can be used as a bridge to unassisted breathing.[40] Prior to and just after extubation, the medical team and patient must formulate specific plans regarding recurrent respiratory failure. Clinicians have two options in this situation: reinitiate mechanical ventilation or initiate aggressive symptom management of dyspnea without ventilatory support. Waiting until the patient de-

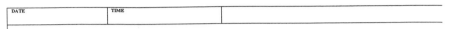

DATE	TIME	

PRINCIPLES FOR WITHHOLDING AND WITHDRAWING LIFE SUSTAINING TREATMENT

1) Death occurs as a complication of the underlying disease. The goal of the comfort care outlined on the reverse is to relieve suffering in a dying patient not to hasten death.

2) Withdrawal of life sustaining treatment is a medical procedure that requires the same degree of physician participation and quality as other procedures.

3) Actions solely intended to hasten death (for example, high doses of potassium or paralytic drugs) are morally unacceptable, however, any dose of pain relieving medication can be used when required to provide comfort even if these doses may hasten death.

4) Withholding treatments is morally and legally equivalent to withdrawing them.

5) When one life sustaining treatment is withheld, strong consideration should be given to withdrawing other current life sustaining treatments and changing the goals of care to comfort.

6) Any treatment can be withdrawn including nutrition, fluids, antibiotics, and blood.

7) Assessing pain and discomfort in intubated, critically ill, patients can be difficult. The following should be assessed and documented in the medical record when increasing sedation: tachypnea, tachycardia, diaphoresis, grimacing, accessory muscle use, nasal flaring, and restlessness.

8) Concerns about hastening death by over-sedating patients are understandable. However, clinicians should be extremely sensitive to the difficulties of assessing discomfort in critically ill patients and should know that many patients develop tolerance to sedative medication. Therefore, clinicians should be wary of under-treating discomfort during the withdrawal of life sustaining treatments in the ICU.

9) Brain dead patients do not need sedation during the withdrawal of life sustaining treatment.

10) Patients should not have life support withdrawn while receiving paralytic drugs as these will mask signs of discomfort. Life support can be withdrawn from patients after paralytic drugs have been stopped as long as clinicians feel that the patient has sufficient motor activity to demonstrate discomfort.

PHYSICIAN SIGNATURE		DATE:	TIME:	RN's SIGNATURE		DATE	TIME
	M.D.				R.N.		

PT.NO.

NAME

D.O.B

COMFORT CARE ORDERS FOR THE WITHDRAWAL OF LIFE SUPPORT IN ADULTS IN THE ICU

Page 2 of 2

Figure 11–1.—Continued

velops respiratory failure to formulate a plan leads to chaotic decision making in the middle of the night with an acutely ill and dyspneic patient. If the patient and family choose not to reinitiate mechanical ventilation, then sedation and other treatment as outlined elsewhere in this chapter are begun, acknowledging that the goal of unassisted breathing is no longer attainable. Clinicians may be tempted to "make sure" the patient still refuses intubation at the time of respiratory compromise, however, intubation need not be specifically offered if the patient has already participated in a decision to withhold it.

Despite clinicians' best efforts to clarify the choices and formulate a prospective plan for patients who develop respiratory failure after extubation, some patients or their families who initially refuse reintubation change their minds. These situations can be harrowing for providers because of the urgency of the decision to choose between reintubation and palliative sedation, and the difficulty in ascertaining which request represents the patient's true wishes. Because mechanical ventilation can be ethically, legally, and humanely withdrawn later, an informed request by the patient for intubation should be fulfilled even when it violates prior requests. Complex and subtle discussions regarding end-of-life treatment choices should never occur at the bedside of a dyspneic acutely ill patient in imminent danger of cardiopulmonary arrest.

Survival despite withdrawal of life-sustaining treatment

Patients who survive the withdrawal of life-sustaining treatments present clinicians with several dilemmas. Families and clinicians can become frustrated and hope for some means to expedite death. These requests should be dealt with honestly and compassionately. Although the evidence suggests that measures are taken to hasten death in the ICU,[16] treatments solely intended to hasten death or increases in sedation that are not necessary to relieve discomfort are not justified under current ethical and legal consensus.[41] Families should be reassured that their loved one is comfortable and that the timing of death is out of the control of the clinical team. It is appropriate to transfer these patients out of the ICU to an area in the hospital with more privacy as long as the family has been prepared for the move. Prolonged survival may cause those involved to question their decision to withdraw life-sustaining treatments. The available data suggest that prolonged survival after a decision to withdraw life support is uncommon.[42] However, these cases are particularly difficult for clinicians who approach family members recently resigned to the death of a loved one to discuss a change in plans. Because so little is known about the timing of death after withdrawal of life support, clinicians should be wary of revising their plans and prognosis on the basis of a perceived delay in the expected timing of death. These changes in plans can have a devastating effect on loved ones and staff.

Coma and brain death

Many of the patients from whom life-sustaining treatments are withdrawn have neurologic impairment.[42] In these cases, the decision to use sedation during withdrawal of life support is complicated by concerns that unconscious patients, by definition, cannot perceive pain and therefore may not require sedation or analgesia. Patients with diminished levels of consciousness also may not be able to manifest signs of discomfort. Studies indicate that physicians do use sedation when withdrawing life support from patients with catastrophic neurologic injury.[43,44] The problem is that we have no gold standard test for perception of pain. While facial electromyography and augmented electroencephalographic techniques may be helpful in determining the level of arousal, they have not been validated in this setting. Given the inherent uncertainty in assessing suffering in neurologically impaired patients, we believe that clinicians should err on the side of administering some sedation rather than withholding it completely. One approach is to select the average adult dose of medication used in a large series of patients receiving withdrawal of life support (diazepam at 10 mg/hr and morphine sulfate at 10 mg/hr) and not adjust this dose unless objective signs of breakthrough suffering are detected.[42] If patients had been placed on sedatives earlier in the course of their critical illness and show no signs of discomfort, we would not reduce this level of sedation for the purposes of withdrawing life support. Obviously, if patients show signs of clinical distress during the withdrawal of life support, then this dose should be increased. We acknowledge the possibility that in using this approach, some comatose patients may experience undetected discomfort while others may have their death hastened without benefit. Brain-dead patients do not need sedation during the withdrawal of life support.

Pharamcologic paralysis

Managing pharmacologic paralysis during the withdrawal of mechanical ventilation presents some unique problems.[45–47] Agents such as pancuronium and vecuronium are used in critically ill patients to improve ventilator synchrony and reduce oxygen consumption. However, they serve no purpose in fulfilling comfort goals during the withdrawal of life support. Although the argument has been made that paralytic drugs ease the family's distress by making the dying patient appear comfortable, they actually prevent clinicians from adequately assessing patients' discomfort and therefore may contribute to the patient's suffering. Paralytic drugs are also problematic because they may hasten death by preventing respiration without offering any beneficial effects to the patient.

The primary concern about withdrawing ventilation in the face of pharmacologic paralysis is its masking effect on patient discomfort. For this reason, paralytic drugs should be stopped as soon as the withdrawal of life-sustaining treatments is considered. Some clinicians may choose to try to reverse pharmacologic paralysis in an effort to restore some of the patient's ability to manifest discomfort to help guide sedation requirements. Unfortunately, after an extended course of these drugs, some critically ill patients will not regain normal neuromuscular function for days or weeks.[48] Some physicians may regard withdrawing mechanical ventilation in a partially paralyzed patient as euthanasia and wish to delay this withdrawal until neuromuscular function returns to normal. We do not feel that this delay is justified. In these cases, neuromuscular weakness is a complication of the patient's critical illness and the drugs used to treat it. Withdrawing life support in the face of treatment complications is justified because the complications, even if iatrogenic, are part of the patient's illness, the complications may not resolve, and continued support imposes an unwanted burden on the patient. Patients receiving pharmacologic paralysis should have it stopped prior to the withdrawal of life-sustaining treatments. Clinicians should wait for the return of sufficient neuromuscular function to detect spontaneous movements and attempts at respiration. Therefore, physicians should stop neuromuscular blocking drugs as soon as the withdrawal of life support is anticipated, but they need not wait for the effects of these drugs to disappear completely before withdrawing life-sustaining treatments.[48,49]

The do not resuscitate (DNR) order

The decision to withhold cardiopulmonary resuscitation has been the focus of much of the literature about limiting life-sustaining treatments. In the hospital, there is a great deal of emphasis placed on whether a patient is a "no-code" or "DNR." Unfortunately, these orders occasionally generate confusion. Should DNR patients be admitted to the ICU? If a patient is DNR, what other life-sustaining treatments should be offered? The simplest remedy for this confusion is for the hospital to apply a very strict definition to the DNR order. These orders should only apply to the use of cardiopulmonary resuscitation (CPR) for an unconscious, pulseless and apneic patient. With this narrow definition, DNR orders do not apply to intubation for impending respiratory failure, to admission to the ICU, or to the use of any other life-sustaining treatments. Because the DNR order carries such symbolic significance, we advocate using a different form or note to communicate decisions about other life-sustaining treatments including intubation, ICU transfer, and blood products. The form that is used to communicate the decision about CPR should not break CPR up into its components. Since CPR and Advanced Cardiac Life Support are designed as an algorithmic intervention and the outcome data on these treatments are derived from their application as a combined package, partial attempts at resuscitation should be avoided unless there is a specific rationale. A "menu" approach to CPR can lead to clinically incongruous selections such as "defibrillation and chest compressions but no intubation" or "chemical code only (medications but no defibrillation)." Following this line of reasoning, patients who refuse a part of CPR implicitly refuse CPR. For example, a patient who refuses intubation or defibrillation has implicitly refused CPR and a DNR order should be written. The converse is not true. Some patients may refuse CPR yet desire intubation, pressors, ICU admission, and cardioversion. In these cases, aggressive life-sustaining treatments may prevent the need for CPR; however, should the patient sustain a cardiac arrest despite these interventions, CPR would be withheld.

Some physicians are reluctant to write a DNR order for patients in the ICU because of concerns that a DNR patient will receive less intense treatment.[50] This concern should be addressed through staff education; it is certainly reasonable and consistent for a patient to forego CPR yet request other aggressive life-sustaining treatments with outcomes that may be better than the 5% survival-to-hospital discharge rate quoted for most hospitalized patients receiving CPR.

Future Directions

Although the withdrawal of life support is increasingly common and currently may account for most deaths in ICUs, practical aspects of this procedure have received little attention in the medical literature or in clinical training. Now that an ethical and legal consensus is forming on the process surrounding the decision to limit life support, we must turn our collective research and educational skills toward improving the delivery of this care. Further research is needed on optimal sedation regimens, palliative nursing care for critically ill patients, devices to assist communication with and pain detection in intubated patients, and outcomes to measure the quality of death. A course "Approach to Withdrawing Life Support" should take a place in the critical care curriculum next to sessions on "Approach to Airway Management" and "Approach to Central Venous Catheterization." The clinician's responsibility to the patient does not end with a decision to limit medical treatment, but continues throughout the dying process. Every effort should be made to ensure that the withdrawal of life support occurs with the same quality and attention to detail as is routinely provided when life support is initiated. By approaching the withdrawal of life support as a medical procedure, clinicians will have a recognizable framework for their actions. A key step in this process is identifying explicit shared goals for the process. Our hope is that by adopting a formal approach to this common procedure, the care of patients dying in hospitals will improve.

References

1. Vincent JL, Parquier JN, Preiser JC, Brimioulle S, Kahn RJ. Terminal events in the intensive care unit: review of 258 fatal cases in one year. *Crit Care Med* 1989; 17:530–533.
2. Vernon DD, Dean JM, Timmons OD, Banner W Jr, Allen-Webb EM. Modes of death in the pediatric intensive care unit: withdrawal and limitation of supportive care. *Crit Care Med* 1993;21:1798–1802.
3. Koch KA, Rodeffer HD, Wears RL. Changing patterns of terminal care management in an intensive care unit. *Crit Care Med* 1994;22:233–243.
4. Smedira NG, Evans BH, Grais LS, Cohen NH, Lo B, Cooke M, Schecter WP, Fink C, Epstein-Jaffe E, May C, et al. Withholding and withdrawal of life support from the critically ill. *N Engl J Med* 1990;322:309–315.

5. Grenvik A. "Terminal weaning"; discontinuance of life-support therapy in the terminally ill patient. *Crit Care Med* 1983;11:394–395.

6. Grenvik A, Powner DJ, Snyder JV, Jastremski MS, Babcock RA, Loughhead MG. Cessation of therapy in terminal illness and brain death. *Crit Care Med* 1978;6:284–291.

7. Fisher MM, Raper RF. Withdrawing and withholding treatment in intensive care. Part 3. Practical aspects. *Med J Aust* 1990;153:222–225.

8. Fisher MM, Raper RF. Withdrawing and withholding treatment in intensive care. Part 2. Patient assessment. *Med J Aust* 1990;153:220–222.

9. Fisher MM, Raper RF. Withdrawing and withholding treatment in intensive care. Part 1. Social and ethical dimensions. *Med J Aust* 1990;153:217–220.

10. Klocke RA. Withholding and withdrawing life-sustaining therapy. Practical considerations. *Am Rev Respir Dis* 1992;145(2 Pt 1):251–252.

11. Simpson T. Nursing considerations related to withdrawal of mechanical ventilatory support. *Am Rev Respir Dis* 1989;140(2 Pt 2):S41–43.

12. Faber-Langendoen K, Bartels DM. Process of forgoing life-sustaining treatment in a university hospital: an empirical study. *Crit Care Med* 1992;20:570–577.

13. Hall JB, Schmidt GA, Wood LDH. Principles of Critical Care. New York: McGraw-Hill, 1992.

14. Brody H, Campbell ML, Faber-Langendoen -K, Ogle KS. Withdrawing intensive life-sustaining treatment— recommendations for compassionate clinical management. *N Engl J Med* 1997;336:652–657.

15. Edwards MJ, Tolle SW. Disconnecting the ventilator at the request of a patient who knows he will then die: the doctor's anguish. *Ann Intern Med* 1992;117:254–256.

16. Asch DA. The role of critical care nurses in euthanasia and assisted suicide. *N Engl J Med* 1996;334:1374–1379.

17. The SUPPORT Principal Investigators. A controlled trial to improve care for seriously ill hospitalized patients. The Study to Understand Prognoses and Preferences for Outcomes and Risks of Treatments (SUPPORT). *JAMA* 1995;274:1591–1598.

18. Weir RF, Gostin L. Decisions to abate life-sustaining treatment for nonautonomous patients. *JAMA* 1990;264:1846–1853.

19. Lo B. Resolving Ethical Dilemmas: A Guide for Clinicians. Baltimore: Williams & Wilkins, 1995.

20. Ruark JE, Raffin TA. Initiating and withdrawing life support. Principles and practice in adult medicine. *N Engl J Med* 1988;318:25–30.

21. Withholding and withdrawing life-sustaining therapy. *Am Rev Respir Dis* 1991;144(3 Pt 1):726–731.

22. Asch DA, Hansen-Flaschen J, Lanken PN. Decisions to limit or continue life-sustaining treatment by critical care physicians in the United States: conflicts between physicians' practices and patients' wishes. *Am J Respir Crit Care Med* 1995;151(2 Pt 1):288–292.

23. Wachter RM, Luce JM, Hearst N, Lo B. Decisions about resuscitation: inequities among patients with different diseases but similar prognoses. *Ann Intern Med* 1989;111:525–532.

24. Cook DJ, Guyatt GH, Jaeschke R, Reeve J, Spanier A, King D, Molloy DW, Willan A, Streiner DL. Determinants in Canadian health care workers of the decision to withdraw life support from the critically ill. *JAMA* 1995;273:703–708.

25. Hanson LC, Danis M, Garrett JM, Mutran E. Who decides? Physicians' willingness to use life-sustaining treatment. *Arch Intern Med* 1996;156:785–789.

26. Truog RD, Brett AS, Frader J. The problem with futility. *N Engl J Med* 1992; 326:1560–1564.

27. Plows CW, Tenery RM, Hartford A, Miller D, Morse L, Rakatansky H, Riddick FA, Ruff V, Wilkins G, Ile M, Munson J, Emanuel LL. Medical futility in end-of-life care—Report of the Council on Ethical and Judicial Affairs. *JAMA* 1999;281:937–941.

28. Gazelle G. The slow code—should anyone rush to its defense? *N Engl J Med* 1998;338:467–469.

29. Diem SJ, Lantos JD, Tulsky JA. Cardiopulmonary resuscitation on television. Miracles and misinformation. *N Engl J Med* 1996;334:1578–82.

30. Nicholson AC, Titler M, Montgomery LA, Kleiber C, Craft MJ, Halm M, Buckwalter K, Johnson S. Effects of child visitation in adult critical care units: a pilot study. *Heart Lung* 1993;22:36–45.

31. Shapiro BA, Warren J, Egol AB, Greenbaum DM, Jacobi J, Nasraway SA, Schein RM, Spevetz A, Stone JR. Practice parameters for intravenous analgesia and sedation for adult patients in the intensive care unit: an executive summary. Society of Critical Care Medicine. *Crit Care Med* 1995;23:1596–600.

32. Truog RD, Berde CB, Mitchell C, Grier HE. Barbiturates in the care of the terminally ill. *N Engl J Med* 1992;327:1678–1682.

33. Faber-Langendoen K. A multi-institutional study of care given to patients dying in hospitals. Ethical and practice implications. *Arch Intern Med* 1996;156:2130–213.

34. McCann RM, Hall WJ, Grothjuncker A. Comfort care for terminally ill patients—the appropriate use of nutrition and hydration. *JAMA* 1994;272:1263–1266.

35. Solomon MZ, O'Donnell L, Jennings B, Guilfoy V, Wolf SM, Nolan K, Jackson R, Koch-Weser D, Donnelley S. Decisions near the end of life: professional views on life-sustaining treatments. *Am J Public Health* 1993;83:14–23.

36. Gianakos D. Terminal weaning. *Chest* 1995; 108:1405–1406.

37. Meisel A. Legal myths about terminating life support. *Arch Intern Med* 1991; 1551:1497–1502.

38. President's Commission for the Study of Ethical Problems in Medicine and Biomedical and Behavioral Research. Deciding to Forego Life-sustaining Treatment. Washington, DC: U.S. Government Printing Office, 1983.

39. Davidowitz M, Myrick RD. Responding to the bereaved: an analysis of "helping" statements. *Death Ed* 1984;8:1–10.

40. Meyer TJ, Hill NS. Noninvasive positive pressure ventilation to treat respiratory failure. *Ann Intern Med* 1994;120:760–770.

41. Wilson WC, Smedira NG, Fink C, McDowell JA, Luce JM. Ordering and administration of sedatives and analgesics during the withholding and withdrawal of life support from critically ill patients. *JAMA* 1992;267:949–953.

42. Prendergast TJ, Luce JM. Increasing incidence of withholding and withdrawal of life support from the critically ill. *Am J Respir Crit Care Med* 1997;155:15–20.

43. Mayer SA, Kossoff SB. Withdrawal of life support in the neurological intensive care unit. *Neurology* 1999;52:1602–1609.

44. Campbell ML, Bizek KS, Thill M. Patient responses during rapid terminal weaning from mechanical ventilation: a prospective study. *Crit Care Med* 1999;27:73–77.

45. Kirkland L. Neuromuscular paralysis and withdrawal of mechanical ventilation. *J Clin Ethics* 1994;5:38–39; discussion 39–42.
46. Rushton CH, Terry PB. Neuromuscular blockade and ventilator withdrawal: ethical controversies. *Am J Crit Care* 1995;4(2):112–115.
47. Truog RD, Fackler JC. Withdrawing mechanical ventilation. *Crit Care Med* 1993; 21(9 Suppl):S396–5397.
48. Segredo V, Caldwell JE, Matthay MA, Sharma ML, Gruenke LD, Miller RD. Persistent paralysis in critically ill patients after long-term administration of vecuronium. *N Engl J Med* 1992;327:524–528.
49. Hansen Flaschen J. Improving patient tolerance of mechanical ventilation. Challenges ahead. *Crit Care Clin* 1994;10:659–671.
50. Henneman EA, Baird B, Bellamy PE, Faber LL, Oye RK. Effect of do-not-resuscitate orders on the nursing care of critically ill patients. *Am J Crit Care* 1994;3:467–472.

Chapter 12

The Role of Critical Care Nurses in Providing and Managing End-of-Life Care

KATHLEEN A. PUNTILLO

A Case Scenario

Mr. Harper was a 56-year-old man with end-stage liver disease. He had been on the liver transplant waiting list for many months before his condition worsened, requiring this current admission to the ICU. His ICU clinical course was very unstable; he was being mechanically ventilated for acute respiratory failure and receiving continuous veno-venous hemofiltration (CVVH) for acute renal failure. On day 25 of his ICU stay, he was taken off the liver transplant waiting list, and his wife was told to prepare for his demise. During that night, Mr. Harper showed a picture of sepsis, with a temperature spike and drop in blood pressure, the latter requiring dopamine support. At this time, the transplant team felt that his aggressive therapies should be continued while his sepsis was treated. During the next day, Mr. Harper's nurse carried out and assisted with the aggressive assessment and treatment interventions that were part of Mr. Harper's care plan. The CVVH was continued, antibiotics were hung, Mr. Harper was suctioned intermittently, a new central line was placed, he had chest X-rays in the morning and after central line placement, and he underwent an abdominal ultrasound to identify sources of infection. As the day progressed, the nurse did frequent hemodynamic assessments, needing to intermittently increase the rate of the dopamine infusion to maintain Mr. Harper's mean arterial blood pressure at 60 mmHg. Noting that Mr. Harper would become agitated during tactile stimulation, his nurse was successful in obtaining a prescription for an IV opioid. Prior to this, Mr. Harper had had no coverage for pain or agitation. During the day, Mr. Harper's condition continued to deteriorate. Many family members and friends arrived at the hospital to say their good-byes. A family conference was held, and a decision was made by all to withdraw CVVH, to taper down the dopamine infusion, and prepare for Mr. Harper's death.

At this time, the actions of Mr. Harper's nurse clearly changed. Now the overriding goal was to prepare Mr. Harper and his environment, so that a peaceful death could occur for him and his family. She provided time for family members and friends to say their good-byes to Mr. Harper and answered their questions. Mr. Harper was bathed, new linens were applied, alarms were turned off, he was administered more opioids for his agitation and suspected discomfort, chairs were brought into his room for family members, lights were lowered, and the CVVH machine was moved away from his bedside. His wife remained at his bedside, telling him that it was all right for him to go now; that he had suffered enough. Mr. Harper expired 18 hours later with his wife present.

Reflection

This patient and family situation is all too familiar in ICUs. Nurses and other health care team members implement aggressive care to improve the prognoses of their patients. Yet, many patients do not survive. Frequently a shift must be made from "cure" interventions to focusing on the dying process, with an emphasis on care that promotes patient and family comfort.[1] Critical care nurses play an essential role in the provision of the best possible care during their patients' end of life. The purpose of this chapter is to describe the unique role of the critical care nurse in providing end-of-life care to dying, critically ill patients and to make specific recommendations for interventions.

The Orientation and Vision of Nursing

Nurses are concerned with the human experiences of others, including birth, health, illness, and death. Foci of nursing care and research include their patients' physical and emotional comfort, discomfort, and pain.[2] Nursing actions may either be directed at providing interventions for patients and their families or be performed away from the patient but on the patient's behalf. These actions encompass management of the patient's care environment as well as interdisciplinary collaboration.[2] Specifically, nurses contribute to the care of these patients in the following ways:

- Incorporating goal setting into the daily plan of care for the patient
- Symptom management
- Identifying and recruiting all members of the health care team that can make a contribution to the end-of-life care of the patient
- Providing care to patients' families.

Goal setting

One of the most valuable steps in the provision of appropriate care to any critically ill patient is setting short- and long-term goals that are specific to the individual patient. This allows for care that is proactive rather than reactive. Setting goals that are relevant and achievable provides clarity to the overall plan. If the goal is cure, then the planning of curative interventions would be most appropriate. However, if the patient is dying, then the most appropriate goal would be to plan palliative, comfort care.[3]

Goal setting should be a conscious, deliberate activity performed by the health care team, patient, and patient's family. Incorporating goal setting into the daily team reports is as, if not more, important as the review of body systems and diagnostic tests. It is a time for the team to step back from the minute-to-minute assessments and interventions that are so much a part of critical care and ask the following questions: "what is best for this patient and his or her family?"; "what can we achieve?"; "how can we go about achieving it?"

Critical care nurses play a major role in setting goals related to end-of-life comfort care. They are unique health care providers for patients because they are frequently with patients for up to 12 hours each day or night. Generally, and optimally, they are in a position to care for a particular patient over a period of time and have learned to "know" the patient and the patient's family. They are the major providers of comfort care for critically ill patients at *all* times. Therefore, it is imperative that critical care nurses advocate when they believe, and the patient's condition indicate, that comfort care should be the primary goal for this particular patient. Thus, a primary nursing activity is to be present during team and family discussions of the patient. The nurses must be direct, clear, and assertive in their communications with physicians and other health care providers. They should encourage a team dialogue that demonstrates respect for others' perspectives about the best plan of care for the individual patient. A team that acknowledges the different perspectives of its members yet works together to develop the best possible plan of care for the patient will be more satisfied with the outcomes and with their working relationships over time.

Often a busy patient assignment may preclude the patient's nurse from participating in the patient or family discussions. At these times, arrangements should be made with other bedside nurses, the charge nurse, or the clinical nurse specialist to provide time for the patient's nurse to participate in patient rounds or family conferences. Incorporating this peer support into unit practice will help all nurses to be active members of the patient's team and ensure that nursing is represented during goal setting for dying patients.

Palliative care and symptom management

Palliative care is comprehensive management of physical, psychological, social, and spiritual needs of patients.[1] Palliative care is provided to lessen the severity of a symptom or clinical process when cure is not an outcome.[4] Some of the most common symptoms experienced by many patients at the end of life include pain and anxiety; agitation, confusion, and altered cognition; dyspnea;

and fatigue.[5-7] For years symptom management has been the essence of hospice nursing.[4] Principles and knowledge from hospice nursing can be adapted to critical care settings since many critically ill patients suffer from these same symptoms. Thus, patient comfort can be enhanced through assessments and interventions directed toward symptom control.

Pain and anxiety

Pain is one of the most prevalent and distressing symptoms of seriously ill patients dying in large teaching hospitals. In a recent study, over 5000 patients or their family members were asked questions about the patients' pain.[6] Almost one-half of these patients reported pain, and almost 15% of those had pain that was extremely severe or moderately severe occurring at least half of the time. While patients with colon cancer had the most pain, many of the patients reporting pain had diagnoses that were not surgery or cancer related (e.g., chronic obstructive pulmonary disease or congestive heart failure). Thus it is important to attend to the assessment of pain in *all* ICU patients. Desbiens and colleagues noted that "in seriously ill patients, pain should be monitored as frequently as vital signs and treated vigorously."[8]

Discussion of pain will be limited here to the monitoring of pain and potential sources of pain since interventions for pain are discussed in Chapter 10. Advances have been made over the past 10 years in the assessment of pain in critically ill patients. Research has shown that many critically ill patients are able to use simple tools to communicate their pain, even if they were mechanically ventilated.[9] Simple numeric or word rating scales, word quality scales, and body outline diagrams can be offered to patients who are able to point to words, numbers, and figures.[10] In a group of seriously ill hospitalized patients who were able to identify the location of their pain ($N = 85$), the pain sites varied considerably.[11] This finding reinforces the importance of determining the location of pain whenever possible so that treatment is guided by accurate information rather than assumptions.

A strong concordance between nurses and patients on the degree of pain felt by critically ill patients can occur particularly when nurses use a structured, systematic method of pain assessment that includes observation of behavioral and physiological signs of pain.[12,13] Bedside pain assessment checklists that include potential pain behaviors and changes in physiological signs can assist nurses into drawing inferences about their patients' pain. Figures 12–1 and 12–2 represent the front and back of a laminated bedside pain assessment tool developed from research findings that is used in ICUs at the University of California, San Francisco.[°]

It is important to acknowledge that patients in pain can also have distress—that is, a psychological response—when they are in pain. In fact, both anxiety

°I am grateful to Hildy Schell, R.N., M.S., Critical Care Pain Taskforce Chairperson, and my other colleagues on the taskforce—Ann Daleidan, Carla Graf, Sheila Gleeson, and Diane Ayers—for their work in developing this bedside chart with me.

Pain

Assess

Intervene

Note (document assessment and response to intervention)

Assess

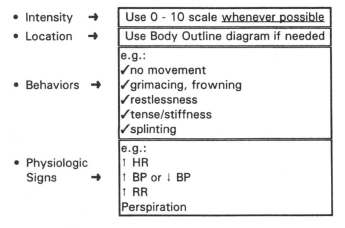

* Intensity ➜ | Use 0 - 10 scale <u>whenever possible</u> |
* Location ➜ | Use Body Outline diagram if needed |

* Behaviors ➜
e.g.:
✓no movement
✓grimacing, frowning
✓restlessness
✓tense/stiffness
✓splinting

* Physiologic Signs ➜
e.g.:
↑ HR
↑ BP or ↓ BP
↑ RR
Perspiration

✳<u>Remember: Absence of pain signs does not mean absence of pain</u>✳

Intervene: Give analgesics as ordered and provide comfort measures.

Note: <u>Document:</u> • Initial assessment of pain
                        • Interventions
                        • Response to interventions

Figure 12–1. Reproduction of front side of bedside pain assessment tool.[36,37] Developed by University of California, San Francisco Medical Center Critical Care Pain Task Force (1996).

and depression have been associated with increased pain and increased levels of dissatisfaction with pain control in seriously ill patients.[6] What is unclear is whether pain worsens distress, whether pain increases as a response to distress, or both.[6] However, assessment of the distress component of pain provides the practitioner with information that can guide the use of specific interventions. Simple pain-related *distress* numeric rating scales can be used to identify how much patients are psychologically bothered by the pain that they are experiencing.

If distress is an important component of the patient's pain, it may appear as

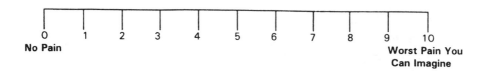

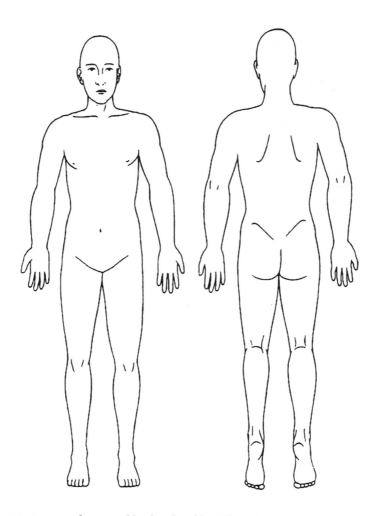

Figure 12–2. Reproduction of back side of bedside pain assessment tool. Developed by University of California, San Francisco Medical Center Critical Care Pain Task Force (1996).

anxiety. Common behavioral or physiological signs of anxiety include trembling, restlessness, sweating, tachycardia, tachypnea, difficulty sleeping, and irritability.[3] The nurse can choose interventions to decrease the pain-related distress or anxiety since pain intensity in seriously ill hospitalized patients can be enhanced by anxiety.[6] These interventions can be as simple as providing information, initiating measures to promote relaxation, and/or suggesting the addition of anxiolytics or antidepressants to the pharmacologic regime.

While the use of self-report measures of pain intensity and distress is the optimal approach to pain assessment, assessment remains problematic in situations when patients have altered levels of consciousness due to disease. Likewise, the use of certain pharmacologic interventions makes it extremely difficult to assess the degree of pain and/or anxiety being felt by the patient. For example, the use of benzodiazepine infusions may make patients too sedated to respond to pain, although it might still be present. On the other hand, use of low doses of the anesthetic agent propofol and use of neuromuscular blocking agents (NMBAs), such as vecuronium, limit or entirely mask the patient's ability to express or show any behavioral signs of pain. It is essential that clinicians understand that low-dose propofol and all doses of NMBAs have no analgesic properties, even though visible signs of pain would be absent during their use. Under these circumstances, the nurse can enlist the assistance of the patient's family members or friends in their evaluation of the patient's discomfort. The nurse can ask them about any chronic pain experienced by the patient or methods used by the patient at home to decrease pain or stress. This information can be incorporated into the patient's care plan. In addition, nurses can use their imagination to identify possible sources of pain by asking the question, "If I were this patient and had intact sensations, what might be making me uncomfortable?"

The assessment of pain is also problematic if the patient has altered cognitive processing. Nurses and patients' family members may ascribe more pain to the agitated patient than is actually present because of their reliance on distress-related behaviors exhibited by the patient.[14] A small sample of patients ($N = 11$) who recovered from agitated cognitive failure (ACF) reported that they did not remember having pain during their ACF phase. However, they had received more doses of narcotics than other patients treated on the unit, which may have kept them pain-free. In addition, absence of memory does not mean that pain was absent. The clinician is encouraged to treat pain whenever there is an indication that pain might be present in a patient with cognitive failure.

Certainly the many diagnostic and treatment procedures performed in critical care units are sources for pain in critically ill patients. Research has shown commonly performed procedures such as central, arterial, peripheral line placements, nasogastric tube placements,[15] chest tube removal, and endotracheal suctioning[16] to be very painful for patients. Discomfort from invasive and painful procedures may be the primary cause of suffering at the end of

life.[15] Other procedures that may be unnecessary, painful, and unpleasant include frequent vital sign assessment, frequent turning, wound debridements,
frequent dressing changes, and use of sequential compression devices.[3] It is of
primary importance to determine the necessity of any and all procedures after
a decision has been made to end life support. Nurses can act as "gatekeepers"
by evaluating the appropriateness of procedures being planned for patients and
advocating for their omission. Helping the patient to avoid iatrogenic suffering
is a fundamental part of palliative care.[15] The only important procedures for
patients to experience at end of life are those that will promote comfort.

Agitation, confusion, altered cognition
There are numerous reasons why patients in ICUs have altered cognition.
Many of the causes are identifiable, such as the effects of drugs, metabolic
alterations, hypercarbia, hypoxia, environmental problems, and pain.[17] Yet, the
cause can often be unknown, as was the case in most (83%) of 47 patients with
cognitive failure who died on a palliative care unit.[14] In another study, 77% of
cancer patients who died in the hospital developed impaired mental status an
average of 9 days before their death.[18] Most of those patients who became
confused died sooner than those without confusion.

Successful detection of confusion requires careful surveillance and screening.[19] Table 12–1 provides guidelines for assessing and treating delirium, confusion, and agitation. Clinicians can attempt to assess the presence of confusion
and, when able, eliminate the source(s) of that confusion. Even when the
causes are unknown, erring on the side of treatment and symptom control may
help to reduce the patient's and family's suffering. Numerous drugs are known
to cause confusion.[5] If drugs are suspected to be the source of confusion, the
challenge is to balance the benefits of the drugs (e.g., pain relief from an
opiate, anxiolysis from benzodiazepines, elevated mood from tricyclic antidepressants) with the potential adverse effects of the drugs. In some cases,
switching from one drug to another in the same category (e.g., from morphine
to fentanyl) may help alleviate the confusion.[19] Confusion can also be due to
pain, constipation, biochemical imbalances, extreme anxiety, and alcohol or
benzodiazepine withdrawal.[5] Each of these potential causes requires careful
assessment and appropriate intervention.

When indicated, nurses can advocate for the addition of psychotropic medications to the patients' treatment regime. Neuroleptics such as haloperidol are
often the first-line treatment for nonspecific agitation[19] and are recommended
as such in guidelines published by the Society of Critical Care Medicine.[20] The
critical care nurse is responsible for monitoring patients' responses to haloperidol including the development of the most serious adverse effects—i.e.,
extrapyramidal side effects and neuroleptic malignant syndrome.[21]

A patient's family can become very concerned about development of confusion in their loved one. They may equate the confusion and agitation with pain
even though pain is not necessarily present during confusion. It is the

Table 12–1. General approach to management of delirium, confusion, and agitation in terminal illness

- Maintain a high index of suspicion for delirium in terminal illness.
- Search for potentially reversible causes of delirium.
- Search for other problems that might contribute to confusion or agitation.
- Remember that multiple potential causes of delirium are usually present in the setting of terminal illness.
- Err on the side of treatment; be willing to palliate confusion.
- Establish a soothing environment to the extent possible; familiar objects, photographs, and familiar music can be helpful.
- Start at the lower end of the dose range of a given pharmacologic agent, but recognize that standard or higher doses may be required.
- Assess treatment response and side effects frequently.
- Aim to provide maximum (ideally complete) resolution of delirium, confusion, or agitation, but recognize that some cases of end-of-life delirium can only be managed with heavy sedation.
- Educate patients and families about delirium and its treatments; patient education may have to wait until delirium clears.

Reprinted from Shuster JL. Delirium, confusion, and agitation at the end of life. *J Palliat Med* 1998;1:117–186, with permission.

nurse's responsibility, however, to institute interventions to promote the patient's comfort.

Patient confusion can develop at any time. Knowing this, the nurse can encourage open communication among the patient and all family members and encourage them to discuss unresolved issues while the patient is cognitively intact.

Dyspnea

Dyspnea is a very complex, subjective sensation of difficulty in breathing that is not necessarily related to exertion.[7] Severe dyspnea was one of the major symptoms reported by patients or their family members in a sample of hospitalized seriously ill patients.[6] Pharmacological and nonpharmacological conditions can be both the causes of and treatments for dyspnea. For example, dyspnea can increase when patients are receiving adrenergic agonists (metaproterenol, albuterol) and theophylline since these drugs can cause severe agitation, anxiety, and tremor.[22] Morphine, however, can directly improve dyspnea by decreasing cardiac preload, and benzodiazepines can indirectly improve dyspnea through their anxiolytic effects. Being in a stifling ICU room surrounded by machines can enhance the feeling of shortness of breath. Placing the patient in a position of comfort (e.g., sitting upright) can help to relieve dyspnea, while use of a bedside fan can provide a cool breeze and make breathing easier. Repeated reassurance is an effective intervention for dyspnea when the patient trusts the professional staff.[6] This reassurance can be more effective if team members give consistent explanations. Alert dyspneic patients can obtain comfort from knowing that they will not be left alone and that they are being provided some degree of control in their care.

Thirst, dry mouth, and dehydration

Thirst and dry mouth can be very uncomfortable symptoms at the end of life.[22] These and other uncomfortable symptoms, such as headache, nausea, vomiting, and cramps, were associated with dehydration in young healthy subjects many years ago by Nadal and colleagues.[23] More recently, 27 of 32 patients who died on a comfort care unit were considered to have had a comfortable death.[24] Before their deaths, they reported that lack of food and fluids in sufficient amounts to balance losses did not cause them suffering as long as they received mouth care and sips of water.

It is important to note that dehydration is not a necessary prerequisite to development of thirst and dry mouth. In a sample of 23 patients with malignant disease, 87% reported dry mouth and 83% felt thirsty in the 2 days before their death.[25] One-third of these patients were not biochemically dehydrated. It is important to identify other pharmacologic causes of thirst and dry mouth, such as opioids, phenothiazines, hyoscine, antihistamines, and antidepressants. In addition, mouth breathing and candidiasis may also cause dry mouth.[25] The patient's mouth should be gently inspected every day with a padded tongue blade and flashlight. Dry mouth and thirst can be helped with meticulous mouth care. Treatment of candidiasis includes the use of oral nystatin suspension 1–2 ml swished in the mouth every 6 hours or systemic ketoconazole or fluconazole.[5] Mouth ulcers can be treated with triamcinolone acetonide dental paste applied every 6 hours.[5] When possible, the administration of small amounts of oral fluids and/or ice chips also helps to minimize thirst and dry mouth.[26,27]

Withholding of or decreasing the amount of fluids administered to a patient at the end of life is a serious issue. There are many beneficial effects to the patient from decreasing or withholding fluids. There may be a greater potential for cough, congestion, and dyspnea when fluids are administered;[18] decreasing fluid administration may help to alleviate those discomforts. Withholding fluids may also help to decrease dependent edema,[25] which can be quite uncomfortable for the patient. It is important to help the patient's family understand that dehydration is not accompanied by physical pain.[4] In fact, Printz[28] has indicated that dehydration may decrease the need for analgesia. The potential explanations for this phenomenon, which has been seen by those who work with the dying[26] are as follows: (1) an altered metabolic state decreases the patient's level of consciousness and, thus, the ability to perceive pain; (2) accumulation of ketones causes loss of sensation; (3) there is an increased production of opioid peptides or endorphins during states of fasting or water deprivation.[28]

In contrast to practices in hospice settings, fluids are seldom withdrawn completely from a dying patient in an ICU. This may be due to the traditional aggressive care approach in ICUs rather than to the thoughtful consideration that fluid withdrawal might be an appropriate consideration in a particular situation. There is no rationale unique to ICUs for continuing fluids and nutrition for critically ill patients when other life-sustaining therapies are stopped. The process of deciding whether and when to institute terminal hydration can be difficult for patients, family members, and health professionals alike. The reader is referred elsewhere.[27,29] for a discussion of ethical considerations and guidelines for the care of patients undergoing terminal dehydration.

Fatigue

Fatigue is probably one of the most frequent symptoms experienced by the general ICU patient population. However, surprisingly little data exist to quantify its prevalence. In a study of seriously ill hospitalized patients, almost 80% of more than 3000 patients or their surrogates reported patient fatigue at the end of life.[6] When cure is no longer the goal in a patient's plan of care, the critical care nurse can help to control the patient's environment and promote patient sleep by implementing a rest-activity schedule for the patient and his or her family.[7] The nurse can cluster care activities, use "do not disturb" signs on patient's doors, consider applying a headset and tape recorder with music preferred by the patient, and turn down or off monitor alarms to promote a sleep environment for the patient.

Other comfort care measures

In addition to alleviating or minimizing the distressing symptoms addressed above, the critical care nurse can also perform other specific hygiene measures that will increase patient comfort. These include the use of lotion on dry skin and ointment on dry lips. If the patient's eyes are dry and/or do not close completely, use of artificial tears or eye ointments can decrease eye discomfort. Patients should be told that these tears or ointments are being used, so that they will understand why their vision is blurred. Fever can be a source of discomfort for patients. The nurse can try to maintain a normothermic body temperature by sponge bathing the patient with lukewarm water, using fans, and applying just enough linen to maintain the patient's privacy. The nurse can be alert for the development of pressure areas, especially over bony prominences, and use massage and turning as appropriate. Often the hair of ICU patients gets matted when unstable patients must lie in one position for long periods of time. Matted hair can also be from body fluids secreted in the area of the head (e.g., blood loss from an internal jugular catheter insertion site). Gentle washing and combing of the patient's hair are hygienic measures that can be soothing to the patient and help to maintain the patient's dignity. During the provision of these comfort measures, the nurse can talk gently to the patients, informing them about what activities are being performed. Part of patient comfort is knowing that their providers care about them and will be with them when needed.

Working with the patient's family

At the end of a patient's life, the patient's family is as important a recipient of nursing care as the patient. There are very specific actions that the nurse can provide for family members. Some relate directly to the patient and the patient's physical environment, while others are directed toward promoting optimal communication. Table 12–2 outlines specific nursing activities that may be extremely helpful to family members. In general, family members should be awarded every opportunity to participate in decision making and in the physical and emotional care of the patient. Family visiting policies must remain extremely flexible, considering the limited time left for being with and saying good-by to the dying patient. Children, even young ones, should be allowed to visit their dying mother or father.[3] It is important, however, that they be accompanied by a family member who can concentrate on the child's response to the situation and intervene accordingly. The family unit is usually the strongest of social units in a person's lifetime. The nurse who appreciates this will provide the necessary support to the patient's family. See Chapter 13 for more detail.

Table 12–2. Nursing activities with family members of dying patients[a]

Activities related to patient and physical environment	Activities that promote optimal communication
Personalize and domesticate the patient's environment through use of family pictures, afgans, religious ornaments, personal pillows, music from home.	Carefully listen to the family member; use clear and understandable language; share information in a timely manner; explain all procedures in understandable, lay terms.
Arrange for time to talk and visit with the patient. Encourage a family dialogue with and about the patient in the patient's room (i.e., tell family stories).	Help the family to understand the implications of prognostic information. Anticipate that family members may respond with anger, emotional outbursts, or temporary inconsolable grief.
Provide for family privacy with the patient so that personal words can be expressed. Provide for tissues and chairs at the patient's bedside. Remain in visual contact, but outside of hearing range, in case the family needs support.	Assist family members to understand, participate in, and accept the transition from aggressive care-saving goals to end-of-life palliative care goals.
Help the family to prepare for the patient's death. This may involve having the family member participate in various aspects of care, e.g., bathing, hair combing, etc.	Coach the family in communicating with various members of the health care team, including physicians, clinical nurse specialists, social workers, pharmacists, clergy.
Involve willing members to assist with postmortem care.	Ascertain whether family members want to be present during withdrawal of treatment, e.g., during terminal weaning or extubation, and advocate for the family's wishes.

[a]Activities compiled from references 3, 5, 6, 34, 35.

Nursing "Systems" Issues

In many institutions, acuity systems are used to determine staffing patterns. Patients receiving aggressive interventions such as CVVH, mechanical ventilation, multiple vasoactive drips, for example, receive more "acuity" points than patients receiving less of these interventions. This method of determining staffing needs provides a barrier to effective nursing care of dying patients. Activities of family communication, provision of comfort care, and interdisciplinary consultations are not reflected well in many acuity systems; yet these activities require substantial nursing time. Research has shown that nursing care requirements of do-not-resuscitate (DNR) patients in an ICU were no less intense than patients without DNR orders.[30] In fact, although the level of required observations decreased, DNR patients required more nursing care because of their intense physical dependency and social and emotional needs. Furthermore, 73% of the 71 DNR patients had various life-sustaining interventions continued after the DNR order was written, necessitating nursing surveillance and manipulation. Since many patients remain in ICUs from DNR order initiation until time of death, critical care nurses need support from hospital systems to have time to provide the type of care that patients and their families deserve. It is inappropriate to transfer a moribund patient from an ICU environment that is familiar to the patient's family, especially if the patient still has intensive care requirements.[3] If financial or bed availability pressures dictate that a dying patient must be moved from the ICU, the nurse can try to ensure that the care environment to which the patient is transferred will meet the needs of the patient and his family. The nurse can help to make the transition to another care setting as smooth as possible so that the patient and family's stress is not compounded.[31] The nurse's continued communication with the patient and/or family after the patient's transfer, either by visits or phone calls, is a way of demonstrating that the nurse remains interested in the patient's welfare.

Providing Care for the Caregiver

Ensuring and promoting care for the caregiver cannot be overemphasized. Our culture does not prepare health professionals adequately for dealing with the discomfort associated with death and dying.[1] Even though many nurses receive much satisfaction from providing good care to their patients at the end of life and even volunteer to care for dying patients, many times this is a stressful situation for them. Staff meetings can be set aside to review stresses that nurses experience in providing end-of-life care.[31] These meetings can provide a setting for involved health professionals to process their own feelings about death and their inability to prevent it.[31] Discussions can focus on the dilemmas they face by working in an environment in which values aggressive, life-saving

Table 12–3. Terms that describe "a good death"[a]

Painless	Family support	Home
Quick	Dignity	No procedures
Agreement	Environment (supportive)	Not being/dying alone
No (patient) fear of dying	Spiritual support	Belief system honored
Peaceful	Own decision when to die	Comfort
Warm, soft	Atraumatic	Not awake; asleep
Patient and family content with death	Time to prepare	Wholeness of body

[a]I am grateful to my 1999 Critical Care/Trauma and Acute Care Nurse Practitioner graduate students at the University of California, San Francisco for their thoughtful consideration of what constitutes "a good death."

care is valued but that also has many dying patients with very different needs. Developing a unit philosophy about care of dying patients can be a concrete method of recognizing the value of such important nursing work. For additional information on this important topic, see Chapter 14.

Summary

Most patients who are seriously ill prefer an approach to care that focuses on comfort, even if this means that their life is shortened.[6] Recently, graduate nursing students in a critical care course were asked to provide terms that would describe "a good death." (See Table 12–3). Although describing "a good death" is often difficult, nurses usually "know it when they see it". Critical care nurses dedicated to promoting a peaceful end of life for their patients may evaluate the care they give to their dying patients according to five outcomes developed by Ruland and Moore.[32] These outcomes are that the patient (1) is not in pain; (2) experiences comfort; (3) experiences dignity and respect; (4) is at peace; and (5) experiences a closeness to significant others or other caring persons. A basic tenet of professional nursing practice has been that nurses, "put the patient in the best condition for nature to act upon him."[33] Promoting and providing optimal end-of-life care to ICU patients provides an exquisite opportunity for nurses to do so.

References

1. Taskforce on Palliative Care. Precepts of palliative care. *J Palliat Care* 1998;1:109–112.
2. American Nursing Association. *Nursing's Social Policy Statement.* Washington DC: American Nurses Publishing, 1995.
3. Campbell ML. *Forgoing Life-sustaining Therapy.* Aliso Viejo, CA: AACN Critical Care Publication; 1998.
4. Gurfolino V, Dumas L. Hospice nursing: the concept of palliative care. *Nurs Clin North Am* 1994;29:533–546.

5. Kaye P. *Symptom Control in Hospice and Palliative Care.* Essex, CT: Hospice Education Institute; 1990.

6. Lynn J, Teno JM, Phillips RS, Wu AW, Desbiens N, Harrold J, Claessens MT, Wenger N, Kreling B, Connors AF Jr. Perceptions by family members of the dying experience of older and seriously ill patients. *Ann Intern Med* 1997;126:97–106.

7. Sheehan DC, Forman WB. Symptomatic management of the older person with cancer. *Clin Geriatr Med* 1997;13:203–219.

8. Desbiens NA, Wu AW, Yaseei Y, Lynn J, Alzola C, Wenger NS, Connors AF, Phillips RS, Fulkerson W. Patient empowerment and feedback did not decrease pain in seriously ill hospitalized adults. *Pain* 1998;75:237–246.

9. Puntillo K, Weiss SJ. Pain: its mediators and associated morbidity in critically ill cardiovascular surgical patients. *Nurs Res* 1994;43:31–36.

10. Puntillo KA, Wilkie DJ. Assessment of pain in the critically ill. In: *Pain in the Critically ill* (Puntillo KA, ed.). Gaithersberg, MD: Aspen, 1991, pp. 45–64.

11. Desbiens NA, Wu AW, Broste SK, Wenger NS, Connors AF Jr, Lynn J, Yasui Y, Phillips RS, Fulkerson W. Pain and satisfaction with pain control in seriously ill hospitalized adults: findings from the SUPPORT research investigations. *Crit Care Med* 1996;24:1953–1961.

12. Puntillo K, Miaskowski C, Kehrle K, Stannard D, Gleeson S, Nye P. Relationship between behavioral and physiological indicators of pain, critical care patients' self-reports of pain, and opioid administration. *Crit Care Med* 1997;25:1159–1166.

13. Stannard D, Puntillo K, Miaskowski C, Gleeson S, Kehrle K, Nye P. Clinical judgment and management of postoperative pain in critical care patients. *Am J Crit Care* 1996;5:433–441.

14. Bruera E, Fainsinger RL, Miller MJ, Kuehn N. The assessment of pain intensity in patients with cognitive failure: a preliminary report. *J Pain Symptom Manage* 1992;5:267–270.

15. Morrison RS, Ahronheim JC, Morrison GR, Darling E, Baskin SA, Morris J, Choi C, Meier DE. Pain and discomfort associated with common hospital procedures and experiences. *J Pain Symptom Manage* 1998;15:91–101.

16. Puntillo K. Dimensions of procedural pain and its analgesic management in critically ill surgical patients. *Am J Crit Care* 1994;3:116–122.

17. Doherty MH. Benzodiazepine sedation in critically ill patients. *AACN Clin Issues Crit Care Nurs* 1991;2:748–761.

18. Bruera E. Issues of symptom control in patients with advanced cancer. *Am J Hospice Palliat Care* 1993;March/April:12–22.

19. Shuster JL. Delirium, confusion, and agitation at the end of life. *J Palliat Med* 1998;1:177–186.

20. Society of Critical Care Medicine. *Practice Parameters for Systemic Intravenous Analgesia and Sedation for Adult Patients in the Intensive Care Unit.* Anaheim, CA: SCCM, 1995.

21. Ziehm S. Intravenous haloperidol for tranquilization in critical care patients: a review and critique. *AACN Clin Issues Crit Care Nurs* 1991;2:765–777.

22. Storey P. Symptom control in advanced cancer. *Semin Oncol* 1994;21:748–753.

23. Nadal JW, Pederson J, Maddock WG. A comparison between dehydration from salt loss and from water deprivation. *J Clin Invest* 1941;20:691–713.

24. McCann RM, Hall WJ, Groth-Juncker A. Comfort care for terminally ill patients: the appropriate use of nutrition and hydration. *JAMA* 1994;272:1263–1266.

25. Ellershaw JE, Sutcliffe JM, Saunders CM. Dehydration and the dying patient. *J Pain Symptom Manage* 1995;10:192–197.
26. Holden CM. Nutrition and hydration in the terminally ill cancer patient: the nurse's role in helping patients and families cope. *Hospice J* 1993;9:15–35.
27. Musgrave CF. Terminal dehydration: to give or not to give intravenous fluids? *Cancer Nurs* 1990;13:62–66.
28. Printz LA. Is withholding hydration a valid comfort measure in the terminally ill? *Geriatrics* 1988;43:84–88.
29. Sutcliffe J, Holmes S. Dehydration: burden or benefit to the dying patient? *J Adv Nurs* 1994;19:71–76.
30. Lewandowski W, Daly B, McClish DK, Juknialis BW, Youngner SJ. Treatment and care of "do not resuscitate" patients in a medical intensive care unit. *Heart Lung* 1985;14:175–181.
31. Danis M, Federman D, Fins JJ, Fox E, Kastenbaum B, Lanken PN, Long K, Lowenstein E, Lynn J, Rouse F, Tulsky J. Incorporating palliative care into critical care education: Principles, challenges, and opportunities. *Crit Care Med* 1999;27:2005–2013.
32. Ruland CM, Moore SM. Theory construction based on standards of care: a proposed theory of the peaceful end of life. *Nurs Outlook* 1998;46:169–175.
33. Nightingale F. *Notes on Nursing: What It Is and What It Is Not.* New York: Dover; 1969, p. 133.
34. Stannard D. *Reclaiming the House: An Interpretive Study of Nurse–Family Interactions and Activities in Critical Care.* Doctoral dissertation, University of California, San Francisco, 1997.
35. Taskforce on Ethics of the Society of Critical Care Medicine. Consensus report on the ethics of foregoing life-sustaining treatments in the critically ill. *Crit Care Med* 1990;18:1435–1439.
36. Analgesia, sedation, NMBA Administration Reference Card. In, ICU Bedside Book. University of California San Francisco Medical Center.
37. Pain Management in Adults. In, University of California San Francisco Medical Center Nursing Policy and Procedure Manual Vol. 1

Chapter 13

Helping Families Prepare for and Cope with a Death in the ICU

SARAH E. SHANNON

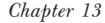

Families play important roles in the critical care environment: they serve as familiar context for the patient, they are often called upon to act as surrogate decision makers, and families are recipients of care themselves. This chapter examines those three roles and suggests strategies to support families facing the transition from curative therapy goals to planning for a comfortable death.

Do Families Belong in the ICU?

Historically, ICUs have not been "visitor-friendly" environments.[1] Family presence at the bedside has been restricted through policies that limit the length of visits, number of visitors, and times of visitation. Structural obstacles have discouraged visitors, including unpleasant waiting rooms, open bay designs that preclude privacy, or a lack of comfortable chairs at the patient's bedside. Rather than working to minimize obstacles to family involvement, care providers sometimes employ strategies that increase families' disenfranchisement from their loved one and the care environment.[2]

Caregivers' tension around the families' presence in the ICU has focused on many issues. Nurses often prefer that families not be present while nursing care is being provided because of convenience for the nursing staff, discomfort at being observed, a desire to work efficiently and without interruption, a belief that witnessing care subjects the family to embarrassment or further trauma, and a need to protect the privacy of other patients in an open ICU setting.[3–7] Physicians also prefer that families not be present at the bedside during examinations, procedures, or daily rounds for many of the same reasons. Physicians may also want to control the timing of when families approach them with questions or concerns.

Are families a problem in the intensive care setting? What is their role? How can healthcare providers support family members? In particular, what do families need when the goals of care have shifted from cure to comfort? To answer these questions, one needs to consider the legal and moral basis for a family's connection to a critically ill person. Families play three crucial roles: they provide a context for the patient, they act as proxy decision makers for the patient, and they are recipients of care themselves. For this chapter, the term "family" will be used inclusively to refer to both legal (close relatives by either blood or marriage) and "chosen" family (the unique constellation of nonmarital partners, close friends, and relatives such as cousins, nephews, or nieces whose lives are interwoven with the patient).

Families as "context"

Osborne, reflecting on death in the intensive care setting, remarked, "Doctors do the doctoring but patients do the dying *in community*."[8] Family and friends are the context, the human community, in which a person lives and dies. The meaning of a person's death to one's spouse, children, parents, siblings, and friends dwarfs the meaning within the narrow context of the critical care unit where the actual death occurs.

Family and friends are often first-line caregivers for ill loved ones. Whether helping someone manage after an acute injury such as a broken bone, cope with a chronic condition like rheumatoid arthritis, or face a terminal diagnosis such as end-stage liver failure, families provide basic care and support. When individuals are released within hours of having ambulatory surgery or leave their doctor's office after receiving the bad news regarding a biopsy result, family and friends are likely to be the ones offering care and support. They have a wealth of knowledge about the individual who is ill: what scares them, what inspires them, what comforts them. A patient's loved ones are experts at being that person's friend, companion, and foil. Patients benefit from remaining linked to the context of their lives during an illness, especially when diminished consciousness makes it difficult for them to communicate their needs and preferences easily or independently.[9,10]

Families as proxy decision makers

Approximately three-quarters of all intensive care patients are unable to participate in health care decision making at the point that difficult decisions must be made.[11–13] When patients cannot make choices for themselves, a surrogate is identified. Overwhelmingly, legally recognized family members (spouse, children, parents, and siblings) or persons who are granted legal status by patients (i.e., Durable Power of Attorney for Health Care, or DPAHC) will act as surrogate or proxy decision makers for decisionally incapacitated patients. Why is this? Clearly, physicians, nurses, social workers, lawyers, and other professionals have specialized knowledge about difficult medical decisions such as withholding or withdrawing life-sustaining therapy. Yet, when individuals are asked whom they would wish to have make medical care decisions for them if they were unable, they usually name family or close friends—moral intimates— rather than professional experts.[14] Decisions about life-sustaining therapies are moral choices, not simply medical decisions. Hence, we seek intimates from our moral communities who share our values, and perhaps history, to speak for us. The legal codes in the United States reflect this selection of moral intimates as surrogate decision makers for health care choices, creating a hierarchy of surrogates based on presumptions of moral intimacy (see Chapter 8.)

To be able to make informed choices for decisionally incapacited patients, surrogates need to fully understand the patient's current situation. This means that surrogates should receive the same information that a patient would be legally entitled to when making autonomous health care decisions such as treatment options, benefits, and risks. In addition to this basic information, surrogates also need to have direct, intimate knowledge of the patient's current experience. How is the patient responding to therapy physically and emotionally? Is the patient suffering? What are the potential benefits and burdens of therapy? To make informed choices, a surrogate needs to understand the patient's *current* quality of life and the prognosis for *future* quality of life.

Surrogates need direct, intimate knowledge of the patient's experience to fulfill their legal and ethical duty to make informed choices for another.[12,15] This includes opportunities to share with the critically ill patient treatment successes and setbacks, restful periods and painful times, calms and crises. A surrogate decision maker's need for moral intimacy encumbers the health care providers with a reciprocal duty to not obstruct access to their loved one.

Families as recipients of care

When a loved one is critically ill, the family should also be viewed as recipients of care from the health care team for three reasons: to benefit the patient, to express compassion, and to meet consumer demand. Treatment of families of critically ill and dying patients is undergoing a transformation similar to that which occurred 30 years ago at the other end of the life continuum—birth— when expectant fathers and other family members became legitimate participants in the delivery room.

Families are often in crisis as they contemplate the loss of a loved one.[16–18] The physicians, nurses, social workers, and others caring for the patient can become an important source of support and assistance for family members because of their proximity to the situation, professional expertise, and knowledge of the culture of critical care and process of dying. This in turn allows the family to be as effective as possible in comforting, supporting, and buffering the patient during the crisis of critical illness.[10,16] Care providers are not "family substitutes"; they are professionals who have a responsibility to assist families to fulfill their unique role as the patient's intimate.

In addition, for many families the death of a loved one is an alien experience—one they are ill prepared for by modern culture. Normal sources of social support, such as friends, neighbors, and co-workers, can be strained by the complexity of critical illness and the difficult choices faced when the goal of care turns from cure to comfort. Hence, family members may turn to the patient's caregivers for the support and comfort they would normally obtain from others.[4,16]

Finally, families are in a position to evaluate the quality of care delivered to their loved one and, as future health care consumers, will make choices and recommendations based on their experiences. Patient and family satisfaction with health care delivery is increasingly important in this era of managed care. Just as consumer demand dictated radical changes in hospital birth practices, family and patient preferences about how to die need to be assessed and accommodated.[19]

Supporting Families of Critically Ill Patients

Support of families in the critical care environment can be divided into four categories: general support during the crisis of critical illness, support for surrogate decision making, support during the dying process, and support following the patient's death (see Table 13–1 for a summary). These categories are intended to be cumulative, meaning that support to families during the dying process should build upon prior general support and support for surrogate decision making. Each category is introduced below with one or more quotes drawn from a study of the experiences of families making surrogate decisions for dying loved ones in the critical care environment.[20]

Supporting families in the critical care setting

Families of critically ill patients may experience insensitivity or compassion, detachment or intimacy from the critical care team.

From a young husband of a woman dying from an overdose:

> I guess the main thing is that they treated her like she was going to wake up any minute; like she was a human being that a lot of people loved, and not just a body lying there almost dead. I think that's the main thing, is that there was that compassion. They didn't know [the patient] from Eve until she showed up in the ICU, but they treated her with respect and compassion, just like she was one of their best friends.[20]

Table 13–1. Strategies for helping families prepare for and cope with death in the ICU

Supporting families in the critical care setting

Treat the patient with respect and compassion.
Allow families to be with the critically ill patient.
Allow families to be present during codes and other invasive procedures.
Identify the intimate community of each patient.
Communicate openly and honestly with the family.

Supporting families in surrogate decision making

When possible, facilitate advance care planning.
Help families to interpret clinical signs accurately.
Cue families to consider what the patient would have wanted.
Create private spaces to facilitate decision making.
Focus on what will be done, not just on what won't be done.

Supporting families during the dying process

Educate the family about what to expect.
Offer your presence.
Assist families in creating rituals to make death meaningful.

Supporting families after the death of a patient

Provide immediate bereavement support.
Provide written materials with information about what families need to do after a death.
Connect with bereavement groups or other services.
Develop a program for contacting families post-death.
Assess family satisfaction with care through a survey.

From the adult daughter of an elderly patient who died 1 week later of end-stage respiratory and cardiac disease:

> I think it was the only day where he could still talk . . . Dad said, "Oh my dinner will be here pretty soon; maybe you can stay and help feed me?" And I said, "Oh, sure. I'll do that." It was a long time before it got there and I just kept waiting and waiting and anyway it finally came in and the nurse said, "Oh, are you still here? . . . I can't do my job when you stay so long." And I didn't think that was necessary. And I said," Well, I just thought I'd stay here and feed him his dinner." And she goes," Well, that's what we're here for." Here he was, he was dying![20]

What can be learned from these family members and from research on the needs of families during the critical care hospitalization of a loved one? At least five lessons can be drawn about how to support families during the crisis of critical illness.

Treat the patient with respect and compassion
It is important to families and patients that health care providers touch patients gently, protect their dignity and privacy, explain what they are doing (even when the patient has severely diminished consciousness), and alleviate the pa-

tient's pain and suffering as much as possible. These simple acts communicate to the family an attitude of respect and compassion.

Allow families to be with the critically ill patient
The foundation for trust, communication, and support of families is built upon the respect for the family's integral role in the patient's life. Communicating that respect requires that families be allowed to be with their loved one. Health care providers do not "own" critically ill patients; they are entrusted to the care of health care providers by the family. As Molter expressed it, "Families are not visitors in the critical care unit."[21] Although nearly three decades of research on the psychological and physiological effects of family visitation on patients have confirmed the positive benefits of having loved ones at the critical care bedside,[1,3,10,22–35] restrictive ICU visitation policies are still common. Fifty years ago, parents were allowed to visit their hospitalized children once a week.[1] Less than 40 years ago, expectant fathers were excluded from the delivery room.[36] Few families, or professionals, would condone such policies today, yet many of the objections that were raised around these issues are echoed in the current debate around allowing families open access to the ICU.

There are three ethical justifications for restricting family visitation: (1) to adhere to the patient's preference for limiting visitors, (2) to protect the privacy of other patients, and (3) to protect the safety of hospital staff. The first situation is obvious but clearly may require skillful handling when patients refuse to see some or all family members. The issue of ensuring patient privacy may be used to justify requesting family members to phone the unit prior to entering but should not be used to justify blanket exclusions (such as policies that do not allow any visitation during nursing change-of-shift periods). The third issue, staff safety, is the most challenging. Hospitals located in high crime areas may prefer to require all visitors to leave the institution between 8 P.M. and 8 A.M. for protection of staff and patients. However, models exist for ensuring safety in other areas such as in newborn nurseries where up to three family members are issued armbands that allow them to be present on the unit. Alternative options need to be explored that do not involve blanket exclusions of family visitors. A final issue that is often cited as an ethical justification for limiting family presence at the bedside is that families can interfere with providing care to the patient. While it is ethical to negotiate with the family around actual obstacles such as space limitations, too often, this reasoning is inappropriately extrapolated to imply that the mere presence of family at the bedside interferes with care. The rare family who truly *does* interfere with the patient's care needs careful assessment to determine what supports are necessary to help them effectively be present at the patient's bedside.

The creation of visitation policies that show respect to the family for their central role in the patient's life is essential for three reasons. First, patients need and want contact with their loved ones in the unfamiliar environment of critical care and during the crisis of illness.[25] This is especially true when the critically ill patient is an infant or child.[37] Second, family members need to be intimately aware of the patient's situation to fulfill their social roles as advisor, sounding board, or cheerleader and, potentially, to fulfill their legal role as surrogate decision makers for incapacitated patients. Third, family members benefit from close contact with the patient.[35,38–40] Demonstrating respect for the family generates a climate of mutual positive regard and trust with the health care team. Many units allow the family unlimited access to the patient once the person is formally recognized as "dying." While this is compassionate, it is also troublesome. This accommodation only serves to confirm the power relationship between the staff and family and to emphasize the capricious nature of the original exclusion.

In addition to changing visitation policies, critical care units can be structurally redesigned to facilitate family presence at the bedside. See Table 13–2 for environmental features that are conducive to family visitation.

Children are also visitors in the critical care unit. Visitation policies should not exclude children except in situations of significant risk of infection.[41] Even if children are not at the actual bedside, they are likely to spend long periods in ICU waiting rooms accompanying adult visitors. All ICU waiting rooms need to

Table 13–2. Features of a supportive environment for family visitation

- Provide chairs at the bedside: Chairs should be comfortable, at a height that allows interaction with the patient, and be movable close to the bedside.[40]

- Provide access to facilities to meet visitors' basic human needs: This includes (1) telephones; (2) bathrooms for visitors that are close to the critical care unit; (3) access to kitchen, laundry, and shower facilities; (4) sleeping areas; and (5) access to healthy snacks and meals.[4,10,41,62,68,69]

- Provide complimentary coffee and tea in the waiting area:[41] Offering refreshments is an almost universally recognized message of welcome.

- Provide a beeper to each family:[4,16] Beepers allow family members to leave the immediate area to exercise, eat, sleep, or pray while remaining in touch with staff and/or family with the patient.

- Provide private spaces for family to gather:[41,65] If several small rooms are not available, redesign large waiting rooms to create smaller spaces where family members can gather to talk and support one another.

- Provide distractions in waiting room areas: A television that can be volume controlled, magazines, puzzles, windows, bird feeders, fish tanks, and other distractions are appreciated. Include play areas for small children and toys and books for older children.[41]

- Provide an attractive, quiet space for spiritual worship:[62] Meditation and prayer are important elements of coping and bereavement in many cultures.

- Provide access to a computer with an Internet link: Many families cope with a loved one's dying by educating themselves about their loved one's condition. Providing access to the Internet links them to sources of information and support. Suggestions for helpful and accurate sites may be useful.

- Provide ancillary or volunteer staff support: Families appreciate a resource desk staffed by volunteers or others to provide information about housing, restaurants, transportation, parking, and the like.

reflect this reality by providing a play area for small children and reading materials, television, or other distractions for older children and adults.

Allow families to be present during codes and other invasive procedures

One or two family members can be routinely invited to witness attempted resuscitations and other procedures from which they are often excluded by hospital staff. Experience suggests that when family members are supported by a liaison staff member, their presence at attempted resuscitations does not interfere with medical procedures and it can be very helpful for some family members.[42-46] While this is true for patients of all ages it is particularly urgent that family members be with pediatric patients. Parents or another family member should be allowed to be present with children during emergency room procedures, anesthesia induction, recovery from anesthesia, and other invasive or frightening procedures.[47]

Allowing family members to be present during codes or other procedures require the support and sensitivity of the health care team. Families need to be coached on how to apply their expertise at soothing their loved one in this new context. Efforts to protect families from painful or traumatic experiences are ineffective and ultimately may backfire when families having unrealistically hopeful expectations are called upon to act as decision makers for incapacitated patients.

Identify the intimate community of each patient

Health care professionals need to complete initial and ongoing assessments of the composition of the patient's intimate community.[16] If the patient is competent, he or she should be asked to name any friends or other nonrelated persons who should be considered "family" for the purposes of visitation (and any family or friends who should be excluded). In addition, the patient should be asked if they wish to have any family members or friends involved in their health care decision making and to provide their names. Those persons should then routinely be included during discussions between the health care team and the patient. Patients need to know who their legal surrogate/s would be, according to state law, should they become incapacitated and be offered the opportunity to complete a Durable Power of Attorney for Heath Care (DPAHC) form if they prefer a different decision maker.

Incapacitated patients also need to have their intimate community identified. Family members should be asked to identify who should be involved in communication about the patient's condition, who should have open access to visitation, who the legal decision maker is, and the like.[4] Families should also help to personalize the "body in the bed." In some critical care units, families are asked to bring in a picture of the patient, which is used to create a poster about the *person*: their likes and dislikes, names of family and friends, names of pets, occupation, nicknames, and any other information that helps health care professionals relate to a loved individual, not just a "sick body."

Communicate openly and honestly with the family

Communication is a "mutual exchange of information between two or more individuals".[48] Clinicians have specialized information about a patient's medical condition, prognosis, and treatment options. Families and other moral intimates have specialized information about patients' previous wishes, emotional responses, and psychological coping. The need for open communication with families is widely accepted yet not routinely achieved.[49,50] The obstacles for the clinician are many: time constraints, competing demands by other patients, difficulty in coordinating rounds with times of family visits, the emotional challenge of confronting intense grief, and medical uncertainty. Yet, these obstacles are weak excuses when weighed against professional and ethical duties.

Two approaches are used to improve clinician communication with families. The first is focused on improving the attitudes and skills of individual clinicians (see Chapter 9). The second is focused on creating a supportive organizational culture (see Chapter 20). Both approaches are crucial for achieving effective clinician-family communication.

Physicians, nurses, social workers, chaplains, and others have identified the need to improve skills at communication for difficult situations such as breaking bad news, responding to patient requests for assistance in dying, requesting an autopsy, responding effectively to angry or distressed family members,[41] and disclosing errors (for examples, see references 6 and 51–58). Strategies to foster a supportive organizational culture address the need to create opportunities for open dialogue. For example, in many settings patient care conferences are used primarily only after conflicts have developed. Hence, they become a symbol of broken communication. To counteract this tendency, some units have policies of proactively scheduling patient care conferences at regular intervals on all patients who can be predicted to require complex care coordination (i.e., patients who have been on mechanical ventilation for longer than 3 days). Similarly, ensuring that families receive consistent messages regarding prognosis from all members of the care team is critical. This is particularly relevant in units where patients share a common diagnosis or treatment regimen, but may experience poignantly different outcomes, such as a bone marrow transplant unit. One strategy is to institute a daily conference for the interdisciplinary team to briefly discuss (1–5 minutes per patient) the current prognosis, treatment plan, and other issues to ensure consistent communication with families.[59] Another strategy for increasing communication between family and staff is to locate all clinical information about a particular patient (e.g., flow sheets, progress notes, lab values, care plan) near the patient's room so that the bedside nurse, medical team, and patient's visitors are in close proximity to one another creating opportunities for interaction.

A foundation for good communication includes (1) opportunities for families to receive information and get questions answered; (2) respect for privacy by ensuring ready access to private areas for team–family communication and intrafamily discussions; (3) family-centered attitudes on the part of the critical care team; and *(4)* a climate of trust and openness among the interdisciplinary team members.

Supporting families in surrogate decision making

Families are often thrust unexpectedly into the role of surrogate decision maker for a loved one. Their experiences are sobering reminders of the enormity and importance of this moral and legal duty.

From a woman in her 60's who missed the last chance to talk with her husband because of miscommunication with the health care team:

> I regret because of what happened afterwards, but I stayed down there with those people instead of going back up to the room where H. was. Although they told us he was back up there, I thought that he would come down. But that was the last time I could have talked to him. Because after the surgery, he lived that whole week with a tube. . . . To not be able to talk, he couldn't ask questions! That was the worst part.[20]

From the parents of a post-transplant patient, recalling the care conference with the medical team that preceded their decision later the same day to withdraw support from their dying daughter:

> Father: I think the way that it was put, that one statement that the doctor said, "You're going to have to sooner or later." I think that kind of pressured me into going with it.
>
> Mother: And then there was one doctor that got up and walked out. Just left the meeting. And I think she was upset because [the patient's father] was shaking his head. He didn't really want to give up.
>
> Father: No. I didn't agree to it right then, no.[20]

Research on surrogate decision making suggests five ways that family members and others (such as DPAHCs) can be supported when they are called upon to act as proxy decision makers for incapacitated patients: facilitate advance care planning, help families to interpret clinical signs accurately, cue families to consider what the patient would have wanted, create private spaces to facilitate family decision making, and focus on what will be done, not just on what won't be done.

Facilitate advance care planning

In some circumstances, ICU patients are able to discuss their specific preferences regarding end-of-life treatment with their family. When clinicians assess that a patient is mentally capable of advance care planning, patients and families appreciate help in recognizing this opportunity.[13,14,49] In addition, clinicians can facilitate patient–family communication regarding end-of-life preferences by offering to facilitate the discussion or to be present to answer questions. There are at least two compelling reasons for helping families and patients to discuss these difficult issues. The first is that surrogate decision makers are frequently inaccurate when they try to predict the patient's wishes.[60,61] Improving communication may improve the surrogate's knowledge of patient wishes. Second, families who eventually need to make decisions for a dying loved one benefit from believing that they did what the patient would have wanted.[62]

Help families to interpret clinical signs accurately
Many families will interpret the appearance of a comatose or obtunded patient as the normal activity of sleeping. Families need help sorting through the clinical signs and information to draw accurate interpretations about their loved one's condition. Allowing families to "see" what the clinician is observing can be very helpful. For example, for families, cold hands and feet can mean too few blankets; dilated, nonreactive pupils can be viewed as unremarkable; slow, irregular breathing can mean deep sleep. Family members need assistance in observing and interpreting the clinical signs that are meaningful to clinicians.[35,63]

Cue families to consider what the patient would have wanted
Too often health care professionals end a discussion with a family faced with making surrogate decisions with the statement, "What do you want us to do?". This is the wrong question. It suggests that the correct stance is for the surrogate to choose what he or she would wish in the same situation. But surrogate decision makers are expected from both an ethical and legal perspective to attempt first to use a substituted judgment standard. We need to cue family and other surrogate decision makers to use this standard by asking, "Given the situation, what do you think your loved one would have wanted?" or "Now is the time to gather together as a family and think about what your loved one would have chosen." If the answer is, "I don't know," then families need to be cued to consider a best-interests standard by asking, "What do you think would be best for your loved one?".

Create private spaces to facilitate family decision making
Decisions to withhold or withdraw life-sustaining therapy involve conversations that are intensely private. Families report that having a private place to gather enhances communication among the family and with the health care team, ultimately facilitating decision making.[41,64] Importantly, families do not consider the patient's bedside an appropriate place to discuss the patient's grim condition, impending death, or decision making around withholding or withdrawing therapy. Families report that these conversations need to occur in a place where they can speak openly without a perceived need to protect the patient from harsh or unpleasant information, regardless of the patient's level of consciousness.[20]

Focus on what will be done, not just on what won't be done
Too often clinicians discuss what will be withdrawn or withheld when the goal of treatment shifts from cure to care without emphasizing what will be done to

promote the patient's comfort and dignity and to support the family. Providing this information prevents the family from feeling abandoned and enables open dialogue with staff about what actions would be supportive for the family.[65]

Supporting families during the dying process

When patients die in the ICU, families have an opportunity to be guided and supported through the death experience.

From the husband of a woman with breast cancer who collapsed at home unexpectedly:

> [The nurses told us things like] "We're going to turn off the Dopamine. We're going to discontinue that." And [the nurse would] say, "We're going to start turning down the respirator." . . . I think that was just basically understanding and appreciating what was going on (crying). . . . And I think that was really helpful.[20]

From the adult son of a woman who died of end-stage lung disease:

> It was like being in a really wonderful restaurant with a great wait staff that knew just when to show up. It seemed like every time we turned around, you know, as we were saying or talking about my mom saying, "Boy, I wonder if they could increase the morphine?" or "I wonder if they'd check this monitor?"—just as we'd said that, we turned around and in walked [a nurse].[20]

In addition to ensuring patient comfort, health care professionals have the opportunity to support families of dying patients in at least three ways: by educating the family about what to expect, by offering one's presence, and by assisting the family to create rituals to make death meaningful.

Educate the family about what to expect

The dying process is unfamiliar to most families. Providing information about what to expect as treatments are withdrawn and as the patient nears death is very helpful to families.[65] They also appreciate understanding what is being done to promote comfort for their loved one.

Offer your presence

Families appreciate that clinicians and, in particular, nurses and chaplains continue to be available during the dying process.[4] Families need to not feel abandoned or negatively judged during this time. Actions such as spending time at the bedside, frequently checking on the family, and providing comfort measures such as chairs, blankets, coffee, or tea are perceived as supportive.

Assist families to create rituals to make death meaningful

Although death in the critical care unit can be as meaningful for families as death in the home environment, families may need permission and guidance to achieve this ideal. Nurses and others can assist families to reflect on what would be best for their family by presenting various options around (1) family presence at the time of withdrawal of life-sustaining treatment (e.g., none, some, all of the family), (2) religious/spiritual or cultural ceremonies prior to withdrawal (e.g., last rites), and (3) family communication for the period after treatment is withdrawn but before the patient's death (e.g., share stories, reminisce, and the like). In addition, many families create time for each family member to speak to the dying person. Some families do this as a group with each person taking a turn to address the patient. Other families prefer that each member have 5 to 10 minutes of privacy with the patient to say good-bye and express their love or perhaps their regrets. Family members who cannot be physically present can still participate by phoning the patient's room and having the receiver placed by the patient's ear for the allotted time.

Supporting families after the death of a patient

After the death of an ICU patient, families may have lasting positive or negative experiences about the health care team.

From the husband of a woman who died 3 days after suffering a cardiac arrest at home:

> I knew this would be the last time I would ever see her as a person. I still remember very clearly the scene as I entered the room where she was. All the equipment was gone and the room was all cleaned and the bedding upon which my honey rested was very neat. She was laying there, raised up, her hair very neatly arranged as if she herself had done it. She looked alive with her eyes closed. It is a picture I shall never forget. I was able to kiss her for the last time. I will always be grateful to the lady on the ward that took care of her and prepared her for the last viewing.[20]

From the adult daughter of a woman who died from an overwhelming infection:

> The physician that did the operation on her stress ulcers actually sent us a letter, probably maybe 10 days after she died. He was out of town and didn't get back until a couple days later. And so you know, expressing his sorrow. And basically agreeing with our decision that extubating her was the right thing [to do]. And because the autopsy results confirmed what they believed was the case. And it just shortened what could have otherwise been prolonged, you know the inevitable. . . . It was helpful to get that letter.[20]

Supporting families after the death of a loved one in the ICU involves attention to at least five different issues: immediate bereavement support, information about what survivors need to do after a family death, bereavement resources for future reference, contact with the family post-death, and assessment of the quality of care the family experienced.

Provide immediate bereavement support

The period immediately following the death of the patient is critical to the family's grief process. What each family needs will depend on cultural and individual characteristics; however, commonalties do exist among family needs that clinicians should be sensitive to.[41] Families often want time with the dead person. Attending to the appearance of the body and the room is important to creating the fewest barriers for the family to view and touch the body. This can include removing equipment and tubes, cleaning the body (particularly the face and mouth), changing the sheets, lowering the bed, and creating soft lighting. Clinicians need to provide opportunities for post-death rituals such as washing the body, prayer, etc. Spiritual counseling should be offered, such as calling the hospital chaplain or facilitating contact with the family's own spiritual counselor. Furthermore, successful bereavement is enhanced through activities such as allowing the family to take pictures of the deceased person if they wish. Parents who lose a child should be offered a "baby box": a collection of a picture of their child, a lock of hair, arm band, and notes from care providers. Similarly, when a child loses a parent, clinicians can offer to create a "parent box," which might include many of the same items. Finally, some families may need a private place within the hospital to gather briefly after the death.

Provide written materials with information about what families need to do after a death
The death of a family member is not only a private experience but a public and legal event involving administrative issues such as obtaining the death certificate, making funeral arrangements, considering an autopsy, and reporting the death to financial institutions. Many ICUs provide families with written materials about these issues including information from their state's department of health on legal requirements.

Connect with bereavement groups or other services
Information on local bereavement groups should be provided to families, including how and when to contact a crisis line. Many hospitals have post-death support groups, some of which are specific to critical care patients.[41] It may be helpful to provide this information again by mail several weeks following the death to both the legal next-of-kin (such as the spouse) and other family members (such as adult children).

Develop a program to contact families post-death
Families often appreciate being contacted by the patient's care providers after the death.[46,66] Contact can take a variety of forms. Medical teams and nursing staff, together or independently, may send a sympathy note after the death, telephone the family within several weeks, follow-up by phone or mail 6 months post-death, and/or send a card on the first anniversary. ICUs can develop a clearly defined procedure for contacting families post-death to ensure that the planned contact actually does occur and that it addresses identified needs of the family.

Assess family satisfaction with care through a survey
Units should seek families' opinions of the care provided to their dying loved one and to the family.[19,46] This information should be collated and shared with

the staff of the unit to build a culture of family-focused care and to guide changes to unit policies.

Summary

This chapter has focused on means of supporting families in their roles as context to the critically ill patient, as surrogate decision makers for mentally incapacitated patients, and as recipients of care themselves. While the emphasis has been on supporting families when the goal of care shifts from a curative to a palliative focus, the support strategies presented here have implications for all critical care patients. A complete shift toward family-focused care in the critical care setting will require major changes in policies, staff attitudes, and available resources for many units.[67] Yet, one has only to recall the tremendous shift in childbirth care that occurred over a relatively short period of time to appreciate that this change is possible.

Clinicians who have experienced serious illness and death within their own families can be important ambassadors in their work places by helping their colleagues to confront the chasm between what "clinicians" would want for themselves and what they offer patients' families. When clinicians relinquish a sense of control, uncertainty and stress ensue. Moving to a family-focused care delivery system also means not being able to escape the constant reminder that admission to the critical care unit is frequently a time of tragedy and crisis for the patient's family. Health care professionals need education and support for developing the necessary counseling skills to meet this challenge. Finally, health care system administrators must recognize that for clinicians to provide family-focused care, they need support such as adequate staffing to allow time for family interaction, resources for making structural changes, and recognition of and support for the stress of being emotionally available to grieving families. In the next decade, family-focused care will become the standard for all patients in the ICU, especially those for whom the goal of care has shifted from cure to comfort.

References

1. Giganti A. Families in pediatric critical care: the best option. *Pediatr Nurs* 1998; 24:261–265.
2. Chelsa C, Stannard D. Breakdown in the nursing care of families in the ICU. *Am J Crit Care* 1997;6:64–71.
3. Simpson T, Wilson D, Mucken N, Martin S, West E, Guinn N. Implementation and evaluation of a liberalized visiting policy. *Am J Crit Care* 1996;5:420–426.
4. Titler MG, Bombei C, Schutte DL. Developing family-focused care. *Crit Care Nurs Clin North Am* 1995;7:375–386.
5. Kirchhoff K, Pugh E, Calame R, Reynolds N. Nurses' beliefs and attitudes toward visiting in adult critical care settings. *Am J Crit Care* 1993;2:238–245.

6. Chesla CA. Reconciling technologic and family care in critical-care nursing. *IM-AGE: J Nurs Scholarship* 1996;28:199–204.

7. Hupcey JE. Establishing the nurse family relationship in the intensive care unit. *West J Nurs Res* 1998;20:180–194.

8. Osborne M. Personal communication. December 1998.

9. Eagleton BB, Goldman L. The quality connection: satisfaction of patients and their families. *Crit Care Nurse* 1997;17:76–80.

10. Leske JS. Needs of adult family members after critical illness. *Crit Care Nurs Clin North Am* 1992;4:587–596.

11. Faber-Langendoen K. Process of forgoing life-sustaining treatment in a university hospital: an empirical study. *Crit Care Med* 1992;20:570–577.

12. Danis M. Improving end-of-life care in the intensive care unit: what's to be learned from outcomes research? *New Horizons* 1998;6:110–118.

13. Tilden V, Tolle S, Garland M, Nelson CA. Decisions about life-sustaining treatment. Impact of physicians' behaviors on the family. *Arch Intern Med* 1995;155:633–638.

14. Coulton C. Research in patient and family decision making regarding life sustaining and long term care. *Soc Work Health Care* 1990;15:63–78.

15. Harvey MA. Evolving toward—but not to—meeting family needs. *Crit Care Med* 1998;26:206–207.

16. Leske JS. Treatment for family members in crisis after critical injury. *AACN Clin Issues* 1998;9:129–139.

17. Covinsky K, Goldman L, Cook E, Oye R, Desbiens N, Reding D, Fulkerson W, Connors AF, Lynn J, Phillips RS. The impact of serious illness on patients' families. *JAMA* 1994;272:1839–1844.

18. Tomlinson PS. Caregiver mental health and family health outcomes following critical hospitalization of a child. *Issues Mental Health Nurs* 1995;16:533–545.

19. Johnson D, Wilson M, Cavanaugh B, Bryden C, Gudmundson D, Moodley O. Measuring the ability to meet family needs in an intensive care unit. *Crit Care Med* 1998;26:266–271.

20. Shannon S. Picker/Commonwealth Scholars Project. the experience of families with proxy decision-making at the end-of-life: comparisons across institutions. In: Picker/Commonwealth Scholars program, The Commonwealth Fund, 1995.

21. Molter N. Families are not visitors in the critical care unit. *Dimens Crit Care Nurs* 1994;13:2–3.

22. Titler MG, Walsh SM. Visiting critically ill adults: strategies for practice. *Crit Care Nurs Clin North Am* 1992;4:623–632.

23. Simon SK, Phillips K, Badalamenti S, Ohlert J, Krumberger J. Current practices regarding visitation policies in critical care units. *Am J Crit Care* 1997;6:210–217.

24. Sickbert S. Coronary care unit visitation and summary of the literature. *J Am Geriatr Soc* 1989;37:655–657.

25. Simpson T. Critical care patients' perceptions of visits. *Heart Lung* 1991;20:681–688.

26. Brown A. Effect of family visits on the blood pressure and heart rate of patients in the coronary-care unit. *Heart Lung* 1976;5:291–296.

27. Simpson T, Shaver J. Cardiovascular responses to family visits in coronary care unit patients. *Heart Lung* 1990;19:344–351.

28. Theorell T, Wester P. The significance of psychological events in a coronary care unit. *Acta Med Scand* 1973;193:207–210.

29. Kleman M, Bickert A, Karpinski A, Wantz D, Jacobsen B, Lowery B, Menapace F. Physiologic responses of coronary care patients to visiting. *J Cardiovasc Nurs* 1993;7:52–62.

30. Schulte D, Burrell L, Gueldner S, Bramlett M, Fuszard B, Stone S, Dudley WN. Pilot study of the relationship between heart rate and ectopy and unrestricted vs restricted visiting hours in the coronary care unit. *Am J Crit Care* 1993;2:134–136.

31. Lazure L, Baun M. Increasing patient control of family visiting in the coronary care unit. *Am J Crit Care* 1995;4:157–164.

32. Prins M. The effect of family visits on intracranial pressure. *West J Nurs Res* 1989;11:281–292.

33. Hendrickson S. Intracranial pressure changes and family presence. *J Neurosci Nurs* 1987;19:14–17.

34. Bay E, Kupferschmidt B, Opperwall B, Speer J. Effect of the family visit on the patient's mental status. *Focus Crit Care* 1988;15:10–16.

35. Walters AJ. A hermeneutic study of the experiences of relatives of critically ill patients. *J Adv Nurs* 1995;22:998–1005.

36. May K, Mahlmeister L. Comprehensive Maternity Nursing: Nursing Process and the Childbearing Family, 2nd ed. Philadelphia: J.B. Lippincott, 1990.

37. Carnevale FA. The experience of critically ill children: narratives of unmaking. *Intensive Crit Care Nursing* 1997;13:49–52.

38. Quinn S, Redmond K, Begley C. The needs of relatives visiting adult critical care units as perceived by relatives and nurses. Part I. *Intensive Crit Care Nurs* 1996;12:168–172.

39. Seideman RY, Watson MA, Corff KE, Odle P, Haase J, Bowerman JL. Parent stress and coping in NICU and PICU. *J Pediatr Nurs* 1997;12:169–177.

40. Simpson SH. Reconnecting: the experiences of nurses caring for hopelessly ill patients in intensive care. *Intensive Crit Care Nurs* 1997;13:189–197.

41. Granger CE, George C, Shelly MP. The management of bereavement on intensive care units. *Intensive Care Med* 1995;21:429–436.

42. Hanson C, Strawser D. Family presence during cardiopulmonary resuscitation: Foote Hospital emergency department's nine-year perspective. *J Emergency Nurs* 1992;18:104–106.

43. Meyers TA, Eichhorn DJ, Guzzetta CE. Do families want to be present during CPR? A retrospective survey. *J Emerg Nurs* 1998;24:400–405.

44. Eichhorn DJ, Meyers TA, Mitchell TGG, Guzzetta CE. Opening the doors: family presence during resuscitation. *J Cardiovasc Nurs* 1996;10:59–70.

45. Post HR, Redheffer G, Brown J. Letting the family in during a code. *Nursing* 1989;19:43–46.

46. Twibell RS. Family coping during critical illness. *Dimens Crit Care Nurs* 1998; 17:100–112.

47. Sacchetti A, Lichenstein R, Carraccio CA, Harris RH. Family member presence during pediatric emergency department procedures. *Pediatr Emerg Care* 1996; 12:268–271.

48. Vincent JL. Communication in the ICU. *Intensive Care Med* 1997;23:1093–1098.

49. Hanson LC, Danis M, Garrett J. What is wrong with end-of-life care? Opinions of bereaved family members. *J Am Geriatr Soc* 1997;45:1339–1344.

50. Hickey M. What are the needs of families of critically ill patients? A review of the literature since 1976. *Heart Lung* 1990;19:401–415.

51. Buckman R. Communication in palliative care: a practical guide. In: Oxford Textbook of Palliative Medicine pp. 141–156. (Doyle D, Hanks G, MacDonald N, eds.) Oxford: Oxford University Press, 1992.

52. Buckman R. How to Break Bad News: A Guide for Health Care Professionals. Baltimore: The Johns Hopkins University Press, 1992.

53. Baile W, Kudelka A, Beale E, Glober G, Myers E, Greisinger A, Bast RC, Goldstein MG, Novack D, Lenzi R. Communication skills training in oncology. Description and preliminary outcomes of workshops on breaking bad news and managing patient reactions to illness. *Cancer* 1999;86:887–897.

54. Lo B, Quill T, Tulsky J. Discussing palliative care with patients. ACP-ASIM End-of-Life Care Consensus Panel. American College of Physicians–American Society of Internal Medicine. *Ann Intern Med* 1999;130:744–749.

55. Novack D, Suchman A, Clark W, Epstein R, Najberg E, Kaplan C. Calibrating the physician. Personal awareness and effective patient care. Working Group on Promoting Physician Personal Awareness, American Academy on Physician and Patient. *JAMA* 1997;278:502–509.

56. Novack D, Epstein R, Paulsen R. Toward creating physician-healers: fostering medical students' self-awareness, personal growth, and well-being. *Acad Med* 1999; 74:516–520.

57. Tulsky JA, Chesney M, Lo B. How do medical residents discuss resuscitation with patients? *J Gen Intern Med* 1995;10:436–442.

58. Tulsky J, Chesney M, Lo B. See one, do one, teach one? House staff experience discussing do-not-resuscitate orders. *Arch Intern Med* 1996;156:1285–1289.

59. Back A. Personal communication. October 1997.

60. Uhlmann R, Pearlman R, Cain K. Physicians' and spouses' predictions of elderly patients' resuscitation preferences. *J Gerontol* 1988;43:M115–M121.

61. Tsevat J, Cook FE, Green ML, Matchar DB, Dawson NV, Broste SK, Wu AW, Phillips RS, Oye RK, Goldman L. Health values of the seriously ill. Am Coll Physicians 1995;122:514–520.

62. Jacob DA. Family members' experiences with decision making for incompetent patients in the ICU: a qualitative study. *Am J Crit Care* 1998;7:30–36.

63. Swigart V, Lidz C, Butterworth V, Arnold R. Letting go: family willingness to forgo life support. *Heart Lung* 1996;25:483–494.

64. Maunder T. Principles and practice of managing difficult behaviour situations in intensive care. *Intensive Critical Care Nurs* 1997;13:108–110.

65. Goetschius S. Families and end-of-life care. *J Gerontol Nurs* 1997;23:43–49.

66. Warren NA. Bereavement care in the critical care setting. *Crit Care Nurs Q* 1997;20:42–47.

67. Levine C. Rough Crossings: Family Caregivers' Odysseys Through the Health Care System. Special Report. New York: United Hospital Fund of New York, 1998.

68. The Picker Institute. New visions for health care: ideas worth sharing. In: Through the Patient's Eyes in a Pediatric Setting. Boston; 1999. Available at http:// www.picker.org/Research/NewVisions/Default.html.

69. Zazpe C, Margall MA, Otano C, Perochena MP, Asiain MC. Meeting needs of family members of critically ill patients in a Spanish intensive care unit. *Intensive Crit Care Nurs* 1997;13:12–16.

Chapter 14

Helping the Clinician Cope with Death in the ICU

SUSAN D. BLOCK

*I*ntensive care unit clinicians confront the challenge of simultaneously preparing for both survival and death as possible outcomes for their patients. While they are striving to rescue their patients from an acute illness or exacerbation of a chronic disease, ICU clinicians also recognize that a substantial proportion will die in the ICU or during this hospitalization. Practically every death in the ICU now involves some degree of withholding or withdrawing potentially life-prolonging treatment.[1] A focus on intensive care and one on palliative support are often viewed as incompatible, as reflected in the common opposition of "aggressive care" and "comfort measures only." But good palliative care can be highly "aggressive," yet aimed primarily at comfort, and fine intensive care attends carefully to the comfort of the patient, regardless of the goals or methods of care. Growing levels of concern from patients about losing control over their dying, greater attention to patient-centered care, and ever-increasing technological support available to keep patients alive have created a new impetus to reexamine the old assumption that the practices of palliative care and intensive care are mutually exclusive.

Palliative care is "comprehensive care, provided by an interdisciplinary team, for patients and families living with a life-threatening or terminal illness, particularly where care is focused on alleviating suffering and promoting quality of life." It focuses on pain and symptom management, discussion and negotiation of treatment goals, psychosocial and spiritual support, and coordination of care.[2] While there are significant similarities between palliative care and intensive care, there are also instructive differences. Almost by definition, every ICU patient has a life-threatening illness and receives care from an interdisciplinary team. However, the ICU team, in contrast to a palliative care team, generally focuses more intensively on biomedical care needs than on psychosocial and spiritual concerns and on the needs of the family. The focus on rescue may override or obscure concerns about comfort and relief of suffering; preserving or improving of quality of life is a long-term goal, but not attended to explicitly in the ICU. Indeed, admission to the ICU often represents a decision to make short-term trade-offs in comfort and well-being in the service of possible long-term gains in quantity and quality of life.

Stressors in the ICU (Table 14–1)

In addition to the extraordinary biomedical expertise required to competently manage life-threatening illness, ICU clinicians are called upon to perform numerous demanding psychosocial tasks. They are expected to assess patient–family relationships, provide appropriate hope, understand and support the patient's values and priorities, negotiate goals of treatment in a setting of intense emotion and frequently of conflict, deal with prognostic uncertainty, support other staff members in providing care, and manage their own emotional responses to disturbing clinical situations and death. Several other features of the ICU contribute to the stress on clinicians. Time pressures are intense, and clinicians must make high-stakes, split-second decisions. A focus on the immediate needs of the patient may make it difficult for clinicians to recognize and respond to the atmosphere of family crisis that an ICU hospitalization represents.

Increasingly, deaths in the ICU are "managed," with clinicians assuming an active role in determining the timing and conditions of death. The patients who are admitted to the ICU may be young and may have experienced catastrophic, and often unusual, events. In some ICUs, traumatic events or illnesses—burns,

Table 14–1. Major Stressors of Caring for the Dying and Manifestations of These Stressors

Major Stressors	Common Manifestations
Communication problems with other health care professionals	Staff conflict
	Depression, grief, and guilt
Communication problems with patients and family members	Distancing, depersonalization, and intellectualization
Inadequate resources or staffing	Anger, irritability, and frustration
Role ambiguity	Helplessness, inadequacy, and insecurity
Role conflict	Job–home tensions
Role overload and role strain	Errors in judgement
Exposure to family distress	Avoidance of patients and families
Personal responsibility for end-of-life decisions	
Exposure to patient suffering	

injuries, infections—have caused terrible deformities that must be confronted in providing care. While many patients are sedated or comatose and may seem somewhat dehumanized to their care providers, those who are awake may be suffering with distressing symptoms—dyspnea, pain, or terror. Frequently, patients die, but there is little time to process, review, or grieve for them. While the clinicians who work in ICUs may become accustomed to this milieu, the ICU is an extraordinary setting, dense with violence and drama, indeed a place of intensive emotion as well as intensive care.

Patients in the ICU challenge the clinician to both deny and attend to their humanity. Patients with whom the clinician might otherwise identify often evoke distancing behavior because closeness and empathy may seem incompatible with the clinician's role of aggressively seeking rescue, often utilizing invasive and painful procedures. On the other hand, patients who are comatose or unconscious may seem "less than fully human" to professionals who have never met them or known them as individuals. The clinician's challenge in this circumstance is to find ways of helping the patient remain human, even in their vulnerable state, but not so human that the clinician feels inhibited in performing the often invasive procedures that are needed to sustain life. Desensitization, while it is adaptive, carries with it the risks of distance and dehumanization.

How Clinicians Cope

The excitement of the ICU—the intense teamwork, the opportunity to use cutting-edge technology, the sense of control over physiological processes that can be achieved at times in the ICU—may mask some of its disturbing psychological effects on clinicians. While there is little systematic research, several reports suggest that nurses are often distressed by the care offered to patients in this setting, and by their exposure to death and dying in the ICU.[3-5] A study of 79 physicians interviewed as part of a study of occupational stress in the care of the dying found that the major stressors were communication problems with other professionals, role overload, role strain, patient–family communication problems, team communication problems, inadequate resources/staffing, role ambiguity, and role conflict. These stressors were manifested in job–home tensions; staff conflict; depresion, grief, and guilt; anger, irritability, and frustration; helplessness, inadequacy, and insecurity; distancing, depersonalization, and intellectualization; errors in judgement; and avoidance of patients.[6] A survey of 598 oncologists about "burnout" showed that 56% reported being burned out and 53% attributed these feelings to continuous exposure to fatal illnesses.[7] A study of 25 pediatric residents explored the relationship between attitudes about death and responses to a clinical vignette about a dying patient. Residents with high death anxiety scores were more likely to adopt the dysfunctional coping strategies of avoidance and denial for dealing with the clinical situation described in the vignette.[8] A British study of general practitioners found that exposure to death and dying was not a major source of stress, but was associated with alcohol use, especially among women physicians.[9] In a recent study of 218 graduating Harvard medical students, Block and Billings (unpublished) found that 63% reported symptoms of post-traumatic stress disorder related to their involvement in the care of dying patients.

Several observers emphasize the role of helplessness and failure as determinants of dysfunctional clinical practices in physicians.[10] Feelings of failure can result in wishing the patient would die (to avoid having to deal with the patient), as well as overtreatment (to ensure that "everything has been done" to save the patient). In addition, clinicians may withdraw or avoid patients who are dying in an effort to deal with feelings of grief. Closeness and empathy with patients may also evoke difficult responses by forcing the physicians to confront their own mortality.[11-13] Grief about the loss of valued and meaningful relationships with patients is a feature of physicians' experience that is commonly acknowledged but little understood.

In general, medical and nursing education provides inadequate preparation for caring for dying patients. Most physicians and nurses have had little training in providing end-of-life care and lack expertise in these aspects of clinical care.[14] Only 6% of ICU physicians and 21% of ICU nurses reported receiving any training in dealing with grief and bereavement, regular features of clinical care in the ICU.[15] In a recent national survey, medical students, residents, and faculty evaluated themselves as inadequately prepared to care for patients at the end of life (mean level of preparation of students = 5.8, of residents = 6.9, and of faculty = 6.6 on a 0-10 scale where 0 = no preparation and 10 = optimum preparation). Critical care physicians reported the same level of preparation to care for patients at the end of life as that of physicians with much lower levels of exposure to this clinical task.[16] Exposure to these tasks does not necessarily guarantee competence in performing them. Nor does competence or confidence in care ensure appreciation of the strain of the work or development of healthy coping strategies.

Strategies for Helping Clinicians Cope with Death in the ICU (Table 14-2)

The combination of the stresses of providing clinical care and the absence of adequate preparation for caring for the dying make the ICU a challenging arena for clinical practice. Yet, many opportunities for improving this environment are present. First, involvement of role models and teachers with expertise in palliative care as well as critical care is likely to broaden the vision of the type of care that the ICU can offer. Palliative care experts can be expected to place special emphasis on comfort, dignity, and recognition of the psychosocial and spiritual dimensions of care, as well as on communication that enhances

Table 14–2. Strategies for Helping Clinicians Cope with Death in the ICU

Specific Coping Strategies

Enlist palliative medicine specialists to teach and model
  Comfort, dignity, and recognition of psychosocial and spiritual dimensions and care
  Communication with patients and families
  Pain and symptom management
  Acute bereavement care

Family meetings early in the ICU course
Regular inter-disciplinary meetings focusing on treatment goals and plans
Involve nursing, social work, psychiatry, pastoral care and other professionals in routine ICU work rounds
Staff support groups and "Balint groups"
Rituals for the staff to mark the death of patients
Bring families back to the ICU after a patient's death to meet with the staff

decision making, patient and family trust, and satisfaction. They can also teach new approaches to pain and symptom management and other topics to their intensivist colleagues. Mastery of these areas of clinical practice—communication about goals of treatment and patient and family values, pain and symptom management, attention to the emotional needs of patients and families, care of the acutely bereaved—may lead to enhanced competence in and coping with end-of-life care among ICU staff.

Clinical leaders in intensive care might consider several approaches to enlarging the scope of care goals to include palliative care. These include attending educational programs designed to teach palliative care content as well as using strategies to promote teaching and institutional practices that favor palliative care approaches. A palliative care specialist can be recruited to provide regular input and consultation to the ICU. Psychiatrists can join ICU teams, providing perspective on the psychosocial dimensions of life-threatening illness. Through these mechanisms, ICU leaders will enhance their own expertise in palliative care and can become role models and leaders of clinical improvement in this domain in the ICU. As ICU clinicians come to broaden their definitions of success to include both rescue and an appropriate, dignified death, the culture of the ICU is likely to change in ways that will make it a better place to receive and provide medical care, thus decreasing stress on patients and families, as well as on clinicians.

Intensive care unit leaders should develop learning experiences for nursing and medical students and residents focused around death and dying in the ICU. Such experiences should concentrate on the clinical issues involved in the management of the patient as well as on the learner's own emotional responses to the patient's illness and death. Such educational experiences have the potential to be an antidote to the development of distancing behaviors[17] and cynicism,[18] which often arise in response to emotionally overwhelming experiences that take place while learners are immersed in intensive care clinical experiences. As long as there is appropriate emotional support, the immediacy and rawness of the emotions surrounding ICU death for patients, families, and clinicians allow learning to take place at a deep level and support new clinical coping processes that help young clinicians tolerate a degree of intimacy and personal engagement that other aspects of medical training may subvert and undermine.

The practice of making family meetings early in the course of a patient's stay in the ICU a routine feature of care has the potential to reduce ambiguity about goals of care, prevent conflict with the family, and reduce intra-staff tension about how aggressive care should be, all of which are frequent sources of stress for staff in the ICU. Clinicians for whom convening family meetings will be a significant responsibility should consider seeking additional training in family dynamics, group process, and negotiation.

Intensive care unit leaders should recognize that conflict around end-of-life decision making is a regular feature of end-of-life care, and they should develop standard formats for preventing and managing conflict among patient, family members, and clinicians. Morning work rounds that include physicians, nurses, social workers, psychiatrists, and other involved clinicians can be a forum for discussing the immediate decisions that bear on the patient's care and can prevent subsequent conflict or tensions that may arise when staff members feel excluded or not listened to in the decision-making process. The existence of a regular forum for case discussion, as well as a standard process to address differences, reduces staff stress[19] and has the potential to lead to enhanced cross-disciplinary respect, the development, over time, of a consensual comprehensive ICU philosophy of care, as well as improved resolution of conflicts with patients and families. While such regular meetings require an investment of time and emotional energy by staff, they are likely to have positive effects on staff morale, enhance teamwork, and lead to improved satisfaction with care.

Opportunities for staff to discuss their own feelings about the deaths of patients should be integrated into the routine of the ICU. In a study in the U.K., a majority of ICU physicians and nurses thought a staff support group should be available.[15] Opportunities to talk openly about emotional reactions to patients with a skilled mental health provider in a support group or a patient-centered discussion format can allow ICU clinicians to cope more effectively with the stresses of their work and to enhance knowledge about challenging experiences that arise in caring for patients (e.g., management of "difficult" patients, dealing with young children of a seriously ill patient) and thus develop some degree of cognitive mastery over the distress of caring for the dying. "Balint-groups,"[20] in which clinicians have a regular opportunity to talk about their own experiences in providing care to dying patients, have been used in oncology and found by many participants to be helpful. These and similar formats can affirm the central importance of the clinician–patient relationship, the doctor's or nurse's role as healer, the value of sharing experiences with colleagues, and how doctoring and nursing can be vehicles for personal growth. A variety of different models for staff support groups have been proposed.[21] In planning a group, ICU leaders should obtain consultation and input from both ICU staff and experienced group facilitators to adapt the support model for the particular needs of their ICU.

Families often have useful feedback to offer staff about the end-of-life care their relative received in the ICU. Yet, ICU providers rarely have an opportunity to hear these perspectives. When family members report that care has been excellent, they appreciate the opportunity to thank providers and clinicians feel a sense of pride and competence in managing these complex clinical situations. In other circumstances, family members may have valuable suggestions to offer clinicians about care processes, communication, and the overall experience of having a loved one die in the ICU. While such feedback can, at times, be difficult to hear, it provides an excellent mechanism for continuous quality improvement. The ICU clinicians who implement changes in unit routines in response to this feedback and notice improved patient and family outcomes often feel an enhanced sense of professionalism and pride.

Similarly, development of appropriate rituals to mark a patient's death in the ICU helps clinicians feel connected to and supported by their colleagues in this demanding work. Hospice and palliative care programs, and even some ICUs, may hold memorial services to remember those who have died in their settings over a period of time.[22] Some invite staff alone; others welcome family members and friends. In general, such rituals have been well received by professional staff and family members. Such rituals help professional caregivers place deaths, which often are seen as routine occurrences in the ICU, within a broader human context, reminding them that an extraordinary event—the death of a human being—has taken place within the ordinariness of the daily routines of the ICU.

Conclusions

Caring for patients in the ICU is stressful for clinicians. The requirement to simultaneously prepare for rescue and death is a major source of strain. The development of new approaches to ensure that pain and other physical symptoms are well controlled and that emotional suffering of the patient and family are appropriately addressed through integrating palliative medicine into routine care in the ICU has the potential to improve the experience of receiving as well as providing care in this setting. Attention to staff support needs that is focused around the strains of caring for dying patients can also improve clinician morale, competence, and teamwork.

I am grateful for thoughtful editorial suggestions from J. Andrew Billings, M.D.

References

1. Prendergast TJ, Luce JM. Increasing incidence of withholding and withdrawal of life support from the critically ill. *Am J Respir Crit Care Med* 1997;155:15.
2. Billings JA. What is palliative care? *J Palliat Med* 1998;1:1:73–81.
3. Asch DA, Shea JA, Jedrziewski MK, Bosk CL. The limits of suffering: critical care nurses' views of hospital care at the end of life. *Soc Sci Med* 1997;45:1661–1668.
4. Foxall MJ, Zimmerman L, Standley R, Bene B. A comparison of frequency and sources of nursing job stress perceived by intensive care, hospice, and medical-surgical nurses. *J Adv Nurs* 1990;14:577–584.
5. Solomon MZ, O'Donnell L, Jennings B, Guilfoy V, Wolf SM, Nolan K, Jackson R, Koch-Weser D, Donnelley S. Decisions near the end of life: professional views on life-sustaining treatments. *Am J Public Health* 1993;83:14–26.
6. Anderson B, McCall E, Leversha A, Webster L. A review of children's dying in a pediatric intensive care unit. *N Z Med J* 1994;107:345–347.
7. Whippen DA, Canellos GP. Burnout syndrome in the practice of oncology: results of a random survey of 1,000 oncologists. *J Clin Oncol* 1991;9:1916–1920.
8. Neimeyer GJ, Behnke M, Reiss J. Constructs and coping: physicians' response to patient death. *Death Ed* 1983;7:245–264.
9. Cooper CL. Rout U, Faragher B. Mental health, job satisfaction, and job stress among general practitioners. *BMJ* 1989;298:366–370.
10. Block SD, Billings JA. Patient requests to hasten death: evaluation and management in terminal care. *Arch Intern Med* 1994;154:2039–2047.
11. Spikes J, Holland J. The physician's response to the dying patient. In: Psychological Care of the Medically Ill: A Primer in Liason Psychiatry (Strain JJ, Grossman S, eds.). New York: Appleton-Century-Crofts, 1975, pp. 138–148.
12. Weissman AD. Misgivings and misconceptions in the psychiatric care of terminal patients. *Psychiatry* 1970;33:67–81.
13. White LP. The self-image of the physician and the care of dying patients. *Ann N Y Acad Sci* 1964;164:822–831.
14. Billings JA, Block SD. Palliative care in undergraduate medical education: status report and future directions. *JAMA* 1997;278:733–738.
15. Granger CE, George C, Shelly MP. The management of bereavement on intensive care units. *Intensive Care Med* 1995;21:429–436.
16. Block SD, Sullivan AM. Attitudes about end-of-life care: a national cross-sectional study. *J Palliat Med* 1998;1:347–355.
17. Faulkner A, Maguire P. Talking to Cancer Patients and Their Relatives. New York: Oxford University Press, 1997.
18. Becker HS, Geer B. The fate of idealism in medical school. *Am Soc Rev* 1958; 23:50–56.
19. Woolley H, Stein A, Forrest GC, Baum JD. Staff stress and job satisfaction in a children's hospice. *Arch Dis Child* 1989;64:114–118.

20. Balint M. The Doctor, His Patient, and the Illness, 2nd ed. London: Pitman Publishing, 1964.
21. Vachon MLS. The stress of professional caregivers. In: The Oxford Textbook of Palliative Medicine (Doyle D, Hanks GWC, MacDonald N, eds.) New York: Oxford University Press, 1998, pp. 919–932.
22. Lederberg MS. Oncology staff stress and related interventions. In: Psycho-oncology (Holland JC, ed.). New York: Oxford University Press, 1998, pp. 1035–1048.

Chapter 15

The Interface of Technology and Spirituality in the ICU

NANCY CHAMBERS

J. RANDALL CURTIS

Case 1

At 5:30 A.M., a Native American woman in her 70's was found unconscious in her home on the reservation and was flown to the regional trauma center. The nurse of the ICU requested a chaplain to assess the spiritual needs of the family. When the chaplain arrived, he found the family willing to talk about their mother. She was a tribal healer and had passed this gift on to several in her family. The family identified themselves as Christian with some Roman Catholic roots.

The daughters began notifying the relatives who were primarily within 200 miles. The two daughters said that many people would be present within the day. It was important for as many relatives as possible to be there.

At 11:45 A.M. the primary nurse asked me, the chaplain on call, for the chaplain who had been with the family, for they were ready. I asked what "ready" meant. The nurse explained that the family wanted to have a ceremonial prayer prior to the withdrawal of life support and requested support from the chaplain. When told he was off duty, the family had said that anyone would be ok. When I arrived, the nurse said that the family had gathered in the room. I went in and found approximately 25 people there. I introduced myself as the chaplain on call for the day and indicated that I knew the situation. A daughter hugged me and started crying. She said they would want a prayer at some point. I asked them to think about things they might want to add to my prayer. Then, as we waited, the patient's older sister started chanting. She took over as the tribal liturgist. She asked a brother to wet a handkerchief and place it on his sister. Then each person present was asked to think of any way that they had harmed or caused pain or grief to the patient. They were asked to touch the handkerchief so that this pain would be washed away. The relatives then prayed using the sign of the cross and their native language. This was followed by the oldest son taking two large bells from a leather bag. He rang the bells for about 2 minutes. Then one by one, each person told how they had been touched by the dying woman: the gifts she had passed on to them, the faith she had in herself and others, the power she used for good. I did nothing but represent the connection with the hospital. Once, when I moved toward the door so the family could be closer, the sister whispered, "Please stay if you can." As the family finished, they opened the doors and asked that the respiratory therapist be summoned to withdraw the mechanical ventilation. I thanked the family for sharing this sacred event with me and said that I felt honored to be included. They smiled and the sister said, "That was why we invited you."

In modern medicine, we strive to address the needs of the patient's body, mind, and spirit. Yet, the spiritual needs of patients are often neglected or, if addressed, are addressed as peripheral. In the vignette above, the spiritual assessment should have begun as soon as possible and it should have continued in parallel to the medical treatment. A single question upon hospital admission pertaining to faith-tradition is not adequate to assess a person's spirituality or spiritual needs. The answer to one question may indicate whether a person identifies with a particular religious practice, but a single question about religious affiliation fails to meet our obligation as health care providers and fails to meet the Joint Commission for Accreditation of Healthcare Organizations (JCAHO) standards for spiritual care. The JCAHO states that patients have "the right to receive care that respects individual spiritual values." In the provision of medical care, it is important that caregivers address and be sensitive to not just religious needs but also spiritual needs. Spirituality is individual in nature—although it encompasses a person's conscious connection to the universe, it also encompasses a person's relationship with him- or herself, with other people, and with life in general. In this chapter, we will define spirituality and discuss spiritual assessment in the ICU setting. We will also explore the interface of technology and spirituality, examine the role of rituals in the ICU, and discuss the importance of the plurality of spirituality in our society.

What Is Spirituality?

As demonstrated in the case described above, spirituality is not synonymous with religion. Religions are external expressions of a belief system. They may include form and structure such as worship, scripture, sacraments, and prayers. Most religious institutions are characterized by a formalized body of doctrine, creeds, or teachings. Spirituality includes religion, but can not be equated with religion, for not all religious needs are spiritual and not all spiritual needs are met by religion. For the purposes of this chapter, we will be using the words "spiritual" and "spirituality" as meant in the most inclusive sense.

What Is a Spiritual Assessment?

In 1978 the National Committee for the Classification of Nursing Diagnosis (NCCND) developed a "Spiritual Diagnosis Taxonomy." Spirituality is defined as "the life principle that pervades a person's entire being, [their] volitional, emotional, moral–ethical, intellectual and physical dimensions, and generates a capacity for transcendent values. The spiritual dimension of a person integrates and transcends the biological and the psychosocial nature."[1] The word "transcendent" means that one's perspective goes beyond the limitations of self, time, and place. Consequently, the statements or questions that are posed to determine spirituality might include:

1. Tell me about the patient. What things did she value?
2. How might he see what is happening? Did you ever talk with him about anything like this?
3. Where or who would she look to for advice, counsel, sense of hope?
4. What support system has he used in the past?

In the ICU, a spiritual assessment should be done not only with the patient but also with the family. In the ICU and the ICU waiting room, spiritual issues that are not addressed can quickly escalate from concern to distress and then to despair.[2] Early interventions can provide an opportunity for a relationship to develop with the patient or family and the staff and can prevent conflict later in the hospital stay.

Any or all members of the health care team can do spiritual assessment. Ideally, the spiritual assessment begins in the primary care physician's office prior to a hospitalization that necessitates a visit to the ICU. A spiritual assessment could be included as a component of discussions about treatment preferences and advance directives. The physician could encourage that family members be included in these discussions and ask about spiritual, religious, and cultural beliefs that might impact care at the end of life. In reality, many patients in the ICU have not addressed these issues with physicians or other healthcare providers. Consequently, the gathering of information often begins at the hospital. Ideally, formal spiritual assessment should be charted by a trained spiritual caregiver, but any member of the health care team can initiate the process by asking some of the questions. There are several potential screening tools that can be used for this purpose.[3-5]

From the chaplain's perspective, getting this information early in the admissions process is important. In the ICU setting, the most effective way to begin to provide spiritual support is for a clinician to mention that spiritual support is available as part of the multidisciplinary health team. It is often the clinician who recognizes his or her own spiritual needs in a similar situation who can easily articulate the possibility of spiritual needs of the patient or family. In the ICU, frequently the patient is not available for much dialogue, so the assessment may begin with the first family members who arrive. Being trained to do

spiritual assessments means having some sense of one's own spiritual preferences, biases, and opinions. The person doing the assessment is then able to
set aside their own issues and listen to the patient or family.

It is important for health care providers to understand the barriers to an
effective spiritual assessment. Initially, when a patient and/or family members
are asked if they want spiritual support in the form of a chaplain or spiritual
leader in a specific faith tradition, thoughts similar to those listed in Table 15–1
may color a patient/family response and act as barriers to a spiritual assessment. People with spiritual concerns such as those in Table 15–1 may say they
have no need for spiritual care when asked. Members of the health care team
should listen for spiritual needs expressed in other ways, such as disconnected-
ness, distress, or failure to make meaning of the crisis situation. Existential
questions about the meaning of illness, injury, or other events may be implicit
signs of spiritual needs, and patients or families with these concerns may benefit from a formal spiritual needs assessment.

Health care providers need to realize that if they show discomfort with
spiritual issues, this discomfort will diminish the effectiveness of the spiritual
assessment. Those members of the health care team who are more comfortable
carrying out a spiritual assessment should perform this task instead of those
members who are uncomfortable with this. It should be recognized, however,
that spiritual care is a necessary component of clinical practice. To become
more comfortable addressing spiritual needs of patients, clinicians need to
learn more about their own biases. Without acknowledging their own cultural
and spiritual biases and interests, clinicians will likely feel uncomfortable and
be less successful assessing someone else's spiritual needs (see Chapter 4 for
additional discussion of addressing attitudes toward death). For clinicians who
would like to increase their awareness of spiritual issues there are a number of

TABLE 15–1. Attitudes of Family Members that May Serve as Barriers to a Spiritual
Assessment

1. My loved one must be dying. I can't face that, so I literally can't face a chaplain (rabbi, priest,
   imam, minister, shaman or a person who represents God, a Higher Power).

2. I am in shock and a spiritual support person will expect me to be strong or talk about it and I
   can't . . . yet.

3. I feel guilty because I haven't been to church (mosque or temple) as often as I should have
   been. Maybe I am being punished. I don't want to have a bunch of guilt laid on me in the
   midst of this nightmare.

4. I haven't gone to church (or other place of worship) since I was a child or since I got married;
   I am not a good or practicing Catholic (Jew, etc.).

5. I need to focus on the concrete information given by the doctors and try to understand the
   medical situation. I don't have the time or energy to talk religion. It is so abstract.

6. What if a chaplain doesn't respect my particular beliefs? I don't need anything else to cope
   with at this point.

resources available.[5,6] Often, as clinicians become more comfortable with their own cultural and spiritual biases, they may grow to appreciate the varied ways that people find meaning through a personal spirituality or find strength within in a particular faith tradition.

It is also important that clinicians know the cultural milieu of their hospital and the faith traditions represented in the local community, as well as some of the community's explicit and implicit spiritualities. This may include the community faith leaders or support people who should be present as a person dies and different cultures' predominant beliefs concerning dying, death, and handling the body after death. Table 15–2 lists some of the major faith traditions and their respective common beliefs and traditions concerning dying and death. For clinicians who practice in an area with an extremely diverse population, a useful resource is *Culture and Nursing Care: A Pocket Guide,*[7] which provides a concise overview of the following areas: cultural/ethnic identity, death rituals, family relationships, spiritual and religious orientation, and illness beliefs. This resource can be particularly helpful in preparing a spiritual assessment and is a useful manual for pastoral care staff and trainees, as well as nurses and physicians.

Technology and Spirituality: Finding Meaning in the ICU

Clinicians should recognize that as members of the ICU team, they have become comfortable with the way a patient in an ICU looks. They recognize the sounds of the machines and the smells of the unit. They have an established routine that works for them in the ICU. Much of this routine may be mandated by protocol or pathways, but it exists and serves, in part, to lower staff anxiety so that they can make meaning of their vocation. Often the rituals of the medical team control the clinical environment.

Clinicians often find comfort in their familiarity with medical technology and the use of this technology enhances their confidence that "everything is being done." Using medical technology provides clinicians with a tool for making meaning out of illness and death.

The patient and family, however, often perceive the medical technology with a certain amount of fear. Most patients and families feel like foreigners in the ICU environment—this is not their vocation. Their senses are bombarded with the unknown: unfamiliar sights, sounds, and smells, and the patient may look quite different from the person the family knows. They have been told that the machines are helping to sustain the patient's life, which is often in a precarious balance, and they try to acclimate to a very uncomfortable situation. When a machine's alarm is set off by a relatively insignificant problem, families fear the worst. The very life and death of their loved one seems to be embodied in this foreign technology.

TABLE 15–2. Selected Religious Beliefs and Traditions Regarding Death and Dying

Faith	Faith leaders	Beliefs	Handling the body	Preparing the body	Viewing the body
Buddhist	The family may ask for a teacher, a member of the Sangha, or a specific monk. Family may bring religious implements, incense, flowers, fruit, prayer beads, and images of Buddha.	No daily practices are dictated, but chanting, meditation, or rituals might help the person attain enlightenment.	Incense is lit in the room. Organ donation may not be permitted.	The family may choose to wash the body. Cremation is preferred.	The family may need significant time with the body.
Catholic	Families/patient may request visitation and the Eucharist. This can be accomplished by a priest, deacon, nun, monk, or Catholic lay persons.	The Sacrament of the Sick may be given only by a priest. This is viewed as mandatory by most Catholics. However, because of the current shortage of priests, this is not always possible. Families may feel abandoned and express frustration and anger when this request is denied. Chaplains, lay leaders, or motivated clinicians may read appropriate sections from the Prayer Book.	Treat the body with respect. Organ donation and autopsy are permitted.	The body is usually buried. However, cremation is acceptable.	Clinicians can make sure that the family and religious leaders are given privacy and quiet for prayer and/or administration of Sacraments. Most families would be pleased to have staff join them in a time of prayer.

Hindu	Visitors may include a priest, family, and friends.	Amputation is a result of prior sin. Continual changing and prayers occur before and after death. Grief is visually displayed. A thread signifying a blessing may be tied around.	A bath is necessary every day. Organ donation and autopsy are acceptable.	The family may wash the body. Cremation is preferred, with ashes scattered in sacred rivers.	Clinicians should inquire which beliefs and practices are important to a specific family and provide privacy as they carry out those practices (prayer, ritual washing).
Islam	Family and friends visit to provide emotional support. Prayer is said five times each day facing Mecca, following ritual washing. Confession takes places prior to death in the presence of the family. The Koran may be read as a person dies. The person reading should be Muslim and be ritually clean.		Treat the body with respect. After death, the body should be moved to face Mecca. Organ donation is acceptable. Autopsy is permissible only for legal or medical reasons.	To prepare the body for burial, it is ritually washed by a person of the same gender, dressed, and positioned toward Mecca. Burial takes place as soon as possible.	
Jewish	Visitors may include family, friends, the rabbi, and perhaps 10 men from the synagogue. Men may wear a *yarmulke* (cap) or use a *tallit* (prayer shawl); prayers for the sick are said.	The Sabbath is from sundown Friday until sundown Saturday. Orthodox and Conservative Jews do not work on the Sabbath. This includes working, driving a car, and cooking. Check with the patient/ family for particular	Treat the body with respect. Autopsy is discouraged. Organ donation is an ethical dilemma that involves the *Torah* and *Talmud* and an interpretation of obligations, duties, and commitments.	The Ritual Burial Society may be called to wash the body. The body is buried as quickly as possible. Embalming is discouraged. Usually someone stays with the body. Cremation not appropriate.	Clinicians should provide privacy for ritual prayers and preparation of the body.

(continued)

TABLE 15–2.—Continued

Faith	Faith leaders	Beliefs	Handling the body	Preparing the body	Viewing the body
		needs regarding holy days and dietary restrictions. Saving a life overrides most religious obligations.			
Native American	Leaders such as a medicine man/woman may be called cousins or uncles. They may be referred to as shaman healers and may practice traditional tribal practices as well as Christian practices. Chants, prayer, singing, and dancing are part of the tradition.	"Creator" is a unifying term often used interchangeably with "God." Sickness may mean being out of balance with nature. Ancestors may guide the deceased. A medicine bag or prayer staff, rattle, feathers, cedar, sage, and pipe may help with rituals.		Preparation may be done by the family.	The body may be considered and empty shell. Some tribes view the body, and may believe the deceased has ancestors.
Protestant	Ministers, elders, deacons, family, and friends may visit and offer prayer, read the Bible, offer communion, or anoint the body.	Health care decisions are usually the individual's responsibility.	Organ donations and autopsy are acceptable. Most protestants permit termination of extraordinary treatment.	Cremation or burial is appropriate.	Ministers and/or chaplains may design a ritual prayer incorporating specific practices.

These are generalizations. Individual members of a given religion may vary in their views and beliefs.

Family members of a critically ill patient confronted with this alienating environment often must struggle to make meaning out of this environment. When people make meaning they search the reservoirs of their history to find ways in which they have made meaning at other times of crisis. They may or may not name these processes explicitly as spirituality. Explicit spirituality may take the form of a specific religious tradition or a cultural ritual. With help, patients and families can find meaning in an alienating environment and thus gain confidence in determining the spiritual aspects of healing or dying in the ICU setting.

All health care workers bring their own sense of spirituality into their relationship with the patient and family. It is integrated into their care of patients in either an overt or covert way. Research suggests that patients and families would like to know how a clinician makes meaning of the crises that are ever present in their work.[8,9] A clinician's spirituality and meaning making are seldom articulated to patients or their families, but they can be shared in ways that patients and families may find helpful. However, if clinicians do share their own sense of spirituality or meaning with patients, it is essential that this be done in a way that does not pass judgment or impose the clinician's views on the patient, family, or dying process.[9] To impose one's own beliefs and values in a hospital room is tantamount to abuse. Even offering to pray with a family may be interpreted as imposing one's views if it is not preceded by a spiritual assessment to determine if such an offer is appropriate.[9] Families and patients are vulnerable and should not be required to defend their belief systems. If caregivers doubt their capacity to self-reveal in an unbiased manner, they should request that a person trained in spiritual assessment be involved.[9]

The Role of Ritual in the ICU

During times of stress, many people turn to a belief system that has worked in the past. This may include, but not be limited to, religious practices such as prayer or chanting, sacred texts, or sacraments that have sustained them through prior crises. Families may try to adapt meaning-making rituals or patterns that comfort them to an intense or traumatic situation. In accepting the spiritual dimension of life, it may become easier to bring some order to and make meaning of the possibility of death in the ICU. A spiritual assessment may help clinicians join together with families on that sacred ground.

Rituals provide ways to make meaning with both that which is familiar and that which is mysterious. For families of all cultures and faith traditions, the miracles of life and the mysteries of death are marked by life-cycle rituals. These nodal events have resulted in both secular and religious ceremonies. Rituals also provide a lens through which we can see our emotional connections to our loved ones enabling us to explore the meaning of our lives and to build and rebuild our family relationships. Rituals "connect us with our past, define our present life, and show us a path to our future as we pass on ceremonies, traditions, objects, symbols, and ways of being with each other that have been handed down from previous generations."[10]

The most effective rituals spring from the depth of human experience. In this age of technologic health care, families struggle to find ways to give form and meaning to the event of dying in the ICU. Some religious traditions have movable rituals, which, when brought to the hospital, may take precedence over the machines that earlier in treatment pointed to the possibility of sustaining life. When families are asked to make the transition from attempting to cure disease withdrawal of life support, families want to know that their loved one will be respected as a person, not just viewed as a body. By supporting rituals for dying or death in the ICU, clinicians can demonstrate this respect.

When treatment is withdrawn, family and friends look for rituals that may symbolically retrieve a sense of dignity for the patient who has been ensconced in and held captive by the technological mysteries of the ICU. "The birthplace of any single ritual is always in a spontaneous, unpremeditated form emerging from an individual's struggle to regain emotional balance, a sense of wholeness."[11] In the ICU setting, we should support those rituals formally sanctioned by a specific religious tradition (i.e., the Sacrament of the Sick, prayers, chanting) as well as those developed outside specific religious traditions, provided that such rituals do not interfere with the care of other patients or families. "Genuine ritual is powerful, profound and deeply religious and requires no contemplation about its efficacy—one knows that one is moved."[11]

Specific ways in which well-trained clinicians can support rituals in the ICU include the following

1. Become more comfortable with the symbolic language of religion, faith, and spirituality.
2. Make certain that spiritual elements of care are addressed as soon as possible in treatment so that the essential pieces can be put in place as needed.
3. Be willing to be present in the midst of existential angst. Assess what support is needed or ask someone who is more comfortable to assist you. Think of the support people you might want with you in this situation and ask the family, "Do you have the spiritual support you need?"

   When people say they have alerted their temple, church, prayer chain, etc., consider whether you could respond, with integrity, "Prayer is good" or "I believe prayer helps" or "Studies show that prayer is helpful." Families want to be doing something to help their loved one and themselves. You can continue to build your relationship with them by acknowledging your acceptance of or alignment with their expression of spirituality.

4. Acknowledge that families are looking for healing by making meaning and regaining balance in the family as the life cycle draws to its conclusion. In some families, this means trying to integrate several religious traditions. Sometimes, because of the tension of family dynamics, people from each tradition may need their own time and space with a dying loved one.
5. Take at least a minute to participate in this life-cycle event. This might be done by saying:
"I know you had been praying for a miracle, we had hoped for one too."
This is especially helpful when a family has failed to accept the probability of impending death.
"It was an honor to have participated in the care of _____."
"I know that this is a painful time for you, and I wish I could make the pain less."

The Plurality of Spirituality in Modern Society

Case 2

A patient was brought into the hospital after experiencing a seizure. A test was run to establish a diagnosis of brain death. In keeping with local hospital policy, a second test was to be run 6 hours later. There was tension in the family as they waited for the results of the second test. After waiting 3 hours, two of the children requested a priest. The priest had left for the day, so another chaplain went to assess the family's and patient's spiritual needs. On initial assessment, it was determined that the patient had been baptized Lutheran, but was not practicing Lutheran; the husband was baptized but not practicing Roman Catholic; three of the adult children wanted administration of the Sacrament of the Sick the the remaining relatives were Pentecostal and did not want pastoral care.

On further assessment, it became clear that the same-sex partner of one of the children was a nurse and was a central figure in the family's interactions with the health care team. She was uncertain what the chaplain might say about her and her partner's relationship, and this tension was initially a barrier to the spiritual assessment.

The family needed a ritual that acknowledged the diversity and complexity of all their spiritual needs. Although the children felt the husband (their stepfather) was not able to see their mother until a decision was made, he asked the Presbyterian chaplain to go with him to offer prayers that would express his love, grief, and readiness to let his wife go. The priest returned to offer the Sacrament to those who wished to participate. The Pentecostal group prayed in tongues but paused as the priest prayed. The scene was a potpourri of expressions of Christian beliefs. The family was able to find a ritual that fulfilled their

specific beliefs while honoring each others' rituals to facilitate healing individu-
ally and as a family.

This case highlights the importance of not reducing families or even individuals to just one faith tradition. There may be several traditions in one family
and individuals may feel connected to more than one tradition. The understanding and honoring of this plurality are important components of spiritual
care in the hospital setting.

Conclusions

Spiritual assessments and the facilitation of spiritual care are important components of providing high-quality end-of-life care in the ICU. The ICU clinicians
should be competent at initiating spiritual assessments and facilitating the spiritual care needed by patients and families. Part of this competence is appreciating how foreign the ICU is for many patients and families and how difficult it
can be to find meaning in this setting. Clinicians should understand the importance of rituals at the end of life and facilitate these rituals whenever possible.
Furthermore, clinicians can play a part in the spiritual care and rituals of patients and their families in the ICU, as needed. Sometimes there may not be
time to stay with a family for a particular spiritual practice or ritual, but when
the time exists, taking these opportunities can result in rewarding experiences
for ICU clinicians and be very meaningful for families. Most families are honored to have staff involved, even if only on the fringes. This involvement is a
concrete way of showing respect and honor to the patient and family.

In many circumstances, the clinician is the primary liaison in helping the
family as they experience the transition from cure to comfort. This should be a
gentle transition, when end-of-life spiritual issues are treated with respect, sensitivity, and compassion. Patients may have their last meal and their last breath
in the midst of technological life support. The goal of good spiritual care is to
help make these final moments have meaning. This may take the form of an-
cient and traditional rituals or of an innovative and spontaneous ritual that
springs fresh from a particular event. How we create comfort in the midst of
technology will impact the memories that loved ones and staff take home with
them.

References

1. Spiritual diagnosis taxonomy. In: National Committee for the Classification of Nursing Diagnosis. Proceedings of the National Committee for the Classification of
   Nursing Diagnosis, Glendale, CA, 1978.

2. Reed P. Spirituality and well being in terminally ill hospitalized adults. *Res Nurs Health* 1987;10:335–344.

3. Maugens TA. The SPIRITual history. *Arch Family Med* 1996;5:11–16.

4. McBride JL, Arthur G, Brooks R, Pilkington L. The relationship between a patient's spirituality and health experiences. *Fam Med* 1998;30:122–126.

5. Puchalski CM. Taking a spiritual history: FICA. *Spirituality Med Connection* 1999;3:1.

6. Elkins D. Spiritual Orientation Inventory. Irvine CA; Pepperdine University Center, 1988.

7. Lipson JG, Dibble SL, Minarik PA. Culture and Nursing Care: A Pocket Guide. San Francisco, CA: UCSF Nursing Press, 1996.

8. Dossey L. Healing Words: The Power of Prayer and the Practice of Medicine. New York, NY: Harper Paperbacks, 1993.

9. Post SG, Puchalski CM, Larson DB. Physicians and patient spirituality: professional boundaries, competency, and ethics. *Ann Intern Med* 2000:132:578–583.

10. Imber-Black E, Roberts J. Rituals for Our Times. New York, NY: Harper Perenial, 1992.

11. Boyle PJ. Ritual obligation. *Park Ridge Center Bulletin* 1998;Aug/Sept:2.

12. Armstrong RD. First the body, then the mind. *Park Ridge Center Bulletin* 1998;Aug/Sept:6.

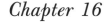

Chapter 16

The Role of the Physician in Sacred End-of-life Rituals in the ICU

STEVEN H. MILES

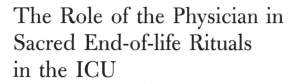

*T*he alien and overwhelming power of the ICU often eclipses a patient's personal identity. Ordinarily this submersion of a patient's personal life in the culture, behaviors, expectations, values, dress, and language of this technical milieu is acceptable for the pursuit of technical healing. Sometimes, however, the ICU is needed to palliate dying or to manage a life support technology–dependent patient as its tools are judiciously removed. In such situations, the overwhelming culture of the ICU can fail to accommodate the ways those patients and their families draw meaning and solace from their personal lives and culture in the face of death. Many people find such strength, purpose, and solace in affirming faiths, rituals, and membership in spiritual communities.[1-3] Physicians must understand why spiritual life should be accommodated in medical settings during dying. They must learn that this accommodation is equally important *and especially difficult* in ICUs. An ICU can accommodate a meaningful death.

The large literature on managing dying during intensive care routinely calls for addressing the alienating aspects of the medical environment. Most advice is well intended, if vague, nostrums: be empathic, respect privacy, and avoid medical jargon. Some is more specific, such as recommendations to waive limited visiting hours or respect advance directives. The sparce content of "living wills," however, does not capture the rich complexity of personal values. Though such advice improves end-of-life care, it does not fundamentally humanize the culture of dying in an ICU.

The core task for humanizing this culture is to create a milieu for personal death. A dying *person* differs from a dying *patient*. The former is defined in terms of his or her own values and relationships. The latter is defined by the role of being under medical care. In personal death, the patient-as-person's lived identity and his or her community identity is in the foreground. In medical death, health professionals play preeminent roles in providing treatment or even waging war against death. In personal deaths, values and community enable intergenerational cultural work and education to occur. A dying person shows family how to die. Personal caregivers comfort the dying person and learn lessons for their own deaths. The youngest generation learns how to care for a dying loved one.

In my own experience as a critical care physician, I have been struck by the importance of the physician's role in facilitating sacred ceremonies carried out by the patient's personal clergy as dying occurs in ICUs and especially as life support is disconnected. There are few accounts of such a role in the medical literature.[4,5] This role goes beyond proposals that physicians identify or respect their patient's religious views.[1,6] Through this role the physician engages more profoundly with family than assuring them that a clergyperson will say final prayers over a dying person. As the case study below shows, this role is connected to the ensuing funeral but differs from the proposal that physicians attend patients' funerals as a way to convey their recognition of the humanity of the death.[7]

Case 1

One morning, a man in his late 70's was admitted to a teaching hospital after resuscitation from an unwitnessed cardiac arrest. Despite significant cardiovascular disease, he was still active in the community. He was an astute retired businessman and was beloved by his wife, siblings, and grown children. On admission to the ICU, he had severe brain damage from a prolonged lack of oxygenation. He was unconscious, and had fixed pupils with no corneal reflexes. A diminished gag reflex was present. He was triggering the ventilator. He had diminished reflexes with diffuse twitching throughout and Babinsky reflexes bilaterally. The exam did not change over 18 hours as his family gathered at the hospital. The prognosis was very poor for neurologic recovery. This patient received medication to decrease the twitching and hypertonicity.

The prognosis and options were discussed at several family conferences. By late afternoon, the family agreed that this man would not want life-sustaining treatment, including the respirator, given his poor prognosis. The patient was Lutheran. We asked the family if they would like their own pastor to be present and said that we were willing to continue life support until the family minister could drive to the hospital from a rural area about three hours away.

The resident and I were paged to the hospital in the early evening. As the family and minister met in a private room, we rearranged the intensive care suite. Bulky, unneeded, and daunting machinery, such as a mattress cooler air compressor, was removed to give the family easier access to the bed. Pressors were stopped and the multiple intravenous bags were replaced with a heparin lock. Distracting video monitors were turned off and alarms for vital signs were silenced. Generally, loved ones want to hold the dying person's hands; so bedrails were lowered and wrist restraints removed. Loved ones also want to behold, caress, or kiss the face and head, so the nasogastric tube and earlobe oximeter were removed. People often weep; so facial tissues were placed on the bed. We first decreased the fraction of inspired oxygen to that of room air and then turned down the ventilator rate to get an idea of what the patient's breathing would be like after extubation. In this case, sedation did not appear to be needed. Hyperpnea can look like distress to the family. If needed for evidence of dyspnea, intravenous sedation can be given to lessen distressing signs.

In the conference room, the resident and I explained how we would remove the respirator. We promised to stay in the ICU to make sure that the patient's needs were met. We talked about Cheynes-Stokes respirations that family sometimes interpret as cyclical gasping for air, respiratory fatigue, and apnea are not evidence of dyspnea. We explained that death sometimes did not immediately follow the removal of ventilatory support. We said that a palliative plan would be set up if longer survival occurred. Family members were offered the option of being present as the respirator was disconnected.

The minister convened the family at the bedside. He began a service with the Lord's Prayer. There was a brief eulogy in which family offered testimonials or spoke to the unconscious man. A Psalm was read and there was a prayer for comfort during the following events. At that point, some family members chose to go to a private lounge as others stayed with the minister at the bedside. The resident stood at the head of the bed and a nurse with an oral suction tube stood on the opposite side. A technician stood at the respirator. I stood with the family and minister at the foot of the bed, softly describing the events. The resident put a small towel over the endotracheal tube, deflated the cuff, extracted the tube under the towel, and stepped back from the bed. The respiratory therapist kept the respirator alarms silent. The nurse suctioned the mouth. The patient's head, face, and arms were now free of devices. The ventilator was removed from the room. Relatives stood next to the bed, taking turns holding his hands and speaking to the unconscious man. The other relatives returned from the lounge. The minister spoke quietly with the family. Ten minutes later, the patient had coarse, moist airway sounds. Family can perceive such persons as "drowning." The resident administered diphenhydramine to quiet these sounds, though scopalamine can also be used. The family and minister stayed with the patient for several hours. The patient died 7 hours after extubation.

Discussion

Sacred end-of-life rituals are best conducted by the patient's own spiritual leader. Such a person may be more likely than a hospital chaplain to better speak the same faith, liturgical, and congregational idiom as the patient and family. They often know the families personally and the families know and have chosen them and their spiritual community. Hospital chaplains can help patients come to terms with a difficult life story, reconcile with estranged loved ones, and prepare for death.[8,9]

The affirmation of spiritual worth and the prayerful context of human mortality can address the conflicted feelings of family who ambivalently want to respect a loved one's preference to not receive life support and who yet feel that forgoing life support is abandoning or devaluing the loved one. For example, one minister offered this prayer to explain how an elderly man who had suffered an immense stroke was at the natural end of life, rather than dying of removing a respirator: "Heavenly Father, we thank you for the life of Earl, our husband, father, brother, and friend. During his life, we realize how often we have taken Your gift of breath for granted. As his spirit now joins you, we are mindful of how each breath and his life was your inspiration."

In several ways, these ceremonies can transform the patient back into a person *before* the treatment is removed. They give a central interpretative role to the familiar and personal leadership of a familiar spiritual leader. They change the language from often poorly understood medical terms to the lay language of values. They give explicit permission for friends and family to play meaningful roles of praying together and comforting one another. Rearrangements in the intensive care suite and the personal ceremony make the deathbed more inviting so that loved ones feel more able to caress the dying loved one.[5] The familiar family and faith make it easier for children to be present. I recall a young boy at a service where life support was withdrawn from his grandmother who was dying of multisystem organ failure. Surrounded by his parents, aunts and uncles, siblings, and his minister, he stepped up to the clean bed of the sedated woman took her hand, and spoke closely to her familiar and unintubated face, "Grandmother, I love you. I just want to tell you that you were the best grandmother anybody could have." These ceremonies usually "rehearse" the prayers and songs that will be said at funeral services. At the funeral, the repetition of portions of the hospital bedside ceremony reinforces the established continuity of passing from patient to person to a remembered loved one.

Earlier in my career, I was reluctant to engage house staff in such ceremonies as they became part of what I did as an attending physician. It is legitimate to debate how to engage house staff in rituals that differ from their own faith perspective. I now believe that the materialism of medical education impoverishes young physicians. Spiritual concerns are important to most patients.[10] Births, deaths, fear, suffering, hope, and joy are part of medicine and summon profound spiritual sentiments. I have heard of similar ceremonies during other medical practices, such as 'ceremonies for life' during bone-marrow infusion or as fertilized eggs are implanted. The thoughtful Jewish resident in the presented case was deeply moved to witness this intimate Christian service and came to appreciate a new dimension to his role as a physician.

Physicians are deeply affected by participating in these ceremonies. We are often strangers to patients and families. We know how to forgo treatment at the end of life, but often inadequately comprehend the social and personal meanings of dying to families. Too often, we approach decision making about ending intensive care as "reverse treatment consents." First, DNR is consented, then decisions to forgo pressors, transfusions, dialysis, or ventilators occur in temporal succession. Performance of a sacred ritual as life support is discontinued affirms the moral significance (or "majesty" as one daughter put it) of death. This is much more than simply acknowledging the futility of life support or of respect for the specific content of an advance directive. Physicians learn important cultural lessons, as these rituals bare the inner life and source of strength of families. I will always remember standing behind an American-Indian family as a healer solemnly chanted the return to the Mother. Such lessons affect the care of future patients by promoting a kind of end-of-life care that is more than simply technically proficient.

Over the last 40 years, there has been increasing attention to managing the end of life in diverse settings. These include freestanding hospices, private homes, nursing homes, hospitals, and ICUs. To some degree, each patient and family will choose a setting for end-of-life care that matches their values. Some will choose to die at home, others as inpatients. Such choices, however, are limited by the abilities of the caregivers, the technology that is needed, and the resources that are available. Good end-of-life care will also require making each setting more responsive to the technical and personal needs of a greater diversity of patients. In this sense, the communal vision of the well-palliated and supported home death, surrounded by friends and family and clergy, that has inspired the hospice concept sends a message all the way to the "opposite" end of the health care universe, to the ICU.

References

1. Barnard D, Dayringer R, Cassel CK. Toward a person-centered medicine: religious studies in the medical curriculum. *Acad Med* 1995;70:806–813.
2. Aries P. The Hour of Our Death. New York: Oxford University Press, 1991.
3. Becker E. The Denial of Death. New York: The Free Press, 1985.
4. Anderson M. Ritual for a dying child. *Park Ridge Center Bulletin* 1998; Aug:8,10.
5. Hochberg T. When a life ends before it begins. *Park Ridge Center Bulletin* 1998; Aug:9.
6. McKee DD, Chappel JN. Spirituality and medical practice. *J Fam Pract* 1992; 35:201–208.
7. Irvine P. The attending at the funeral. *N Engl J Med* 1985;312:1704–1705.
8. Wagner JT, Higdon TL. Spiritual issue and bioethics in the intensive care unit: the role of the chaplain. *Crit Care Clin* 1996;12:15–27.
9. Derrickson BS. The spiritual work of the dying: a framework and case studies. *Hospice J* 1996;11(2):11–30.
10. Koenig HG. Religious attitudes and practices of hospitalized medically ill older adults. *Int J Geriatr Psychiatry* 1998;13:213–224.

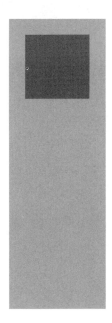

Part IV

Societal Issues

Chapter 17

The Roles of Ethnicity, Race, Religion, and Socioeconomic Status in End-of-Life Care in the ICU

MARION DANIS

*T*he way one experiences illness and death is profoundly influenced by race, cultural and religious background, and socioeconomic status. When patients and clinicians have common backgrounds, these influences can provide a shared understanding and framework for coping with these experiences. When a patient and clinician come from different cultural or religious backgrounds, grappling with the differences can be very difficult. The essence of good medical practice involves recognizing that differences are a universal reality and appreciating that both the physician and the patient are bound by beliefs, customs, experiences, prejudices, rules, and responsibilities.[1] In respecting a patient whose background is different from that of the clinician, the clinician must accept cultural diversity and recognize that human dignity transcends these differences.

In this chapter I will discuss how patients of differing ethnic and socioeconomic classes *wish* to be treated during severe and terminal illness, and how they are *actually* treated during such illnesses. Most importantly, I will review recommendations from the medical literature about how clinicians might *best* address the needs and wishes of critically ill and dying patients whose backgrounds differ from their own.

The compelling need to address this issue becomes apparent when one reviews demographic trends. The relative growth of minority populations in the U.S. between 1980 and 1990, for example, indicates that ethnic diversity has increased dramatically. While the population of the U.S. as a whole increased by 10% during this period, particular groups outpaced this rate: the number of African-Americans increased by 13%; Native Americans by 38%, Asian and Pacific Islanders by 108%, and Americans of Hispanic origin by 53%. The population of refugee groups in the U.S. increased even more dramatically over a comparable time period: the Afghani population increased 5-fold, the Ethiopian population increased 7-fold, the Iranian population increased 36-fold, and the Russian population increased 110-fold.[2] This trend of increasing ethnic diversity is occurring in many countries and needs to be addressed by critical care practitioners worldwide.

This increase in ethnic diversity, in the U.S. and other countries, is accompanied by another demographic trend that has an impact on the experience of ethnic identity: intermarriage among ethnic groups, currently comprises 4% of all marriages in the U.S.[3] Consequently, the number of individuals who do not view themselves as having a single, identifiable ethnic identity has increased. These dynamic trends are reflected in the changing cultural backgrounds, beliefs, and experiences of patients. Also, as Koenig has pointed out, in an increasingly plural society, cultural diversity among health care workers increases.[4]

Definition of Terms

In any discussion involving race and ethnicity, these terms warrant clarification. The biological concept of race has become scientifically outmoded since it is based on inaccurate assumptions about genetic differences. Race is poorly correlated with any biologic or cultural phenomena and yet the term remains commonly used. As Sheldon and Parker write:

> Modern biologists and anthropologists have rejected the scientific basis of such a categorization, for, although it must be true that phenotypic variation has a genetic basis, the point is that there is no consistent categorization across characteristics. Geographical variation in gene frequency is gradual and not qualitative; populations merge into one another. The complex and polygenic determination of human phenotype ensures that there are no typical members of groups, and the amount of variation within any ethnic group is larger than that between groups . . . Although human variation is self-evident, the existence of definable groups or races is not. However, race is still commonly used in medical research.[5]

Thus even though the concept of race may not have a sound scientific basis, a provider's perception of a patient's race may influence the kind of care or any bias in the care given. In addition, patients' perception's of their own racial or ethnic identity may relate to a variety of attitudes about illness and death.

As the concept of race has been discredited, the term *ethnicity* has been increasingly used to refer to shared cultural characteristics and national identity.[5] *Culture* refers to the totality of socially transmitted behavior patterns, arts, beliefs, institutions, and products of human work and thought characteristic of a community or population. It is useful to avoid thinking too simplistically about culture, as Koenig writes:

It is not a simple "trait," an objective, unchanging variable, located within the individual. Culture does not "determine" behavior under certain specified circumstances. Most importantly, culture is constantly recreated and negotiated within specific social and historical contexts . . . Seemingly simple . . . calls for "culturally competent care" ignore the dynamic nature of culture. Moreover, in a complex postmodern world, culture can no longer be simply mapped onto a geographically isolated ethnic group. One cannot assume that a patient or family from Southern China will approach decisions about death in a certain culturally specified fashion.[4]

While it is important to appreciate the complexity of culture, a more succinct definition may be useful: "[Culture] encompasses beliefs and behaviors that are learned and shared by members of a group."[6]

Empirical Evidence

Influence of race, ethnicity, religion, and socioeconomic status on patients' attitudes toward end-of-life care

Ethnicity, religion, and socioeconomic status have strong influences on how patients wish to be treated at the end of their lives.[1,7] To fully document these influences would require an encyclopedic approach. The purpose here is rather to make clinicians aware of how powerfully these influences can affect patient and family attitudes about death and care at the end of life as a prerequisite to providing a useful strategy for helping patients and families of any background.

Ethnicity
As Koenig states, "Cultural conceptions of the self and personhood, the location of the individual within a social group such as the family, orientation to the future, openness about discussing death, and ideas about what constitutes appropriate behavior by healers, are all directly relevant to end of life decisions."[4] The following scenario, to which we will return at the end of the chapter, illustrates the influence of culture on end-of-life care and how understanding of their influence can facilitate care.

A 20-year-old young man from Peru had end-stage lymphoma that was no longer responsive to therapy and was in the ICU because of respiratory failure. The staff thought it was appropriate to withhold cardiopulmonary resuscitation and wanted to speak with the patient about writing a do-not-resuscitate order. His parents, however, did not want this discussion to take place. They felt that a discussion about the reason for the DNR order would involve discussing his terminal prognosis, and in their culture, patients should not be told their prognosis because it causes patients to lose hope.

In a wonderful article that provides case studies of terminally ill patients of various ethnic origins, Klesig outlines several themes that are useful to bear in mind when practicing cross-cultural medicine (Table 17–1).[8] These themes are used to categorize particular developments in the course of an individual's experiences and can become apparent in their beliefs, behaviors, relationships to the family and providers, and in their medical expectations.

Several textbooks exploring the relationship between culture and bioethics have shown that ethical approaches, particularly the importance placed upon the values of beneficence, autonomy, and community, differ among cultures.[9,10] Studies have also been conducted that explore the way people from different cultures approach death.[6,7,11]

Race

As noted in the definitions outlined above, the term, *race* has commonly given way to *ethnic group*. Nonetheless, the concept of race is still often used, particularly with regard to African-Americans, who have had such a harsh experience because of racism. The views of African-American patients regarding medical treatment have been the focus of several studies. They are generally reported to be more inclined to use life-sustaining treatments than non–African-Americans. For instance, African-American patients with HIV infection have been reported to be more likely to want aggressive care but are less likely to communicate these preferences to their doctor.[12] Another study shows that African-Americans living in a nursing home want cardiopulmonary resuscitation (CPR) more often than non–African-American residents.[13] African-Americans are less likely to prepare a living will.[14] To attribute the inclination to use life-sustaining treatments to a fear of discrimination is to oversimplify the African-American experience. As with any ethnic group, the explanations are richly complex. As Cheryl Sanders writes:

> First, the African-American ethos is holistic and nondualistic, emphasizing that most matters are better understood in terms of "but-and" rather than "either-or." Second, it is inclusive, not exclusive, accepting of difference rather than seeing difference as grounds for discrimination or exploitation. Third, it is communalistic, not individualistic, especially valuing family and community over the individual in moral importance. Fourth, it is spiritual, not secular, rejecting any ultimate dichotomy of the sacred and the secular, acknowledging the pervasive presence and power of the unseen realm over and against what is seen. Fifth, it is theistic, not agnostic or atheistic, affirming not only the existence of God but also the relevance of belief to every aspect of life. Sixth, its basic approach or method is improvisational, not forced into fixed forms; it has an openness to spontaneity, flexibility and innovation, particularly in the realm of music and art. Seventh, it is

Table 17–1. Major Themes in the Practice of Cross-cultural Medicine

Experience

Life experience

Historic events such as political upheaval, political torture, war, traumatic losses, and migration may have a profound and lasting impact on the lives of immigrants.

Illness and death

Experience and expression of pain, attitudes in the face of poor prognosis, and response to grief and loss may vary from culture to culture.

Emotions

Patients may retain long-term mental health effects from their life experiences. Depression, apathy, and somatization may result.

Attitudes and beliefs

Cause of illness and practice of medicine

Understanding about the causes of illness and how to heal them may vary from culture to culture.

No matter how acculturated a person appears, during stress such as illness or death, early-learned ideas may resurface and structure responses.

Patient-family relationships

The family is pivotal and the patient may not be viewed as separate from it.

Physician-patient relationship

Disclosure of personal information is not always considered appropriate on first meeting a new health care practitioner.

Bioethical pluralism

There are fundamental differences in the ways that the role of the sick person and family in medical encounters are conceptualized in American medicine.

The assumption that the person experiencing illness is the one to make decisions is not shared by all cultures.

Medical pluralism

Patients may wish to seek alternative cures or therapies to cure spirits, ancestors, sand or behavioral impropriety. Often Western medical treatments and alternative or native therapies are not viewed as mutually exclusive.

Behavior

Emotions are often not openly expressed or talked about.

Emotional expression may vary in culturally appropriate ways.

Family business or "secrets" may be kept from the outside world. Decision making, receiving and disclosing news, and orchestration of care are concerns and responsibilities of the group.

Problems can develop if roles are reversed, especially within immigrant families. This can occur when children are put in positions of authority over parents or older adults, for example, in translating during medical encounters or when children are more acculturated to American life.

Modified from Klesig.[8]

humanistic, not materialistic, valuing human life and dignity over material wealth or possessions.[15]

Socioeconomic status

Educational background and level of income can be related to patients' attitudes toward end-of-life care. In a study of elderly Medicare recipients,[16] individuals with less education were more inclined to want life-sustaining treatments. One can only speculate that individuals with less education may be less aware of the limitations of medical technology, or that a life that affords fewer opportunities makes individuals more eager to try any opportunity to prolong life.

Nationality

Lynn Payer, an American journalist who studied differing views of the practice of medicine in the United States and several Western European countries, has described how varied the understanding of illness is across these countries.[17] At the risk of overgeneralizing, she reports that Germans, for example, are prone to attribute illness to a weak heart, while the French are more inclined to be concerned about liver ailments. These views have tangible consequences, as illustrated by the fact that the use of digitalis is 10-fold higher in Germany than in the United States. Aside from differing beliefs about the pathophysiology of illness, there are different views about the proper style of medical practice. European critical care physicians are much less likely than physicians from the United States to use a collaborative decision-making style with patients and families and are more inclined to use a style that would be considered paternalistic in the U.S.[18]

If perceptions of illness vary among countries as closely linked culturally and politically as those in Western Europe and North America, it is not surprising that attitudes among more diverse nationalities are even more disparate. Blackhall and colleagues studied attitudes toward patient autonomy, particularly the desire for medical information and participation in decision making, among individuals residing in the U.S. who were of various national origins. Korean-Americans (47%) and Mexican-Americans (65%) were less likely than European-Americans (87%) and African-Americans (85%) to believe that a patient should be told about a diagnosis of metastatic cancer or about a terminal prognosis and were less likely to believe that a patient should make a life-sustaining treatment decision (28% vs. 41% vs. 60% vs. 65%).[19] Klesig has reported that the inclination to use, withhold, or remove life-sustaining treatments varies among U.S. residents of different cultural or national backgrounds.[8]

Religion and spirituality

Religious persuasion is reflected not only in beliefs but also in practices (see Chapter 16). Whether an individual believes in an afterlife, whether it is acceptable to tamper with the body after death, donate organs, or observe ritual practices around the time of death varies among religions.[20] Attitudes toward illness and, consequently interactions with the medical team can be profoundly influenced by one's spirituality. Kaldjian et al. reported that HIV-infected individuals who perceived HIV infection as a punishment were less likely than those who believed in God's forgiveness to have had discussions about resuscitation.[21] Individuals who reported praying daily and those who reported that God helped them when thinking about death were more likely to have a living will. Those who viewed HIV infection as a punishment or who felt guilty about having the infection were more likely to be afraid of death. Those who attended church regularly or read the Bible frequently reported being less afraid of death.[21]

Despite these reported associations, it is important to be cautious about assuming that an individual's background necessarily predicts attitudes or behaviors. For example, Whittle and colleagues report that while African-Americans were less likely to say that they would undergo cardiac revascularization procedures, familiarity with procedures was a much stronger predictor of differences in desire for coronary artery bypass graft than race or ethnicity. When knowledge about the procedure was taken into account, the influence of ethnicity became insignificant.[22] Similarly, while patients of various backgrounds may differ in their desire to have their families participate in decision making on their behalf, the accuracy of surrogate decision makers—their ability to predict patients' preferences—is not correlated with ethnic background.[23]

Influence of race, ethnicity, religion, and socioeconomic status on treatment of dying patients in the ICU

The medical literature provides evidence that minority and socioeconomically disadvantaged individuals generally have less access to medical care and have poorer health status.[24] It should be noted that the lack of access to medical care does not entirely explain the discrepancy in health status.[24] Often, lower rates of medical intervention do not lead to worse outcomes. For example, African-Americans have been shown to undergo fewer cardiac procedures (33% less cardiac catheterizations, 42% less coronary angioplasties, and 54% less coronary artery bypass grafts), and yet this difference in treatment was associated with better short-term survival and equivalent intermediate survival rates compared to those for whites.[25] Conversely, even when access is corrected for, health status remains worse, which suggests that poor health status is a function of many adverse factors and that medical care does not correct for them.

The use of life-sustaining treatments tends to follow this overall pattern. African-Americans have been shown to have slightly shorter lengths of ICU stay, although this difference is not associated with any difference in risk-adjusted hospital mortality rate.[26] They have also been shown to have lower rates of organ transplantation, which may be related to lower rates of organ donation. African-Americans have been shown to have lower rates of survival following CPR (odds ratio, 0.31; 95% CI, 0.15–0.68) even after adjusting for age, sex, initial cardiac rhythm, diagnosis of pneumonia, serum creatinine level, and Acute Physiology and Chronic Health Evaluation (APACHE) score.[27] Lower rates of treatment are not the result of less desire for treatment, since studies indicate that African-Americans are generally more inclined to utilize them. For example, African-Americans have fewer DNR orders in nursing homes—an indication that they are less inclined to forgo resuscitation. These studies of health services utilization raise persistent concerns about discrimination.

Aside from having diverse views on life-sustaining treatments, different ethnic groups have also been shown to have different attitudes and behaviors in response to pain and pain management.[28] Given the importance of pain management in palliative care, critical care providers should be aware that individuals of different cultures may not express their experience of pain in the same way. Whether it is for this or other reasons, minority patients tend to receive less adequate pain relief than non-minority patients.[29–31]

Suggestions for ICU Care of Patients with Diverse Backgrounds

When critical care providers help dying patients whose backgrounds differ from their own, they would do well to bear in mind that patients of varying backgrounds may have different views about the care they want at the time of death. Ironically, the literature cited above suggests that the care that patients receive does differ, and yet not in the way patients might wish. It behooves critical care practitioners to avoid using (1) discriminatory biases that may lead to care that is contrary to patient wishes and (2) stereotypes and presumptions of what care patients will want. Rather, clinicians can provide optimal care by being prepared to communicate and negotiate carefully with patients and families and by tailoring the care they provide to the unique needs of each patient and family.

Differences in values can exist between any two individuals, but these differences are even more likely to occur when people differ in terms of their gender, age, religion, culture, political affiliation, or socioeconomic class. In considering suggestions for care of patients with diverse backgrounds, the discussion will focus in particular on cross-cultural differences, since these pose the greatest dilemma. For while differences may exist among different groups within a given culture, it is generally argued that groups within the same culture can at least express their differences through a common language and moral vocabulary. Although this assumption may be somewhat simplistic, it is safe to assume that individuals of different cultures have the greatest divide between their cultural repertoires. As Jecker and colleagues note, "[c]ross-cultural debates often seem to introduce moral anarchy because people lack shared cultural standards or vantage points from which to communicate and resolve value differences."[32] Similarly, Ware and Kleinman suggest that "[c]ross-cultural conflicts may be more deeply rooted, for such differences embody not just different opinions or beliefs, but different ways of everyday living and different systems of meaning."[33]

Relationships between health care providers and patients are generally unequal ones in which the clinician plays a dominant role.[34] Much of the agenda of medical ethics over the last several decades has been an extremely valuable effort to accord as much respect to the patient's perspective as possible. This attention to respect for patient preferences is particularly important when providers and patients differ in their views about what is important and valuable to them. Ironically, this valuable approach, developed in Western bioethics, to respect patient autonomy by honoring the patient's right to self-determination, may prove to be complicated in the setting of cross-cultural care. Other cultures may view the focus on the patient as an individual to be contrary to their view of the individual as inseparable from the family or community. They may also prefer a less explicit communication style than is typical of American medical practice.

A key to making less ethnocentric health care decisions—decisions that do not presume the superiority of one's own culture—is developing an understanding of differences among cultures in the use of language.[35] This requires an appreciation that the way one uses language may affect one's perception of reality. Navahos, for example, prohibit the telling of bad news because they believe that this may lead to the occurrence of a bad event.[36] Thus the truth about bad news, which might be required to make informed treatment decisions in standard U.S. medical practice, may be perceived as disrespectful or dangerous.

In light of the importance of language, to patients and their families and caregivers, the role of interpreters can be crucial. They are not merely translators, rather, they can be a source of cultural information; facilitate care; create trust among providers, health care institutions, patients, families, and communities; improve continuity of care; improve access to care; mediate misunderstandings and disagreements; and act as advocates and counselors.[35] Given the pivotal role of interpreters, clinicians should learn to work effectively with them. Clinicians should speak directly to the patient or family even when utilizing an interpreter and should be aware of the quality of the interpreters at their institution. The clinician should be aware that when having family members serve as interpreters, the patient's privacy may be breached and the family member is likely to filter the conversation, which may or may not be acceptable to the patient.

In attending to the needs of patients of diverse cultural backgrounds, clinicians need to recognize that the ways that patients experience pain and wish to have their pain treated can vary according to this background.[28,37] Clinicians and patients of various cultures may differ in their views of the appropriate way to express pain and treat pain. Patients will receive the best pain management when these differences are acknowledged and addressed.

When critically ill patients do die, families of differing cultural backgrounds may also have different bereavement practices.[38] While the prevailing North American view of grieving is that of an isolated, individual experience involving detachment from the dead, other views of the grieving process may not look like this. Acceptance of this difference is helpful in supporting families through their bereavement.[39] When a patient dies, the family must adjust to new events in the family life cycle and learn to function in the patient's absence. To help families, caregivers need to support them in a manner that fits both their unique circumstances as well as the bereavement expectations of their community and culture.[39]

A particularly useful general approach to caring for patients whose cultural background differs from that of their provider comes from the family practice literature. The *Teaching Framework for Cross-Cultural Health Care*, developed by Berlin and Fowkes,[40] provides a valuable strategy for working with patients from different cultural backgrounds, regardless of how ill they are:

LEARN

L *Listen* with sympathy and understanding to the patient's perception of the problem.
E *Explain* your perception of the problem.
A *Acknowledge* and discuss the differences and similarities.
R *Recommend* treatment.
N *Negotiate* agreement.

Specific strategies for the care of critically and terminally ill patients

The series of questions listed in Table 17–2, which were prompted by the individualized approach suggested by Koenig and Gates-Williams, can serve as an outline for attending to the diverse needs of critically ill dying patients.[41] The clinician should pay attention to the patient's language, religion, social context, beliefs, decision-making style, and social support in the process of getting familiar and working with the patient. These suggested questions can serve as reminders of what the clinician should learn about the patient in each of these domains.

A practical approach to dealing with disagreements about informing the patient

When it is not clear how much information a patient wants to hear, or when there is disagreement about how much information to disclose, Freedman has proposed a strategy for informing patients about their disease called "offering truth."[42] He argues that a patient's desire for knowledge about his or her dis-

Table 17–2. Questions for attending to diverse needs of critically ill patients

Language

What language do the patient and family prefer to use to discuss illness and disease?
How openly do they wish to discuss diagnosis, prognosis, and death itself?

Religion

What is their religious background and how avid is their religious affiliation?
What do the patient and family think about the sanctity of life and how do they conceive of
   death?
Do they believe in miracles?
Do they believe in an afterlife?
Do they believe the body should be handled in a certain way after death?

Social, political, and historical context

Do any of the following factors affect the attitudes of the patient and family: the patient's status
   in the family, country of origin, or experiences such as poverty, refugee status, past discrimination, or lack of access to care?

Beliefs

What do they believe are the causal agents in illness, and how do these relate to the dying process?

Decision-making style

Who makes decisions about matters of importance in the family?
Are the patient and family fatalistic about the course of events or do they wish to take active
   control of events?

Social support and resources

What resources, including community and religious leaders, family members, and language translators, are available to aid in the complex effort of interpreting cultural dimensions of a patient's illness?

Adapted from the work of Koenig and Gates-Williams.[41]

ease is not all-or-nothing; rather, it runs along a continuum. In the spirit of respect for patient autonomy, patients are asked how much they want to know. The discussion begins by asking them what they know about their situation. If they ask why they are being queried about their knowledge, they might be told that knowing their understanding of their illness might save time that would otherwise be wasted on telling them what they already know. When teaching someone, it is important to have an idea of what they know in order to teach them most effectively. As Freedman suggests:

> The important thing is to begin to generate a dynamic within which the patient is speaking and the physician responding, rather than vice versa. Only then can the pace of conversation and level of information be controlled by the patient. The structure of the discussion, as well as the content of what the physician says, must

reinforce the message: We are now establishing a new opportunity to talk and to question, but you as the patient will have to tell us how much you want to know about your illness.[42]

A practical, ethical approach to dealing with different perspectives on patient care

Once the clinician is familiar with the patient's and family's perspective on handling disease, it can be useful to have a practical, ethical approach for finding a care plan in the face of different perspectives. Jecker and Carrese have suggested that such a plan should include the following actions:[32]

1. Identify goals.
2. Identify mutually agreeable strategies.
3. Meet ethical constraints.

The treatment choices should be consistent with the health care provider's beliefs and compatible with the patient's values. If there is conflict, the clinician should reexamine his or her personal values and consider reinterpreting, reordering, or changing them in light of the case. If there is persistent disagreement, it should be adjudicated through a fair process that reflects a nonjudgmental stance.

While we have focused on the attitudes and behaviors that the individual clinician should espouse, the clinician does not and cannot operate optimally in a vacuum. Several recommendations are useful for creating a supportive institutional setting.[43]

1. Bicultural providers, translators, and others who are cognizant of the cultures of patients often seen in the health care organization should be an integral part of the organization.
2. Community leaders should be involved in policy development at the organization and community levels.

The value of these suggestions for the care of patients with diverse backgrounds is exemplified in the care of the Peruvian patient with leukemia described earlier. The ICU staff responded to his family's request by having a conversation with them. After hearing the family's concerns, they formulated a plan to tell the patient the minimum amount of information that would allow him to understand and participate in the DNR decision without destroying his hope. The staff explained to him that sometimes a person's heart stops and resuscitation is performed. But, the staff told him, in his type of case, cardiac resuscitation is not a helpful treatment so they were not planning to use it. No discussion about prognosis was offered and the patient did not ask any further questions. Being satisfied that the patient was sufficiently informed about his care plan, the staff could then write a DNR order. The use and value of strategies outlined above can be seen in this case. The staff listened to the family and explained their concerns. After acknowledging the family's perspective, the staff recommended and negotiated a communication strategy that was mutually acceptable from the patient and family's cultural perspective as well as from the caregivers' perspective.

Conclusion

This chapter has emphasized the influences of ethnicity, religion, and socioeconomic status on patients' experiences of and preferences about critical and terminal illness. It is crucial to bear in mind that *(1)* individuals within any group vary widely; *(2)* a given individual may identify with a number of groupings; *(3)* the degree of affiliation with a culture may vary from person to person; and *(4)* group affiliation may have little predictive value about a given individual's views. It is therefore particularly important to avoid stereotyping individuals. While it is important to respect and understand an individual's culture, religion, nationality, or socioeconomic background, clinicians are likely to provide the best care by being respectful of the unique qualities and attentive to the particular needs of each individual patient.

References

1. Surbone A, Zwitter M. Learning from the world: the Editiors' perspective. *Ann N Y Acad Sci* 1997;809:1–6.
2. Barker JC, Cultural diversity—changing the context of medical practice. *West J Med* 1992;157:248–254.
3. Fletcher M, Interracial marriages eroding barriers. *The Washington Post* 1998, Tues, Dec. 28:A1–A4.
4. Koenig B, Cultural diversity in decisionmaking about care at the end of life. In: Approaching Death: Improving Care at the End of Life (Field M, Cassel C, eds.). Washington, DC: National Academy Press, 1997, pp. 363–382.
5. Sheldon T, Parker H. Race and ethnicity in health research. *J Public Health Med* 1992;14:104–110.
6. Galanti G-A. Caring for Patients from Different Cultures: Case Studies from American Hospitals. Philadelphia: University of Pennsylvania Press, 1993.
7. Kalish RA, Reynolds DK. Death and Ethnicity: A Psychosocial Study. New York: Baywood, 1976.
8. Klesig, J. The effects of values and culture on life-support decisions. *West J Med* 1992;163:316–322.
9. Veatch RM. Medical Ethics. Boston: Jones and Bartlett, 1989.
10. Pellegrino E, Mazzarella P, Corsi P. Transcultural Dimensions in Medical Ethics. Frederick, MD: University Publishing Group, 1992.
11. Irish D, Lundquist EA. Ethnic Variations in Dying, Death, and Grief. Washington, DC: Tayor and Francis, 1993.
12. Mouton C, Teno JM, Mor V, Piette J. Communication of preferences for care

among human immunodeficiency virus–infected patients. Barriers to informed decisions? *Arch Fam Med* 1997;6:342–347.

13. O'Brien LA, Grisso JA, Maislin G, LaPann K, Krotki KP, Greco PJ, Siegert PEA, Evans LK. Nursing home residents' preferences for life-sustaining treatments. *JAMA*, 1995;274:1775–1779.

14. McKinley ED, Garrett JM, Evans AT, Danis M. Differences in end-of-life decision making among black and white ambulatory cancer patients. *J Gen Intern Med* 1996;11:651–656.

15. Cheryl J. Problems and limitations of an African-American perspective in biomedical ethics: a theological view. In: African-American Perspectives in Biomedical Ethics (Flack H, Pellegrino E, eds.) Washington, DC: Georgetown University Press, 1992, pp. 165–172.

16. Garrett JM, Harris RP, Norburn JK, Patrick DL, Danis M. Life-sustaining treatments during terminal illness: who wants what? *J Gen Intern Med* 1993;8:361–368.

17. Payer L. Medicine and Culture: Notions of Health and Sickness in Britain, the U.S., France, and West Germany. London: V. Gollancz, 1990.

18. Vincent JL, European attitudes towards ethical problems in intensive care medicine: results of an ethical questionnaire. *Intensive Care Med* 1990;16:256–264.

19. Blackhall LJ, Murphy ST, Frank G, Michel V, Azen S. Ethnicity and attitudes toward patient autonomy. *JAMA* 1995;274:820–825.

20. McQuay JE. Cross-cultural customs and beliefs related to health crises, death, and organ donation/transplantation: a guide to assist health care professionals understand different responses and provide cross-cultural assistance. *Crit Care Nurs Clin North Am* 1995;7:581–594.

21. Kaldjian LC, Jekel JF, Friedland G. End-of-life decisions in HIV-positive patients: the role of spiritual beliefs. *Aids* 1998;12:103–107.

22. Whittle J, Conigliaro J, Good CB, Joswiak M. Do patient preferences contribute to racial differences in cardiovascular procedure use? *J Gen Intern Med* 1997;12:267–273.

23. Sulmasy DP, Terry PB, Weisman CS, Miller DJ, Stallings RY, Vettese MA, Haller KB. The accuracy of substituted judgments in patients with terminal diagnoses. *Ann Intern Med* 1998;128:621–629.

24. Adler N, Boyce T. Socioeconomic inequalties in health. *JAMA* 1993;269:3140–3145.

25. Peterson ED, Wright SM, Daley J, Thibault GE. Racial variation in cardiac procedure use and survival following acute myocardial infarction in the Department of Veterans Affairs. *JAMA* 1994;271:1175–1180.

26. Williams JF, Zimmerman JE, Wagner DP, Hawkins M, Knaus WA. African-American and white patients admitted to the intensive care unit: is there a difference in therapy and outcome? *Crit Care Med* 1995;23:626–36.

27. Ebell MH, et al. Effect of race on survival following in-hospital cardiopulmonary resuscitation. *J Fam Pract* 1995;40:571–577.

28. Martinelli A. Pain and ethnicity. *AORN J* 1987;46:273–281.

29. Todd KH, Samaroo N, Hoffman JR. Ethnicity as a risk factor for inadequate emergency department analgesia. *JAMA* 1993;269:1537–1539.

30. Todd KH, Lee T, Hoffman JR. The effect of ethnicity on physician estimates of pain severity in patients with isolated extremity trauma. *JAMA* 1994;271:925–928.

31. Cleeland C. Pain and treatment of pain in minority patients with cancer. *Ann Intern Med* 1997;127:813–816.

32. Jecker NS, Carrese JA, Pearlman RA. Caring for patients in cross-cultural settings. *Hastings Cent Rep* 1995;25:6–14.

33. Ware NC, Kleinman A. Culture and somatic experience: the social course of illness in neurasthenia and chronic fatigue syndrome. *Psychosom Med* 1992;54:546–560.

34. Friedson ET. Professional Dominance. New York: Atheneum Press, 1970.

35. Kaufert JM, Putsch RW. Communication through interpreters in healthcare: ethical dilemmas arising from differences in class, culture, language, and power. *J Clin Ethics* 1997;8:71–87.

36. Carrese J, Rhodes L. Western biothics on the Navajo reservation: benefit or harm? *JAMA* 1995;274:286–289.

37. Walker AC, Tan L, George S. Impact of culture on pain management: an Australian nursing perspective. *Holist Nurs Pract* 1995;9:48–57.

38. Rosenblatt P, Walsh R. Grief and Mourning in Cross-Cultural Perspectives. New Haven: HRAF Press, 1976.

39. Shapiro E. Family bereavement and cultural diversity: a social development perspective. *Fam Process* 1996;35:313–332.

40. Berlin EA, Fowkes WC Jr. A teaching framework for cross-cultural health care. Application in family practice. *West J Med* 1983;139:934–938.

41. Koenig B, Gates-Williams J. Understanding cultural differences in caring for dying patients. *West J Med* 1995;163:244–249.

42. Freedman B. Offering truth. One ethical approach to the uninformed cancer patient. *Arch Intern Med* 1993;153:572–576.

43. Hern HE, Jr, Koenig BA, Moore LJ, Marshall PA. The difference that culture can make in end-of-life decisionmaking. *Camb Q Healthcare Ethics* 1998;7:27–40.

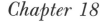

Chapter 18

Legal Liability Anxieties in the ICU

MARSHALL B. KAPP

*L*egal principles and procedures regarding medical decision making and the implementation of treatment strategies in the ICU are considerably more developed and defined in the United States (and in other western democracies as well) at the end of the millenium than they were only a decade earlier.[1-3] Nonetheless, a high degree of confusion and free-floating anxiety persists among health care professionals about possible adverse legal consequences—i.e., criminal prosecution, civil liability, and/or regulatory sanctions—of actions or omissions taking place within this context. This pervasive anxiety sometimes drives provider behavior in directions that serve patients poorly near the end of life.[4]

Much of the legal anxiety influencing suboptimal treatment for dying patients is fueled by misunderstanding and misinterpretation. For example, legal experts interviewed by the U.S. General Accounting Office indicated that, when an individual's wishes are clear, difficulties in getting requests to withhold or withdraw artificial nutrition and hydration honored by health care providers typically arise from confusion about the legal ramifications, rather than because any serious legal impediment actually exists.[5] By late 1998, 31 states had statutes, regulations, and/or formal guidelines providing criminal, civil, and disciplinary immunity for physicians engaged in justifiable, aggressive pain management practices using opiates, but physician worries still persist.[6] Additionally, health care professionals occasionally cite fear of unwanted legal entanglements as a pretext or justification for conduct that is really determined more by other forces, such as the ICU rescue culture,[7] professional education and socialization, clinical biases about what "works" best,[8] shortcomings or discomfort in communicating with patients and/or families about end-of-life matters, financial incentives, or physicians' tendency to define medical success in bare terms of survival rather than meaningfulness or quality to the patient.[9]

However weak the factual foundations, the law-related anxieties expressed by health care professionals—whether sincere or pretextual—are palpable, powerful influences on the quality and humanity of medical care actually provided to vulnerable ICU patients and the support available to their families. Adverse effects may take the form of overtreatment (e.g., inappropriate resuscitation attempts or artificial feeding), undertreatment (e.g., insufficient pain control), and impaired interaction with patients and families. The problem exists even for physicians and others who understand intellectually that their own legal exposure is minimal when their conduct is medically and ethically proper. The very fact that physician conduct in this most delicate of areas could conceivably be publicly questioned in a legal setting is sufficient to alter behavior. Physician Jack McCue correctly urges, "[t]he exaggerated fears of liability risks that pressure physicians and nurses to withhold palliative treatment or continue futile therapy in patients near the end of life must be addressed in a forthright fashion."[10]

This chapter aims to address that challenge. Following a modest attempt to put end-of-life legal risks into some realistic perspective, I outline the most salient legal considerations in a number of specific ICU scenarios. I conclude with the admonition that proper end-of-life care in the ICU basically requires fundamental ethical, medical, and communication, more than legal risk management, responses to the challenges posed.

Putting Legal Risks into Perspective

Legal scholar Alan Meisel has observed, "[t]he proportion of deaths from foregoing life-sustaining treatment that is litigated is . . . very small. Somewhere between 0.2% and 0.5% have been litigated at all, and between 37 and 55 in 10 million have been litigated to the point of yielding an appellate decision."[11] This statement is consistent with the American Hospital Association's claim, in its *Cruzan* case[12] *amicus curiae* (friend of the court) brief, that 70% of the 1.3 million Americans who die in health care institutions each year die only after a decision to forego some form of medical treatment has been made and implemented. In the highly publicized Study to Understand Prognoses and Preferences for Outcomes and Risks of Treatments (SUPPORT) sponsored by the Robert Wood Johnson Foundation,[13] over 11,000 in-hospital patient deaths were investigated, and none of them entailed any after-the-fact legal claims against providers relating to treatment decisions or actions.[14]

In practical terms, these statistics mean that in the overwhelming majority of situations in which decisions need to be confronted about the initiation, continuation, withdrawal, or withholding of life-sustaining medical treatments (LSMTs) for a critically ill patient, a resolution is reached and carried out on the basis of a process of discussion and negotiation involving the patient (where able to participate), family or significant others, physician, other members of the health care team, and perhaps some form of institutional ethics committee (IEC). In most of these situations, decisions and their sequelae quite properly occur without asking the courts to intervene.

In some cases, however, the informal, extrajudicial decision-making process breaks down and the parties elect to go to court to initiate a judicial ruling. The courts are requested to supply equitable relief—i.e., to order parties to do or refrain from doing things other than paying money damages. An equitable order, for example, might forbid a prosecutor from bringing a criminal prosecution for the withholding or withdrawal of particular interventions or might authorize a specific relative to authorize treatment abatement for an incapacitated patient. Judges are asked to decide these questions not because they possess any special expertise or wisdom, but because it is perceived that only the courts have the official power in our society to prospectively provide health care professionals with legal immunity for their actions.

It is important to remember that fewer than a half dozen "right-to-die" legal cases have originated in the procedural posture of a malpractice suit seeking monetary damages from health care providers for improperly abating LSMT for a dying patient. This is quite understandable in light of the four elements that a plaintiff in any civil negligence case (i.e., the category into which all medical malpractice cases except those alleging intentional harm fall) must establish by a preponderance of the evidence, namely: *(1)* a duty owed, defined by the applicable standard of care; *(2)* breach or violation of that duty; *(3)* harm or injury to the plaintiff of the sort that tort law is intended to compensate, and *(4)* a connection of direct or proximate causation between the defendant's deviation from the acceptable standard of care and the plaintiff's injury. In the case of a patient who was inevitably dying with or without aggressive medical intervention, it would be exceedingly difficult for a plaintiff suing for negligence on behalf of a deceased patient or in his or her own right as a survivor to prove these elements to a jury's satisfaction; in such cases, as plaintiffs' attorneys who work on the basis of contingency fees realize, it is the patient's illness or injury that proximately causes death, not any substandard care on the physician's part. (Conversely, there have been a number of malpractice actions filed where there is persuasive evidence that the withheld or withdrawn medical intervention would realistically have cured and restored the patient to good health.)

From the lawsuits requesting equitable orders, as well as the few dealing with after-the-fact complaints seeking monetary damages, a body of case law has evolved since the landmark Karen Quinlan decision in 1976 regarding medical care at the end of life.[15] The various courts that have been confronted by these issues have achieved a high degree of consensus on the major points, although there remains diversity among jurisdictions on a number of secondary questions. Congress and the state legislatures have also gotten involved, mainly by enacting legislation intended to promote and facilitate timely advance health care planning by individuals. Additionally, individual hospitals often choose to adopt internal policies and procedures binding on their medical staffs that go beyond the requirements imposed by the federal and state governments as a matter of law.

Specific Scenarios (Table 18-1)

Brain death

There is no distinction between clinical and legal death; a person is either alive or dead, for all purposes. Providers' common use of language that implies otherwise (e.g., "Your loved one is brain dead, so we would like permission to remove the feeding tubes so that we can declare him legally dead") is ignorant, confusing, and even cruel to family members and others. Once a person is dead (for all purposes), all LSMT may and should be discontinued (unless organs are being maintained for a short period of time for transplantation purposes).

In 1981, a Presidential Commission issued a comprehensive report analyzing this subject and recommended that state legislatures adopt a Uniform Determination of Death Act (UDDA) that stated, "Any individual who has sustained either (a) irreversible cessation of circulatory and respiratory functions, or (b) irreversible cessation of all functions of the entire brain, including the brain stem, is dead."[16] All the states have adopted a version of the UDDA, either by statute or judicial decision.

The President's Commission recognized that, whereas establishing the standards for defining death is a proper function of the legal system, determining the clinical criteria or tests to be used in applying those legal standards to any particular patient is a matter best left to the medical profession. Following this reasoning, the UDDA states that "[a] determination of death must be made in accordance with accepted medical standards." All current state statutes on this subject concur with this approach.

The so-called Harvard Criteria for determining brain death[17] have been widely recognized and accepted in clinical practice. Under these criteria, a permanently nonfunctioning brain (i.e., patient death) could be accurately diagnosed on the basis of four factors:

1. Unreceptivity and unresponsivity
2. No spontaneous movements or spontaneous breathing
3. No reflexes and the absence of elicitable reflexes
4. As a confirmatory measure only, flat electroencephalograms (EEGs), taken twice within at least a 24-hour intervening period.

These 1968 criteria have been updated regularly in light of continuing advances in medical knowledge and technology.[18]

TABLE 18–1. Decision-making scenarios

Patient	Decision maker	Criteria
For decisions about autopsies and organ donation		
Dead	Patient's wishes expressed while alive and decisionally capable	Substituted judgment
	Guardian or family member, in priority order in state statute	
For decisions about removal of artificial life support		
Dead	No decision to be made	No decision
Capable patient	Patient	Patient's wishes
Incapacitated patient with authorized proxy	Authorized proxy	Substituted judgment Best interest
Incapacitated patient with *de facto* proxy	*De facto* proxy	Substituted judgment Best interests
Incapacitated patient without proxy	Patient, if an instruction directive exists	Instruction directive, if any
	Public or volunteer guardian	Substituted judgment
	Institutional Ethics Committee	Best interests
	Physician	

The physician must become and remain knowledgeable about any relevant formal policies on this subject adopted by the particular hospital in which ICU care is being provided. Since the law leaves to clinical discretion the performance of specific tests to confirm a patient's death, individual hospitals frequently have developed their own policies to guide—loosely or tightly—physicians declaring death within the facility. Thus, for example, a particular hospital may choose as a policy matter to require a Xenon blood flow as a confirmatory test for death, even though neither this nor any other specific procedure is required by the state or federal government as a matter of law.

Once a patient satisfies the clinical criteria, and therefore meets the legal definition, the physician is obligated to make a declaration of death. Once the criteria are met, there also is an obligation to respect the family's request to discontinue any further LSMT and to release the body, or else liability for emotional distress may be imposed on the health care institution.[20]

Decisionally capable patients and refusal of life-sustaining medical treatments

There is virtually universal agreement that every decisionally capable adult patient has a right to make personal medical treatment decisions, including the right to accept or refuse LSMT.[21] Predicated on the ethical principle of autonomy or self-determination, the capable patient's right to choose has several firm legal underpinnings,[22] namely: the liberty interest protected by the Due Process clause of the Fourteenth Amendment of the U.S. Constitution; respective state constitutions; state statutes and regulations; and the common law principle of respect for bodily integrity that undergirds the doctrine of informed consent. Under any of these theories, it is now universally accepted that a capable patient need not be terminally ill (i.e., imminently dying) for the "right to choose" to be relevant and that there is no meaningful legal distinction between withholding LSMT initially, on the one hand, and withdrawing current LSMT, on the other. Similarly, the U.S. Supreme Court in *Cruzan* made it clear that decisions about artificial mechanisms of feeding and hydration are to be thought through according to the same legal criteria used when other forms of medical intervention (e.g., mechanical ventilation, antibiotics, dialysis, resuscitation) are under consideration.

The legal and ethical consensus notwithstanding, critical care physicians frequently take actions directly contrary to patients' direct, expressed wishes regarding end-of-life treatment.[23] One important factor driving such physician behavior in many cases is fear—almost always overblown or without any realistic foundation—of relatives who are imagined as potential plaintiffs in lawsuits brought against the physician for following a patient's wishes in the absence of concurrence by the family.[24]

Incapacitated patients

A critically ill patient who is mentally or physically incapable of making and expressing rational decisions regarding the initiation or continuation of LSMT may have a legally authorized proxy. An examination of case law and state statutes reveals guidelines for (*a*) identifying authorized proxy decision makers for an incapacitated patient and (*b*) identifying appropriate substantive decision-making criteria for use by the proxy.

A person may be given legal authority to serve as a proxy in making health care decisions on behalf of another in several different ways. One may be appointed a guardian or conservator of the person (exact terminology varies among jurisdictions) by a court, and given explicit responsibility to make health care decisions on behalf of the incapacitated ward. An individual (the principal or maker), while still decisionally capable, may execute a written durable power of attorney or health care proxy document (forms of advance proxy directives) to take effect ("spring") in the event of the principal's subsequent incapacity, delegating decisional authority to the principal's named agent or attorney-in-fact; statutes in 48 states explicitly authorize such legal instruments. The principal may name contingent agents to have decision-making authority in the event that the originally named agent(s) is (are) unavailable to fulfill that role. In the absence of a guardian or advance proxy directive, statutes in over 30 states authorize other persons (family and friends), in a stated priority order, to make health care decisions—including those pertaining to LSMT—on behalf of a patient whom the attending physician has found to be decisionally incapacitated. Many of these statutes are based on the National Conference of Commissioners on Uniform State Laws' Uniform Health-Care Decisions Act.

The priority order set forth in particular state statutes varies to a small degree. However, Illinois Revised Statutes ch. 755, §40/25 is rather typical: guardian of the person, spouse, adult child, parent, adult sibling, adult grandchild, close friend, and guardian of the estate.

Even when none of these formal mechanisms for transferring decision-making authority apply, the longstanding medical custom has been to involve and defer to an incapacitated patient's *de facto proxies,* who ordinarily are family members or close friends. Indeed, the state statutes alluded to in the previous paragraph essentially represent a codification, rather than a modification, of this custom. Unless providers are aware of a conflict of interest that would interfere with a *de facto* proxy's trustworthy fulfillment of duty, this custom of informally "bumbling through" works well and without negative legal repercussions.[25]

Health care proxies, both legally appointed and *de facto,* ought, where possible, to be guided by the substituted judgment standard of decision making. Under this evidentiary standard, the proxy is expected to act in accordance with what would be the patient's own autonomous preferences if the patient currently could make and express those preferences. The legal presumption is to rely on patient choices that have been unambiguously and repeatedly stated by the patient while able to make and express autonomous choices. When such evidence is unavailable, however, most states permit and indeed encourage proxy decision making on the basis of whatever reasonable inferences about the patient's preferences may be drawn by piecing together the patient's prior informal statements and accumulated life decisions.

Only a few states place limits on such inferential interpretation of a patient's preferences. In Missouri, even when the patient is permanently vegetative, proxy decisions to abate LSMT are legally permissible only when there exists clear and convincing evidence (see Table 18–2) that the withholding or withdrawing of medical interventions would be consistent with the patient's wishes. In New York,[26] Michigan,[27] and Wisconsin,[28] the courts allow withholding or withdrawal of LSMTs for patients who are neither terminally ill nor permanently vegetative only upon a clear and convincing showing of the patient's wishes.

When even inferential evidence of a patient's substituted judgment is missing, the strongly prevailing legal position is to defer to the proxy's opinion about the course of care that will most likely promote the patient's best interests, as those interests would be viewed from the patient's perspective. Although some would argue that aggressive LSMT is always in any patient's best interests,[29] the much more widely held position is that a patient's quality of life may be so hopelessly diminished that the burdens of treatment dispropor-

TABLE 18–2. Decision-making standards and burdens of proof

Bases of Decisions by Proxies

Substituted judgment

What the individual would have chosen for himself/herself if currently able to engage in a rational, autonomous decision making process, determined by either
  a. The patient's own explicit prior statements; or
  b. Inferences drawn from non-explicit prior statements of the patient and/or earlier decisions
     and actions taken by the patient during his/her life.

Proof of what the incapacitated person would have chosen may be established, in most states, by
a preponderance of the evidence—that is, proof that one interpretation of the patient's wishes
is *more probable or likely than not (i.e., at least 51% likely)*.

In New York and Missouri, proof of the patient's intent to limit treatment must be by *clear and
convincing evidence (i.e., much more probable or likely—at least 75%—than not)*.

Best interests

What the substitute decision maker feels would be best for the patient, viewed from the patient's
perspective, as determined by weighing the relative likely risks and benefits of the contem-
plated alternatives for the patient.

tionately outweigh any benefits and hence that death is an acceptable, and
maybe preferable, objective alternative. The idea of weighing respective burdens and benefits, both broadly construed, has largely replaced earlier, confusing language about "ordinary" and "extraordinary" or "heroic" treatments.

Some decisionally incapacitated patients with neither legally authorized nor
known *de facto* proxies may be encountered in the ICU. Health care providers
should consult the hospital's social service department about identifying and
involving any local public or volunteer guardianship programs that might supply proxy decision makers. In theory, only court appointment of a guardian
provides absolute legal certainly regarding proxy decision making for the incapacitated patient. In reality, though, such formality is the exception rather than
the rule. Practical considerations (e.g., time, financial expense, staff inconve-
nience, the lack of anyone suitable for the court to appoint) and the fact that
guardianships rarely actually provide wards with any meaningful added protection if all parties are acting in good faith strongly discourage the initiation of
guardianship proceedings in most cases. Ordinarily, treating physicians—acting
in consultation with medical colleagues, other members of the ICU staff, and
the hospital's ICU—make and implement decisions in these sorts of cases on
the basis of their honest assessment of the patient's best interests, without any
negative legal consequences.

Certainly, efforts should be exerted to try to determine if the patient, while
earlier capable, executed an advance instruction directive (e.g., 48 states authorize living will instruments) that was intended to guide future decisions.

Health care professionals may need to invoke external assistance when
challenged by a situation in which individual family members sharply and

strongly disagree among themselves about the proper course of medical action and counseling and educational efforts are ineffective in reconciling the family's internal dispute. Confusion, consternation, and certainly court involvement should not occur if the patient, while decisionally capable, named a particular relative—or non-relative, for that matter—to act as decision-making agent under a durable power of attorney for health care; indeed, one of the main reasons for executing an advance proxy directive is precisely to avoid judicial involvement. Nonetheless, even in the presence of a durable power of attorney instrument or applicable family consent statute, a loudly protesting relative with no legal authority may so intimidate the health care providers that they ask the courts to intervene before they will act on any family member's desires.[30]

Using the IEC as a forum within which family members may safely vent their feelings, ask questions, and hear the perspectives of others may be valuable. If courts are petitioned by the hospital or family members to become involved in what usually are private matters, because of irreconcilable family differences (or an obvious, serious conflict of interest between the presumed decision maker and the patient), courts are better equipped to choose the most appropriate proxy than to make the treatment decision itself. In just a very small number of cases have judges themselves actually made or approved the LSMT choice itself or held that judges ought to be involved routinely in the direct decision-making process.

A disgruntled family member would have no basis for an after-the-fact malpractice claim against the physician for abating LSMT unless that family member had the legal authority to demand that specific LSMTs be provided (authority conferred by a court order, durable power of attorney, or state family consent statute) and there is evidence that the requested intervention likely would have cured the patient. In the absence of those factors, plaintiffs' attorneys, who get paid only if and when their clients collect on a judgment or settlement, discourage the filing of such unwinnable civil claims by family members. Hence, the threats and acrimony that may accompany this kind of tragic family discord end up in court beforehand with requests by a particular relative for equitable relief (i.e., "Judge, appoint me rather than my brother to be guardian") or not at all. There has been one, widely publicized and routinely miscited, case in which a malcontent nurse convinced a confused family to provoke a state prosecutor to bring a criminal prosecution against two physicians for discontinuing LSMT for a patient in a permanent vegetative state; there, the court dismissed all charges before the case went to trial, with a stern rebuke to the prosecutor about the impropriety of his actions.[31]

Providing life-sustaining medical treatment against patient/family wishes

Providers' legal anxieties regarding ICU treatment of dying patients center mainly on perceived risks for undertreatment (i.e., improperly withholding or withdrawing some form of intervention). At least one attempt by a family to hold physicians and a hospital liable for malpractice (specifically, committing a battery) for overtreating a dying patient has been rejected by the courts on the grounds that support of continued life, regardless of its quality, is not the sort of injury or damage for which the tort system was designed to provide a remedy.[32] Nonetheless, lawsuits complaining of unwanted life support continue to be brought, and some of these claims have resulted in substantial jury verdicts or settlements against the overtreating health care providers.[33] Providers' legal exposure for inflicting unconsented-to LSMT on a dying patient may turn out to be more real than the perceived risks associated with withholding or withdrawing LSMT.[34]

Liability for insufficient palliative care

As already explained, providers' legal anxieties regarding treatment of dying patients may influence behavior in two opposite directions. These fears may effectively encourage overtreatment in the form of inappropriate commencement of certain LSMTs and/or refusal to abate LSMTs that may or may not have been proper when initiated. At the same time, ironically, many of the same health care providers who are using LSMTs excessively are reluctant to provide adequate analgesic treatment to dying patients who are experiencing pain. Physicians are particularly concerned about potential criminal or administrative liability under federal and state controlled-drug prescription laws. Many are under the impression that they are risking punishment if they provide their patients with pain relief consistent with the ethical principle of beneficence.

The legal anxiety surrounding drug prescription for palliative purposes is not totally without foundation. For example, many states not only require special prescription forms or multiple original prescriptions for certain controlled substances but also limit the total number of pills or the dosage that may be prescribed.[35] Nonetheless, as noted earlier, a majority of states now have statutes, regulations, and/or guidelines giving providers immunity against criminal and civil liability for prescribing and delivering adequate pain medication to suffering patients near the end of life. The American Medical Association and the National Federation of State Medical Boards have firmly endorsed and encouraged adequate pain control at the end of life. Moreover, respected legal commentators suggest that the U.S. Supreme Court has at least implicitly recognized a dying patient's constitutional right to receive appropriate pain medication.[36]

Futile treatment

Sometimes patients or families demand that the physician provide the patient with forms of LSMT that, in the physician's opinion, are "futile" or nonbeneficial for that patient. Such demands for aggressive medical interventions occur even in the face of dismal survival and quality-of-life prospects. These demands may create a clash at the bedside between patient autonomy (asserted personally or through a proxy), and a physician's own conscience. Such a clash can inspire legal apprehension.

The issue of whether a physician has a legal obligation to effectuate a patient's or family's demand for LSMT that the physician believes to be futile is unclear at the present time. This situation exists despite the venerable legal maxim, *"lex neminem cogit ad vana seu inutilia peragenda!"*—"the law compels no one to do vain or useless things!" and the AMA's opinion[37] that physicians "are not ethically obligated to deliver care that, in their best professional judgment, will not have a reasonable chance of benefiting their patients. Patients should not be given treatments simply because they demand them."

Using cardiopulmonary resuscitation (CPR) as their focus, Marsh and Staver argue persuasively that a physician has no enforceable duty to provide, or even to discuss, a futile intervention.[38] However, actual case law in what one set of commentators[39] has termed the "right to live" area is still quite sparse. Treatment decisions and conflict resolution about futile demands today must take place in the context of a lack of judicial consensus.[40]

Several cases involve requests by either physicians or family members for judicial clarification before any treatments were withheld or withdrawn. In one case,[41] a probate court continued the appointment of the 87-year-old patient's husband as guardian, knowing that he was demanding ventilator support and artificial feeding for his wife despite her status for more than a year in a permanent vegetative state following CPR. The patient's physicians initiated a request for the court to switch guardians on the grounds that the husband was not acting in the patient's best interests. The patient died despite aggressive treatment before an appeal could be pursued.

In another case,[42] brought before any treatment had been withheld or withdrawn a teenage patient's parents disagreed about treatment, a court ordered the physicians to provide LSMT to a patient in a condition "between a stupor and a coma." In another case[43] initiated prospectively, a court used the federal Emergency Medical Treatment and Active Labor Act (EMTALA) to order a hospital emergency department to attempt resuscitation and ventilator support for an anencephalic infant in the event her mother brought her to the emergency department in cardiac arrest. In a decision running in the opposite direction, one court[44] replaced a patient's son, who demanded doing "everything" to save his father, as guardian with someone else who was willing to consent to a "No Code" order.

Only a couple of legal cases in this area have arisen as after-the-fact malpractice lawsuits brought by unhappy families against involved physicians. In one,[45] a jury totally exonerated a physician and hospital who had entered and acted on a No-Code order, over an adult daughter's protests, for a permanently vegetative patient. In another,[46] a malpractice suit was remanded, per state procedural law, to a Medical Review Panel, but with instructions to the Panel that "[a] finding that treatment is 'medically inappropriate' by a consensus of physicians practicing in that specialty translates into a standard of care." The court added in a footnote:

> Also, if, as in this case, a surrogate decision-maker insists on life-prolonging treatment which the physician believes is inhumane, then the usual procedure is to transfer the patient or go to court to replace the surrogate or override his decision. The argument would be that the guardian or surrogate is guilty of abuse by insisting on care which is inhumane.

Until some more unambiguous legal guidance and societal consensus about delineating futile versus beneficial treatment come about, physicians should act carefully, both legally and ethically, in defining benefit in its most expansive sense and erring on the side of respecting the patient and family as the best evaluators of whether LSMT will be worthwhile for them. When in doubt, the physician probably should presume that the patient would want an intervention whose benefits are uncertain. Concurrently, though, physicians and other members of the intensive care team should be aggressive in explaining to the patient and/or family their point of view concerning an intervention's futility, using information and reason to move toward a responsible choice; few (albeit some) patients and/or families are likely to persist in insisting on truly burdensome, nonbeneficial medical assaults if they trust the physician and hospital.

Conclusion

This chapter has briefly sketched out the basic legal parameters that frame the making and implementation of decisions about the initiation, continuation, withholding, or withdrawal of LSMT for patients in the ICU. Health care providers must be cognizant of these parameters, and especially of any idiosyncracies embedded in their particular state's law. When needed, providers ought to seek out advice on applying those parameters to particular, factual circumstances from the institution's legal counsel, risk manager, and IEC. It should be borne in mind, however, that legal interpretation is no more (and often far less) an exact science than is medical practice; lawyers and risk managers may disagree in their advice when—as is often true—the law on a particular point is presently unsettled or unclear. Moreover, the primary duty of institution-based attorneys and risk managers is to protect their employer against potential liability; this orientation quite frequently will bias the advice they supply toward what they consider (accurately or not) to be a "hyper-defensive" posture.[47]

Within the pertinent legal parameters, there almost always exists a wide range of clinical options. Ultimately, ethical principles and reasoning processes should play a major role in selecting among those legally acceptable options and providing and documenting good care to patients in their final hours and days of vulnerability.

References

1. Kapp MB. Legal issues in critical care. In: Principles of Critical Care, 2nd ed. (Hall JB, Schmidt GA, Wood LDH, eds.). New York: McGraw-Hill, 1998, pp. 47–56.
2. Norton ML, Finch JS, Norton EV. High-Intensity Care: Medical, Administrative, and Legal Issues. Rockville, MD: Aspen Publishers, 1989, pp. 231–256.
3. Raffin TA, Shurkin JN, Sinkler W III. Intensive Care: Facing the Critical Choices. New York: W.H. Freeman and Company, 1989, pp. 145–171.
4. Kapp MB. Treating medical charts near the end of life: how legal anxieties inhibit good patient deaths. *Univ Toledo Law Rev* 1997;28:521–546.
5. U.S. General Accounting Office. Patient Self-Determination Act: Providers Offer Information on Advance Directives But Effectiveness Uncertain. Washington, DC: 1995, p. 16.
6. Choice in Dying. Right to Die Law Digest (Map of State Laws Regarding Intractable Pain). Washington, DC: Choice in Dying, 1998.
7. Kaufman SR. Intensive care, old age, and the problem of death in America. *Gerontologist* 1998;38:715–725.
8. Freed GL, Kauf T, Freeman VA, Pathman DE, Konrad TR. Vaccine-associated liability risk and provider immunization practices. *Arch Pediatr Adolesc Med* 1998; 152:285–289.
9. Gilligan T, Raffin TA. Whose death is it, anyway? *Ann Intern Med* 1996;126:137–141.
10. McCue JD. The naturalness of dying. *JAMA* 1995;273:1039–1043.
11. Meisel A. The 'right to die': a case study in American lawmaking. *Eur J Health Law* 1996;3:49–74.
12. *Cruzan v. Director, Missouri Department of Health,* 497 U.S. 261 (1990).
13. The SUPPORT Principal Investigators. A controlled trial to improve care for seriously ill hospitalized patients: the study to understand prognoses and preferences for outcomes and risks of treatments. *JAMA* 1995;274:1591–1598.
14. Personal communication from SUPPORT investigator Joan Teno, M.D. (December 16, 1998).
15. *In re Quinlan,* 355 A.2d 647 (N.J.), *cert. denied* 429 U.S. 922 (1976).
16. President's Commission for the Study of Ethical Problems in Medicine and Biomedical and Behavioral Research. Defining Death. Washington, DC: Government Printing Office, 1981.
17. Ad Hoc Committee of the Harvard Medical School to Examine the Definition of Brain Death. A definition of irreversible coma. *JAMA* 1968;205:337–340.
18. American Academy of Neurology, Quality Standards Subcommittee. Practice parameters for determining brain death in adults. *Neurology* 1995;45:1012–1014.
19. Williams MA, Suarez JI. Brain death determination in adults: more than meets the eye. *Crit Care Med* 1997;25:1787–1788.
20. *Strachan v. JFK Memorial Hospital,* 538 A.2d 346 (N.J. 1988).
21. American College of Physicians. Ethics manual (4th ed.). *Ann Intern Med* 1998;128:576–594.

22. Meisel A. The Right to Die, 2nd ed. New York: John Wiley & Sons, 1995.

23. Asch DA, Hansen F-J, et. al. Decisions to limit or continue life-sustaining treatment by critical care physicians in the United States: conflicts between physicians' practices and patients' wishes. *Am J Respir Crit Care Med* 1995;151(Pt1):288–292.

24. Kapp MB. *Our Hands Are Tied: Legal Tensions and Medical Ethics.* Westport, CT: Auburn House, 1998, pp. 65–96.

25. Hesse KA. Terminal care of the very old: changes in the way we die. *Arch Intern Med* 1995;155:1513–1518.

26. *In re Westchester County (O'Connor),* 531 N.E.2d 607 (N.Y. 1988).

27. *In re Martin,* 538 N.W.2d 399 (Mich. 1991).

28. *In the Matter of Edna M.F.,* 210 Wis.2d 557, 563 N.W.2d 485 (1997).

29. Bopp J Jr, Avila D. The sirens' lure of invented consent: a critique of autonomy-based surrogate decisionmaking for legally incapacitated older persons. *Hastings Law J* 1991;42:779–815.

30. Kapp MB. Anxieties as a legal impediment to the doctor–proxy relationship. *J Law Med Ethics* 1999;27:69–73.

31. *Barber v. Superior Court,* 195 Cal. Rptr. 478 (Cal. Ct. App. 1983).

32. *Anderson v. St. Francis-St. George Hospital,* 671 N.E.2d 225 (Ohio 1996).

33. Crane M. The latest malpractice risk: saving your patient's life. *Med Econ* 1998;75:226–241.

34. Peters PG Jr. The illusion of autonomy at the end of life: unconsented life support and the wrongful death analogy. *UCLA Law Rev* 1998;45:673–731.

35. Rhymes JA. Barriers to effective palliative care of terminal patients. *Clin Geriatr Med* 1996;12:407–416.

36. Burt RA. The Supreme Court speaks—not assisted suicide but a constitutional right to palliative care. *N Engl J Med* 1997;337:1234–1236.

37. American Medical Association, Council on Ethical and Judicial Affairs. Code of Medical Ethics: Current Opinions and Annotations. Chicago: AMA;1997.

38. Marsh FH, Staver A. Physician authority for unilateral DNR orders. *J Legal Med* 1991;12:115–165.

39. Middleditch LB Jr, Trotter JH. The right to live. *Elder Law J* 1997;5:395–406.

40. Johnson SH, Gibbons VP, Goldner JA, Wiener RL, Eton D. Legal and institutional policy responses to medical futility. *J Health Hosp Law* 1997;30:21–36.

41. *In re Wanglie,* No. PX-91-283, Hennepin Co. Probate Ct., Fourth Judicial Dist. (Minn. July 1, 1991).

42. *In re Jane Doe,* C.A. No. D-93064 (Ga. Super. Ct. 1991).

43. *In re Baby K,* 16 F.3d 590 (4th Cir. 1994).

44. *In re Mason,* 41 Mass. App. Ct. 298, 669 N.E.2d 1081 (1996).

45. *Gilgunn v. Massachusetts General Hospital,* No. 92–4820 (Mass. Sup. Ct. Civ. Action, Suffolk Co., April 22, 1995).

46. *Causey v. St. Francis Medical Center,* 719 So.2d 1072 (La. App.2 Cir. Aug. 26, 1998).

47. Kapp MB. As others see us: physicians' perceptions of risk managers. *J Healthcare Risk Management* 1996(Fall);16:4–12.

Chapter 19

Economics of Managing Death in the ICU

PETER PRONOVOST

DEREK C. ANGUS

$C$are of patients who die in the ICU requires significant resources, prompting many investigators to apply economic analyses to the cost of care for critically ill patients.[1] However, the application of standard economic analyses to costs incurred for care of the dying patient is problematic. Although the costs of treatment for critically ill non-survivors has been evaluated, formal cost-effectiveness analyses have been limited to life-preserving and life-saving therapies in near-death situations, and the valuation of a "good," as opposed to a "bad," death has not been quantified. Yet, without formal economic analyses, the value of end-of-life care remains subjective, and the ability to justify the allocation of health care resources to end-of-life care may be impaired.

In this chapter, we review the basics of economic evaluation, discuss studies on the cost of dying with emphasis on death in the ICU, review cost-effectiveness studies of life-prolonging therapies in critically ill patients, and outline the requirements for cost-effectiveness studies of palliative care.

Types of Economic Evaluations

There are four types of economic evaluations: cost-minimization, cost-benefit, cost-effectiveness, and cost-utility analyses. While these analyses all have costs in the numerator, they differ in the denominator (Table 19–1). In general, economic analyses are used to compare two or more alternatives, such as two different antibiotics for the treatment of sepsis.

Table 19–1. Types of economic analyses

Type of study	Numerator	Denominator
Cost-minimization	Cost (dollars)	None
Cost-benefit[a]	Cost (dollars	Cost (dollars)
Cost-effectiveness	Cost (dollars)	Specific measure of effectiveness (years of life saved)
Cost-utility[a]	Cost (dollars)	A common utility metric (quality adjusted life years)

[a]Because cost-benefit and cost-utility analyses produce a common metric, they can be used to compare studies that evaluate different outcomes.

Methodological Issues in Cost-Effectiveness and Cost-Utility Analyses

Marginal cost-effectiveness

Cost-effectiveness and cost-utility analyses aid in decision making and are always used to compare treatment alternatives.[2,3] Here we will use cost-effectiveness analysis to refer to both cost effectiveness analysis and cost-utility analysis. A cost-effectiveness analysis evaluates the marginal cost-effectiveness, or the cost-effectiveness of switching from one treatment to another. Average cost-effectiveness ratios are generally not helpful, since they do not allow the comparison of alternatives.[3,4]

Perspective: who is paying?

Most parties are concerned only with the costs for which they are at risk. Therefore, costs are seen differently by different parties, and we need to explicitly state from whose perspective we are evaluating costs. In health care, the usual parties are the payer (insurance company or employer), hospital, patient, or society.[3,5]

The numerator: costs

The terminology in cost-effectiveness analysis is highly variable and confusing. As a result, it is often difficult to compare different cost-effectiveness analyses, since they frequently use different definitions for costs and outcomes. In an attempt to reduce this variation, the U.S. Public Health Service and the National Institutes of Health Panel on Cost-Effectiveness in Health and Medicine (PCEHM) made recommendations for the conduct and reporting of cost-effectiveness analyses.[6-8] In general, we need to consider only those costs that we believe to be relevant and likely to differ between the treatment and control groups.[6]

Discounting and inflation

A dollar today is worth more than a dollar a year from now, and interest rates typically reflect a person's preference for having goods sooner rather than later.[6] This preference for a dollar today is called the *time preference of money*. Because of this, we must discount future costs to an index year. Before discounting, all costs should be adjusted for inflation.

The denominator: the value of health consequences

The value of health consequence is usually reported as a quality-adjusted life year (QALY). A QALY is simply the weighted average of the value of the health-related quality of life during the time of increased survival where optimal health has a value of 1 and death has a value of 0.[9-11]

Estimating effectiveness

The data for estimating effectiveness can come from a variety of sources. The goal for the researcher is to select the estimation of effectiveness that is valid for the population under study. While data from clinical trials are generally the least biased, cost-effectiveness analyses based on clinical trial data can overestimate the treatment effect for a number of reasons, including high adherence and close monitoring.[12,13]

Robustness and uncertainty

The estimates of costs, effectiveness, and preferences that make up a cost-effectiveness analysis are subject to both systematic and random error, and this error can affect the conclusions of the cost-effectiveness analysis. Because of this, most cost-effectiveness analyses incorporate a sensitivity analysis to estimate the degree to which the study may be influenced by error in measurement or estimation.

The Costs of Dying in the ICU

Beyond the intangible costs of dying in the relatively hurried, congested ICU environment, there are also considerable direct and indirect health care costs. It is estimated that end-of-life care consumes 10% to 12% of all health care expenditures and 27% of Medicare expenditures. Furthermore, the number of enrollees in Medicare will grow considerably in the next 20 years, raising considerable concerns over the anticipated costs of dying and providing care to an increasing elderly population.[14] As we practice medicine under increasing fiscal scrutiny, many will question the value of this investment of resources.[15]

In addition to health care reform initiatives being put in place to control escalating costs, there are also changing societal attitudes towards patient autonomy, including an increased use of advance directives. Together, these factors and others may be leading to a change in the way death is managed in the ICU. The extent to which this is influencing cost, however, remains unclear.

The costs of hospitalization for patients with advanced stages of nine serious illnesses did not change between 1989 and 1994, and the carefully crafted Study to Understand Prognosis and Preferences for Outcomes and Risks of Treatment (SUPPORT) intervention did not alter those costs.[16] Furthermore, the SUPPORT study demonstrated that increasing the use of advance directives was not associated with a reduction in hospital resource use.[17] Emanuel reviewed the available literature on potential cost savings through the use of hospice and advance directives and lower use of high-technology interventions in the care of terminally ill patients. He estimated that the use of hospice and advance directives could save 25% to 40% in the last month of life, but the savings decreased to 10% to 17% over the last 6 months and 0% to 10% over the last 12 months. It is possible that increased use of palliative care may increase costs of hospital care by increasing nursing hours to provide patient care and increasing pharmacy costs to administer analgesics and sedatives.

Although managed care organizations have been associated with reduced hospital resource utilization for patients in general, the evidence suggests that overall, managed care has had little, if any, impact on ICU resource utilization.[19] Nevertheless, health care reform has led some investigators to attempt to limit care for patients who have a high probability of dying. It was estimated that up to 7% ($5 million) of total annual charges at an academic medical center were potentially avoidable by judicious selection of patients whose care could be limited on day 5 of ICU care.[20] This model proposes that we can use severity-of-illness modeling to identify and limit care for patients who have a high likelihood of dying. Through risk adjustment models we are able to estimate the probability of death for a population of patients but, in general, we cannot accurately predict death in individual patients.[21,22] Therefore, it seems prudent that predictions of death from risk adjustment models be used only as one piece of information along with physician estimates[23] of likely outcome, the patient's and family members' values and desired goals of therapy.

Cher and Lenert explored whether changing reimbursement strategies has an impact on the use of health care resources for patients at the end of life in the ICU. They suggested that managed care physicians may do a better job at limiting unnecessary end-of-life care,[24] although concerns have been raised regarding the study design. In addition, although costs appeared to be lower, the data suggest that some beneficial care was withheld from managed care patients who demonstrated an 8% excess in mortality at 100 days.[25,26] The authors' findings suggest that costs, rather than quality of life, have become the important outcome.[24]

We would anticipate managed care to have little direct impact on ICU care, including end-of-life care. However, managed care may indirectly affect end-of-life care in the ICU by requiring that ICU patients be cared for by critical care physicians. There is an emerging body of evidence which suggests that critical care physicians reduce mortality and resource utilization, and managed care organizations and health care purchasing groups are beginning to require that ICU patients be cared for by critical care physicians.[27,28] We anticipate that this trend will continue, and since the decisions and practices of critical care physicians affect end-of-life care, managed care may indirectly have an impact on end-of-life care in the ICU.[29]

If managed care does influence end-of-life care in the ICU, it is unclear how this will affect patients. Managed care may provide a system for managing death by developing innovative care programs and accountability for care standards.[30] Lynn et al. suggest that end-of-life care under fee for service is frequently deficient, and managed care organizations may be more likely to introduce hospice care and other community programs to improve end-of-life care. On the other hand, managed care organizations may pay less attention to palliative care, such as hospice, since it is unclear that the use of palliative care reduces costs.[18] The financial incentive under managed care is to use less health resources, and this incentive may result in less emphasis on palliative care. Additionally, one of the benefits of managed care is that health care resources are allocated within a fixed budget for a defined population. Under such a restriction, cost-effectiveness analyses are potentially of more value, and hence more likely to influence resource allocation decisions. However, there have not been any studies on the cost-effectiveness of end-of-life care—a problem that must be addressed if we are to justify the allocation of resources to end-of-life care.

Cost-effectiveness of Life-Prolonging Treatments in Critically Ill Patients

Although end-of-life care has not undergone cost-effectiveness analysis, there have been economic evaluations of therapies targeted at critically ill patients at grave risk of death. In a study of the initiation of renal support for seriously ill ICU patients who further develop acute renal failure, the SUPPORT investigators determined that initiating dialysis was associated with a cost-effectiveness ratio of $128,200 per QALY and $274,100 per QALY for the worst prognostic category.[31] The cost-effectiveness of a cardiopulmonary resuscitation (CPR) program was estimated to be $225,892 (range $181,286 to $537,088) per QALY.[32] In addition, the cost per survival to discharge after having in-hospital CPR was $117,000 for a rate of survival of 10%, $248,271 for a rate of survival of 1%, and $544,521 for a survival rate of 0.2%.[33] In general, these ratios are high. Conventionally, health care initiatives are deemed cost-effective if the ratio is less than $100,000 per life saved. Nevertheless, there is little attempt to restrict CPR programs and there are no formal guidelines in the U.S. limiting

hemodialysis in the critically ill. Indeed, a recent study of workforce requirements in nephrology anticipated the need for more nephrologists because of an
anticipated expansion in the number of elderly patients requiring hemodialysis.[34]

There are also examples to suggest that the cost-effectiveness ratio for therapies in the critically ill can be very sensitive to the gravity of a patient's condition prior to treatment. Projections of the likely cost-effectiveness ratio of an
anti-endotoxin therapy in sepsis suggested that the ratio was exquisitely sensitive to the underlying mortality rate, with ratios degenerating markedly when
patients were more seriously ill prior to therapy.[35,36] Similarly, Mark et al.
showed that the cost-effectiveness ratio for thromboplastin in the treatment of
acute myocardial infarction was much worse for older patients with more severe myocardial infarctions at greater risk of death.[37] In both these examples,
the problem was that treatment effects are often diminished in patients at high
risk of death, perhaps because the patient's condition simply overwhelms any
single intervention.

These data raise important issues in the care of the gravely ill. It is quite
conceivable that a therapy may be approved for use at a given institution yet be
restricted to one patient with sepsis and denied to another. This "front-line"
demonstration of resource distribution may cause significant discomfort for clinicians, regardless of its appropriateness.

Cost Effectiveness of Palliative Therapies

There are a variety of new approaches to managing death for the critically ill,
including options within the ICU and other settings. Options within the ICU
include end-of-life consults, additional social and pastoral support services, and
pain management guidelines. Options outside the ICU include alternative care
units,[38] or discharge to hospices or to home with formal support. Furthermore,
new educational programs developed to improve the level of expertise of
health care providers in the care of the dying, as well as patient and societal
interventions to promote use of advance directives and advanced care planning,
may all impact how death is managed in the ICU. All of these approaches have
costs, and arguably, may have better or worse outcomes. However, assessing
the relative "value" of each program and intervention is complicated.

Estimation of the numerator, or costs, in a cost effectiveness analysis of
end-of-life care would be similar to that of other cost-effectiveness analyses. It
would need to include the cost of the therapy, including personnel costs, and
the related costs associated with any change in therapy. For example, the intervention may decrease ICU length of stay but may increase hospice use. The
unrelated costs and future costs would likely be insignificant, since the patient's
life expectancy would be relatively short and likely distributed evenly between
the treatment and control groups, thus potentially eliminating the need to measure these costs.

The approach to estimating the denominator, however, requires significant modification from that currently endorsed by the U.S. PCEHM.[6-8] In the current cost-effectiveness analysis, the QALY is the unit of analysis. In this metric, death is usually the anchor with 0 QALYs, while a year in perfect health is 1 QALY. If all death is valued at 0, we will never be able to differentiate between a "good death" and a "bad death." Intuitively, most would agree that efforts to manage death have value, and most people would prefer a good death over a bad death. Indeed, Patrick et al. have demonstrated that patients view some health states, such as prolonged mechanical ventilation, as worse than death.[39]

Let us say that we have a utility scale that rates a good death as 0.5 utilities and a bad death as 0.01 utilities. Current cost-effectiveness analyses would not differentiate between the two because we would multiply both utilities by 0 (the patient died). With this methodology, we would never be able to justify on the basis of economic analyses, investing resources into palliative care or end-of-life care, since they would always produce 0 QALYs. Therefore, cost-effectiveness analysis of end-of-life care will need to anchor the utility scale with states worse than death rather than just death. Even if we assigned death a value greater than 0, we may need to change the time scale, since most people will live less than a year, and thus the QALYs for end-of-life care will always be low. For example, if we use a palliative therapy at the end of a patient's life for 2 days in the ICU and the utility of these days is 0.5, this would provide 1 quality-adjusted life day, or 0.0027 QALYs. If we assume an average ICU cost of $3,000 per day, we would obtain a cost-effectiveness ratio of $2,222,222 per QALY—far in excess of what is viewed as cost-effective and thus, unlikely to be funded.

Estimation of the measure of effectiveness will also need to change. We will need to evaluate different end-of-life therapies and decide how to put in place the construct of a "good death." Should the outcome variable for a good death be dichotomous, interval, or continuous? From what conceptual model will we evaluate effectiveness? Both professionals and patients see a need to improve end-of-life care,[40] and we need to develop a conceptual framework to evaluate the quality of end-of-life care. Three expert panels have published conceptual frameworks for quality of end-of-life care from the physician's perspective.[41-43] Moreover, the conceptual model for quality of end-of-life care from the patient's perspective differs significantly from models developed using the physician's perspective.[44] The quality of end-of-life care ought to be evaluated from the patient's perspective or that of society.

Therefore, before we can assess the economic value of different ways of managing death, we must achieve two steps in the quantification of the denominator. First, we must be able to discriminate a good from a bad death. This will allow cost-effectiveness analyses that compare different end-of-life management strategies. Second, we must be able to express the marginal gain of a good over a bad death in some form of utility. This will allow economic comparison of end-of-life strategies to other interventions that improve quality-adjusted survival. Even if we overcome these methodological hurdles, we are still left with the value judgement of how to allocate scarce resources. Our society and health care system place a high value on "rescue" therapy rather than preventive therapy. As such, it is unclear how society will value end-of-life therapy relative to rescue therapy. Forming this value judgement will require dialogue involving political, moral, religious, economic, and medical perspectives.

Summary

Economic analyses are used to help make decisions between two or more therapies when resources are constrained. However, these decisions are value judgments. In this chapter, we reviewed the various types of economic analyses, including cost-minimization, cost-benefit, cost-effectiveness, and cost-utility. We also reviewed the cost of dying and how health care reform has, or may, affect these costs. Finally, we discussed cost-effectiveness studies of life-prolonging therapies and the unique issues associated with cost-effectiveness studies of palliative therapy, with emphasis on the problem of calculating a cost-effectiveness ratio when there is no good metric for valuing the quality of death.

As the national debate about health care costs, access, and quality continues, and as more Americans are enrolled in managed care organizations that deliver care within a fixed budget, we will increasingly turn to economic analyses to help make resource allocation decisions. Cost-effectiveness analysis will continue to be the most popular form of economic analysis, since it combines the results (effectiveness of treatment) with the costs of achieving the results. However, methods for cost-effectiveness analysis in health care are evolving, and current measures of both results and costs are imprecise.[45] We must be aware of the limitations of cost-effectiveness analysis and the need for value judgments when using such analyses to inform health care decisions. We look forward to the application of cost-effectiveness analyses to end-of-life care and the further development of cost-effectiveness methods for palliative therapies.

References

1. Schapira DV, Studnicki J, Bradham DD, Wolff P, Jarrett A. Intensive care, survival, and expense of treating critically ill cancer patients. *JAMA* 1993;269:783–786.
2. Detsky AS, Naglie IG. A clinician's guide to cost-effectiveness analysis. *Ann Intern Med* 1990;113:147–154.
3. Petitti D. Meta-analysis decision analysis and cost effectiveness analysis. In: Methods for Quantitative Synthesis in Medicine. (Petitti D, ed.). New York: Oxford University Press, 1994, p. 171.
4. Pauker SG, Kassirer JP. Decision analysis. *N Engl J Med* 1987;316:250–258.

5. Weinstein MC, Fineberg HV. Clinical Decision Analysis. Philadelphia: W.B. Saunders, 1980.
6. Weinstein MC, Siegel JE, Gold MR, Kamlet MS, Russell LB, for the Panel on Cost-Effectiveness in Health and Medicine. Recommendations of the panel on cost-effectiveness in health and medicine. *JAMA* 1996;276(15):1253–1258
7. Russell LB, Gold MR, Siegel JE, Daniels N, Weinstein MC. The role of cost-effectiveness analysis in health and medicine. Panel on Cost-Effectiveness in Health and Medicine. *JAMA* 1996;276:1172–1177
8. Siegel JE, Weinstein MC, Russell LB, Gold MR. Recommendations for reporting cost-effectiveness analyses. *JAMA* 1996;276:1339–1341
9. Patrick DL, Erickson P. Health Status and Health Policy: Quality of Life in Health Care Evaluation and Resource Allocation. New York: Oxford University Press, 1993.
10. Torrance GW, Feeny D. Utilities and quality-adjusted life years. *Int J Technol Assess Health Care* 1989;5:559–575
11. Kaplan RM, Anderson JP. A general health policy model: update and applications. *Health Serv Res* 1988;23:203–235
12. Wennberg DE, Lucas FL, Birkmeyer JD, Bredenberg CE, Fisher ES. Variation in carotid endarterectomy mortality in the Medicare population: trial hospitals, volume, and patient characteristics. *JAMA* 1998;279:1278–1281
13. Ellwein LB, Drummond MF. Economic analysis alongside clinical trials. Bias in the assessment of economic outcomes. *Int J Technol Assess Health Care* 1996;12:691–697.
14. Iglehart JK. The American health care system—Medicare. *N Engl J Med* 1999;340:327–332.
15. Lubitz JD, Riley GF. Trends in Medicare payments in the last year of life. *N Engl J Med* 1993;328:1092–1096
16. SUPPORT Principal Investigators. A controlled trial to improve care for seriously ill hospitalized patients: the Study to Understand Prognoses and Preferences for Outcomes and Risks of Treatments (SUPPORT). *JAMA* 1995;274:1591–1598.
17. Teno J, Lynn J, Connors AFJ, Wenger N, Phillips RS, Alzola C, Murphy DP, Desbiens N, Knaus WA. The illusion of end-of-life resource savings with advance directives. SUPPORT Investigators. Study to Understand Prognoses and Preferences for Outcomes and Risks of Treatment [see comments]. *J Am Geriatr Soc* 1997;45:513–518.
18. Emanuel EJ. Cost savings at the end of life. What do the data show? *JAMA* 1996;275:1907–1914.
19. Angus DC, Linde-Zwirble WT, Sirio CA, Rotondi AJ, Chelluri L, Newbold RC, III, Lave JR, Pinsky MR. The effect of managed care on ICU length of stay: implications for Medicare. *JAMA* 1996;276:1075–1082.
20. Esserman L, Belkora J, Lenert LA. Potentially ineffective care. A new outcome to assess the limits of critical care. *JAMA* 1995;274:1544–1551.
21. Lynn J, Harrell FJ, Cohn F, Wagner D, Connors AFJ. Prognoses of seriously ill hospitalized patients on the days before death: implications for patient care and public policy. *New Horiz* 1997;5:56–61.
22. Angus DC, Pinsky MR. Risk prediction: judging the judges. *Intensive Care Med* 1997;23:363–365.
23. Knaus WA, Harrell FEJ, Lynn J, Goldman L, Phillips RS, Connors AFJ, Dawson NV, Fulkerson WJJ, Califf RM, Desbiens NA, et al. The SUPPORT prognostic

model. Objective estimates of survival for seriously ill hospitalized adults. Study to understand prognoses and preferences for outcomes and risks of treatments. *Ann Intern Med* 1995;122:191–203.

24. Cher DJ, Lenert LA. Method of Medicare reimbursement and the rate of potentially ineffective care of critically ill patients. *JAMA* 1997;278:1001–1007.

25. Lynn J. Potentially ineffective care in intensive care. *JAMA* 1998;279:652–654.

26. Curtis JR, Rubenfeld GD. Aggressive medical care at the end of life. Does capitated reimbursement encourage the right care for the wrong reason? *JAMA* 1997; 278:1025–1026.

27. Pronovost PJ, Jencks M, Dorman T, et al. Organizational characteristics of intensive care units related to outcomes of abdominal aortic surgery. *JAMA* 1999;281:1310–1312.

28. Asch DA, Hansen-Flaschen J, Lanken PN. Decisions to limit or continue life-sustaining treatment by critical care physicians in the United States: conflicts between physicians' practices and patients' wishes. *Am J Respir Crit Care Med* 1995;151:92.

29. Prendergast TJ, Luce JM. Increasing incidence of withholding and withdrawal of life support from the critically ill. *Am J Respir Crit Care Med* 1997;155:15–20.

30. Lynn J, Wilkinson A, Cohn F, Jones SB. Capitated risk-bearing managed care systems could improve end-of-life care. *J Am Geriatr Soc* 1998;46:322–303.

31. Hamel MB, Phillips RS, Davis RB, Desbiens N, Connors AFJ, Teno JM, Wenger N, Lynn J, Wu AW, Fulkerson W. Tsevat J. Outcomes and cost-effectiveness of initiating dialysis and continuing aggressive care in seriously ill hospitalized adults. SUPPORT Investigators. Study to Understand Prognoses and Preferences for Outcomes and Risks of Treatments. *Ann Intern Med* 1997;127:195–202.

32. Lee KH, Angus DC, Abramson NS. Cardiopulmonary resuscitation: what cost to cheat death. *Crit Care Med* 1996;24:2046–2052.

33. Ebell MH, Kruse JA. A proposed model for the cost of cardiopulmonary resuscitation. *Med Care* 1994;32:640–649.

34. Neilson EG, Hull AR, Wish JB, Neylan JF, Sherman D, Suki WN. The Ad Hoc Committee report on estimating the future workforce and training requirements for nephrology. The Ad Hoc Committee on Nephrology Manpower Needs. *J Am Soc Nephrol* 1997;8:Suppl-4.

35. Schulman KA, Glick HA, Rubin H, Eisenberg JM. Cost-effectiveness of HA-1A monoclonal antibody for gram-negative sepsis. Economic assessment of a new therapeutic agent. *JAMA* 1991;266:3466–3471.

36. Linden PK, Angus DC, Chelluri L, Branch RA. The influence of clinical study design on cost-effectiveness projections for the treatment of gram-negative sepsis with human anti-endotoxin antibody. *J Crit Care* 1995;10:154–164.

37. Mark DB, Hlatky MA, Califf RM, Naylor CD, Lee KL, Armstrong PW, Barbash G, White H, Simoons ML, Nelson CL. Cost effectiveness of thrombolytic therapy with tissue plasminogen activator as compared with streptokinase for acute myocardial infarction. *N Engl J Med* 1995;332:1418–1424.

38. Fins JJ, Miller FG, Acres CA, Bacchetta MD, Huzzard LL, Rapkin BD. End-of-life decision-making in the hospital: current practice and future prospects. *J Pain Symptom Manage* 1999;17:6–15.

39. Patrick DL, Starks HE, Cain KC, Uhlmann RF, Pearlman RA. Measuring preferences for health states worse than death. *Med Decision Making* 1994;14:9–18.

40. Anonymous. Good care of the dying patient. Council on Scientific Affairs, American Medical Association. *JAMA* 1996;275:474–478.
41. Lynn J. Measuring quality of care at the end of life: a statement of principles. *J Am Geriatr Soc* 1997;45:526–527.
42. Fields MJ, Cassel CK. Approaching Death, Improving Care at the End of Life. Washington DC: National Academy Press, 1997
43. Emanuel EJ, Emanuel LL. The promise of a good death. *Lancet* 1998;351:Suppl-9.
44. Singer PA, Martin DK, Kelner M. Quality end-of-life care: patients' perspectives. *JAMA* 1999;281:163–168.
45. Hildred W, Watkins L. The nearly good, the bad, and the ugly in cost effectiveness analysis in health care. *J Econ Issues* 1996;30:755–774.

Chapter 20

Organizational Change and Improving the Quality of Palliative Care in the ICU

BARBARA J. DALY

*T*he purpose of this chapter is to address organizational features of critical care units as they affect the provision of palliative care. The premise of the chapter is that an important part of the explanation for the current inadequacies in care of the dying in general and in critical care in particular is failure to appreciate the extent to which the environment of practice influences care providers and processes.

There is ample evidence that critical care practitioners, both doctors and nurses, are not well prepared in the provision of specific components of palliative care. Previous reports have documented such problems as inadequate pain relief, rigid enforcement of restrictions in visiting to the detriment of family support, and lack of knowledge and inconsistency in treatment withdrawal techniques.[1-3] These data are particularly surprising in that, for many issues, it is not the case that we do not know what should be done and what outcomes we want to achieve—we simply cannot accomplish them. Despite the concerns of health professionals themselves about the use of inappropriate, aggressive, and futile interventions, physicians and nurses report frequently providing care that goes against their conscience.[4]

The two best examples of our institutionalized failure are pain management and decision making. For example, Puntillo[5] found that pain, its treatment, and communication about pain were significant problems for a substantial portion of the ICU patients in her sample. Tittle and McMillan[6] similarly found a pattern of undermedication, inadequate assessment, and underreporting of pain in both an ICU and a general surgical ward. The Study to Understand Prognoses and Preferences for Outcomes and Risks of Treatment (SUPPORT) confirmed that, even with a well-planned intervention of specially trained ICU nurses and very precise, reliable prognostic data, investigators were unable to affect such outcomes as time in ICU, pain in the last days of life, adherence to instructions in advance directives, and use of complex technology in terminal states.[7]

The Problem

As with treatment of any problem, designing "curative" approaches to address these issues begins with an understanding of the etiology. Critical care practitioners are subject to the same sociological forces as is American society and the health professions in general. Much has been written about the "death-denying" culture in the United States, which is no where more in evidence than in acute care.[8,9]

A second feature of critical care culture is the supremacy of the 'technologic imperative." This imperative serves as a default principle which specifies that if a technology is available, it must be used.[10] Thus the question, "Can we?" always takes precedence over "Should we?" to the point that evaluation of the rationale for intervention is often ignored. This norm continues to exist despite the recognition that an intervention is justified only if there is reason to believe that the intervention is likely to accomplish a defined goal and the burdens of the intervention are outweighed by the benefits, as evaluated by the patient or the patient's proxy.

It is quite understandable that these two justification criteria were taken for granted in the early days of critical care. The range of options for saving lives were limited, the *raison d'etre* for the existence of the ICU was precisely to provide specialized life-saving treatment, and the burdens of attempting to save life were at least circumscribed in that they either worked or did not and the patient died fairly soon. Neither of these features is present today. Patients often do come to the ICU to have their life saved at all costs, but sometimes they come only for trials of advanced technology and sometimes just because a particular support intervention, such as a ventilator, is not available on the general wards. Once in the unit, however, the range of options is almost limitless. And, as our success in treating the most acute crises has improved, we have created a population of patients who are actively but slowly dying and unable to be cared for on the general wards.

The original orientation of critical care units is perhaps most in evidence in the assumption that survival at all costs is the goal. This is sometimes evident in critical care staff's questioning of the appropriateness of having a patient admitted to the unit after a do-not-resuscitate (DNR) decision has been made. Again, when attempts to resuscitate in the event of a sudden arrest were all that the ICU had to offer many patients, it was reasonable to equate DNR decisions in the ICU with inappropriate use of scarce critical care resources. Today, however, we know that treatment limitation decisions are much more complex than dichotomous all-or-nothing decisions. Rather, treatment limitation is best understood as existing on a continuum of aggressiveness, with the level or extent of limitation stemming from individual patient goals. In many cases patients may choose to receive all available interventions, although a cardiac arrest in this context will be understood as an indication that treatment is not being successful and resuscitative efforts will therefore be withheld. The use of standard treatment limitation levels, such as DNR with all other treatments, DNR and withholding of specific treatments, and DNR with withdrawal of specific treatments reflects the recognition of this continuum.[11,12]

Similarly, with the proliferation of treatment options, patients more often have the opportunity to express preferences to receive some interventions and reject others. Mechanical ventilation and hemodialysis, for example, are interventions that some patients will refuse, while still wishing to receive all other treatments in the hope that the need for ventilation can be forestalled.

The origins of these characteristics are quite apparent. The more important question is why, given the evolution of our understanding of treatment limitation, a body of research on reliable prognostic systems that establish the futility of interventions in specific clinical situations, and the decades of court cases establishing the right of competent persons to refuse any and all treatments,[13] problems with decision making and symptom management of the terminally ill persist. The recalcitrance of practice norms to overwhelming need for change demonstrates the power of the environment to influence practice.

Environment

Reflection on the history of critical care in the United States suggests an interesting pattern. The opening of the first units in the 1950s and 1960s was sparked by the recognition that greater efficiency and effectiveness could be achieved by creating a specialized environment that facilitated provision of quality care through concentrating people with unique expertise and specialized equipment in one place. This approach to the organization of critical care units has been almost universally adopted, with progressive degrees of specialization. Throughout this period of specialization, however, "environment" has primarily been understood as referring to the clinical specialization of providers along diagnostic or clinical service lines (e.g., medicine, surgery, cardiovascular).

In comparison to the obvious benefits of being able to concentrate staff with special expertise in specialized procedures and use of high-tech interventions, the extent to which the environment itself contributes to or detracts from care processes has received less recognition. For the most part, "environment" has been understood simply as the physical structure. The importance of such features as lighting, noise, privacy, and provision for family visiting are clearly important, but represent only one aspect.

A number of studies have documented differences in practice that accompany the development of separate and specialized units. Seamark and colleagues used review of medical records to compare the care provided to terminally ill patients in 12 regular community hospital wards with that provided by a designated hospice unit.[14] Patients on the hospice unit were more likely to be admitted for pain and symptom control and less likely for terminal nursing care, and to have half the length of stay (8 vs. 16 days). Most importantly, community hospital patients had greater use of laboratory tests and radiation and chemotherapy treatments. This study confirmed the earlier results of the National Hospice Study.[15]

Several authors have reported a similar finding after establishing separate units for patients requiring long-term mechanical ventilation. Elpern and colleagues demonstrated positive clinical and financial outcomes when patients who required intensive pulmonary management were grouped together in a noninvasive respiratory care unit rather than in a traditional ICU.[16] As found with palliative care units, Gracey and colleagues also reported improved patient outcomes when ventilator-dependent patients were transferred out of the ICU to a chronic ventilator unit.[17]

Why is it that placing patients in a different place changes the care processes? Physical features cannot be the entire explanation. Concentrating people who are expert in a particular type of care explains some of the differences that occur, but it appears that the same people function better in a different environment. According to proponents of organizational theory, the quality of work is a function of the whole environment. So for example, if we only change the people, or change their skill level, but leave the processes the same, we are unlikely to accomplish much real improvement. Within the persistent debate about how best to conceptualize organizational environment,[18] sociotechnical theory offers a perspective that is particularly suited to efforts to redesign critical care units in order to improve palliative care processes.

Passmore has described organizational environments as encompassing both social systems and technical aspects.[19] Social systems consist of the people who work in the organization and "all that is human," including their attitudes and beliefs, their understanding of their responsibilities, traditions, group norms, hierarchies, and political forces. The technical system consists of the tools and techniques, as the term suggests, but also the methods, choices about how tasks are performed, and patterns and procedures by which work is accomplished. The function of technology is to enhance the quantity and quality of work performed and thus also includes features of the environment, such as reward systems, supervisory techniques, role descriptions, flexibility, and variety of work.[20]

Applying this theoretical framework to the ICU, we can categorize the attitudes, knowledge, and preferences of staff, the communication patterns, and decision hierarchy as part of the social system. The methods of assigning nurses to patients, routines for daily rounds, presence or absence of interdisciplinary conferences, and the numbers and types of equipment represent some of the technical aspects.

To improve the efficiency and effectiveness of organizations, both the social and technical aspects of the organization need to be addressed. This means recognizing human needs and factors that enable people to perform better, such as the preference for autonomy, the need for learning, growth and creativity, and the opportunity to see the long-range effects of work. In addition, the following questions should be asked: Are caregivers able to complete and identify with the whole task? Is equality maximized and subordination minimized? Are workers allowed to set standards? Have human resources been fully developed?[19] To address the technical system factors, the processes that foster or impede goals need to be analyzed, as well as how goals are set, how the tasks and responsibilities are understood, what the criteria of success are, and whether systems to monitor effectiveness are present.

Environmental Change

Organizational and structural options

Consideration of how to improve palliative services for patients often begins with the questions of where to care for such patients and who should care for them. There are three general organizational and structural approaches to addressing these questions: create a physically separate unit, designate a given number of beds and/or staff in an existing unit, or establish a palliative care consultation service. Table 20–1 lists these options, the factors that must be taken into account in choosing a strategy, and some of the major decisions that are contingent on the choice. If organizational or structural changes are not possible or justified, then steps should be taken through education and continuous quality improvement to raise the overall standard of end-of-life care. Strategies for this are addressed below.

The well-documented success over time of palliative care units and hospice in general reflects the advantages of creating a new, separate environment.[21–23] As with any critical care specialty, there are obvious benefits to having a separate unit where the goals of care are uniform and staff can be specially trained in appropriate palliative care techniques. However, in most instances, the ability to create such a unit is determined more by the many practical considerations than by preference. A proposal to establish a palliative care unit must first establish feasibility. The average census of patients appropriate for such a unit must be documented, as well as the actual availability of space. The expense of supporting a small unit that averages only four or five patients at any one time will usually rule out this strategy. Given the fixed costs of overhead and the loss of some staffing flexibility, operating two small units will generally be more expensive than operating one large unit. In addition, support for admitting patients to this unit by physicians must be considered.

Equally important in evaluating feasibility are staffing considerations. In order to operate a palliative care unit, there must be sufficient staff (medical,

Table 20–1. Practical determinants of organizational structure

Option	Determinants	Contingencies
Separate unit	Available location Patient census (average number of palliative care patients) Willingness of medical staff to transfer patients to the unit	Necessary modifications to site (monitoring, bathrooms, conference room, etc.)
Designated beds within unit	Ability to segregate beds Patient census (average number of acute patients and palliative care patients) Staffing demands	Which beds, and how many Designated staff (staff attitudes and preferences)
Consultation team	Availability of palliative care experts Financial support for the service Willingness of medical staff to refer patients	Composition of the team Reimbursement mechanism

nursing, and support services) who are interested in working in such a unit. Recruitment strategies can assist in identifying nurses who would find such a unit an attractive workplace, but opening any new unit needs to begin with the availability of at least a small core of staff committed to the project.

If it is neither possible nor justifiable to open a separate unit for palliative care patients, then patients with these needs must either be integrated among the unit's population or segregated within the unit, such as by designating certain beds as hospice or palliative care beds or by creating a palliative care team among the regular staff. As with the decision to open a distinct unit, the usefulness of designating specific beds or staff depends in large measure on feasibility issues.

Less concrete and perhaps more important than the relatively apparent practical constraints is the rationale for the organization of care. If, for example, the major roadblock to providing effective palliative care is lack of recognition of when it is appropriate to change the goal of care to palliation, then creation of a separate unit will be of no use, and may make it less likely that clinicians recognize the need. Many ICUs have a strong foundation in the provision of aggressive, life-prolonging therapies, are highly specialized, promote the use of very sophisticated technologies, and typically recruit staff who enjoy the fast pace and relatively short stay of patients. In some institutions it may simply be more efficient to designate a different environment for the provision of palliative care than to attempt to address all the features of this environment that would need to be changed. In a survey of 468 critical care nurses' views of end-of-life care Asch and colleagues noted that "the most compelling concept expressed by the nurses was that the environment of critical care is often insufficiently responsive" to patient suffering.[24] The authors concluded that some ICUs might simply be unable to foster the compassion needed to support appropriate care of the dying.

One important disadvantage of creating a separate palliative care unit is that it supports the myth that palliative care, with its intensive symptom management, periodic reassessment of goals, and concentrated attention to the psychosocial needs of patients and families, is only needed by dying patients. The availability of special units for the dying thus has the unintended effect of minimizing the importance of these elements of care for all patients. Fisher and colleagues noted this danger of restricting care of the dying to just hospice personnel.[22] Since hospice, or any specialized palliative care service, will never be able to assume care of all dying patients, this approach runs the risk that others will not have appropriate training, skill, and experience.

Health care managers are sometimes concerned that it is just too difficult to expect any critical care staff to be skillful in providing both aggressive life-saving care for some patients and care oriented toward enabling a peaceful death for others. Although there are some differences within any specialty, segregating patients into different kinds of care does not relieve staff of any need to be knowledgeable, and some central skills, such as assessment and caring, cut across all specialties. For example, Samarel, using ethnographic participative observation to study nurse–patient interactions on a hospital unit designated for both hospice care and acute care, found no differences in how nurses interacted with hospice versus acute care patients.[25] She postulated that highly developed attitudes of caring resulted in gentle, appropriate models of caring strategies for both groups of patients. Contrary to Asch's findings, she concluded that it is possible for some nurses to deal with dichotomous populations effectively. Similarly, Mathew and co-workers reported on the successful integration of hospice beds into an active medical teaching service; in fact, house staff in this study reported feeling more comfortable dealing with terminally ill patients as a result of their hospice experience.[26]

A last alternative that has demonstrated promise in the care of terminally ill patients is the use of palliative care teams that serve as consultants to the primary team and, in some instances, assume responsibility for directing care. The model at Detroit Receiving Hospital is among the best known of these.[27,28] Through this kind of service, ongoing assistance and education can be provided to staff. The availability of this service obviates the need to transfer palliative care patients out of the unit and to demonstrate the provision of improved symptom management.[29] As with the other alternatives, the feasibility of this model is primarily determined by practical factors, such as the availability of clinicians with specific expertise in palliative care and a sufficient workload to make such a service economically sound.

Assessing strengths and needs

As can be seen, regardless of which alternative is chosen, changing the environment begins with accurate assessment of both the social and technical aspects of the current environment. This is particularly important if organizational changes are not possible and efforts must be made to implement change within a given environment. Table 20–2 lists some of the more important aspects to investigate prior to planning changes. The purpose of the assessment is to identify those features that may act as barriers to changing the effectiveness of the care provided.

In some ways, the social aspects—characteristics of the staff—seem the most important, and typically garner the most intention. Attitudes and beliefs of the nursing and medical staff are certainly significant and can be readily assessed through use of surveys and tests. The Frommelt Attitude Toward Care of the Dying, for example, is a short 20-item Likert scale survey that can provide helpful information about general attitudes toward palliative care.[30] There are also a number of tools available that can be used to assess knowledge and beliefs about pain management.[31,32] It is often helpful to add several questions to any standardized assessment tool to seek information about staff preferences and perceptions about the environment, such as "How well do you think we do in caring for the dying," or "What is the most frustrating aspect of caring for a patient who is dying in the ICU?" Information such as this can be used in several ways. Summaries of responses are very powerful prompts for group discussions and can be helpful tools for general discussions as part of team-building exercises. Questions such as these can also elicit hidden issues among staff members that have not previously been identified by managers. The data from such surveys are most helpful in identifying whether there are educational needs or attitudinal issues behind problems with standards of care. Finally, these questions can be used to generate baseline data for demonstrating and measuring change, as part of evaluating the effectiveness of organizational initiatives.

Table 20–2. Organizational assessment

Component	Element	Method
Social components	Attitudes of staff	Survey
	Knowledge of staff	Tests
	Orientation program	Content review
	Continuing education offerings	Review offerings
	Preferences of staff	Survey, team meeting
Technical components	Statement of philosophy of care	Content, theme analysis
	Expectations	Role descriptions
		Evaluation tool
		Reward system
	Documentation system	Review forms, standards
	Assignment pattern	Review patterns

There is a tendency in the health care professions, particularly in academic centers, to assume that the answer to changing behavior always lies with providing more education. While continuing education is often needed, attitudes and preferences play an equally strong role and must not be ignored. It is nonetheless helpful to review the education that has already been provided for the staff to identify factors contributing to inadequate palliative care. For example, if the initial ICU orientation does not address palliative care or pain management and none of the staff development activities involve concepts of palliative care, it is understandable that many staff will be lacking current knowledge in this area.

The tendency to focus on the knowledge base of personnel also contributes to a lack of attention to the technical aspects of the environment. These features are critically important in influencing behavior and must be carefully addressed. As indicated in Table 20–2, a good place to begin is with a statement expressing philosophy of care. Most critical care units do not have this kind of statement because it is assumed that the mission of the unit is clear—to save lives. A very helpful activity when initiating a process of change is to ask the staff to write a brief statement, four or five sentences, of the philosophy of that unit, specifying the mission and values. This is an unusual activity for most critical care personnel, but it can be very effective as an initial assessment tool, as an intervention to help the staff gain insight into the process of change, and as a baseline from which to measure change at a later point. In particular, given the assumptions of an organizational theory such as the sociotechnical theory, that workers, like managers, are motivated by a sincere desire to accomplish good work, this exercise provides useful information about how the staff feel about what they do and how they envision their contribution to patient welfare.

All environments are replete with features that communicate the expectations for behavior to staff. These are sometimes subtle and sometimes overt, but they always require modification to accomplish change. Role descriptions and evaluation tools should be examined for any explicit statements describing the desired behaviors. This might include such things as "coordinates multidisciplinary plans of care for dying patients," or "individualizes plan of care to meet the unique needs of dying patients and their families."

As managers, we know that expectations directly influence behavior, but we sometimes apply this principle only to our verbal expressions and neglect the many ways through which expectations are communicated. Another way in which expectations are conveyed is through reward systems. For nurses, these rewards might include such formal steps as promotion on a career ladder, or informal signs, such as receiving positive anecdotal notes in a personnel folder, being provided with some paid time for writing up care plans, or using work time to attend a conference on palliative care. Meir and colleagues argue for the importance of financial support for physicians, clinical and programmatic research, professorships, and the availability of teaching mentors in creating a positive climate for palliative care.[33]

In sociotechnical theory analysis, attention must also be paid to the routines and procedures in the environment that can act as barriers or facilitators to the desired work processes. Typically, there are many features in a critical care unit's operations that have strong effects on how work is accomplished, but two of the most significant for nurses are the assignment pattern and documentation system. Another obvious but frequently ignored principle is that consistency in care providers is an essential feature of quality. Because most patients in an ICU are there for only short periods of time, systems to ensure consistency, such as primary nursing, have not been well developed. For most patients, this does not have significant effects on their care. However, for the dying patient and the family, the establishment of personal, intimate relationships with caregivers and having confidence that the caregiver knows the plan of care and understands what is important in these last few days are absolutely critical. Clearly, there are multiple factors that have to be taken into account in making patient assignments on any one day, such as skill level, learning needs, and preferences of the staff, but consistency of care must be added to the list. Some units have adopted a pattern of forming "primary teams" to deal with the problems inherent to the use of 12-hour shifts, which tend to increase inconsistency over time.

The documentation system can also be either a barrier to or a facilitator of good-quality care, because physicians and nurses spend a large amount of time documenting or recording care processes. Quite simply, if critical care staff are to pay attention to certain aspects of care, requiring that these aspects be documented is a straightforward way to reinforce this behavior and provides a tool for monitoring. Although it is not a simple matter to alter documentation systems and habits without adding unrealistic expectations for cumbersome, redundant charting, it is possible to make some minor modifications that help guide staff in the desired direction. For example, if pain management is an issue, the addition of a column on the flow sheet for regular recording of the pain level, using a 1–10 scale, reminds staff to assess pain hourly. Voight and colleagues confirmed the effectiveness of this in their program to improve pain management in patients undergoing cardiac surgery.[34] Using a pre–post design, the researchers found a significant decrease in the average pain levels experienced by patients after the addition of a pain flowsheet to the standard documentation system.

Use of preprinted forms to document discussions and decisions made at a multidisciplinary team conference ensures that all staff are aware of plans. Display areas on computer screens can be designed for recording the name of a primary nurse and inputting automatic 7-day reminders to update care plans, with designated areas for documenting level of treatment limitation and approaches to pain and dyspnea management.

It is particularly useful to have preprinted forms that require specification of the goal of treatment for all decisions regarding treatment limitation. This prompts staff to evaluate the decision to withdraw or withhold specific interventions, such as mechanical ventilation or vasopressors, in light of the goal of care. The aim of this is to decrease the likelihood that such decisions will be arbitrary and more related to professional biases than being part of a coherent plan. For example, if the goal is to facilitate a peaceful and inevitable death, withdrawal of all life-prolonging interventions may be indicated. If, on the other hand, the goal is to maximize the chance of returning the patient to home once more without adding to the current burdens of treatment, withholding additional interventions might be indicated whereas withdrawing treatment and monitoring may not.

Consideration of documentation systems also involves evaluating the place of standardized care plans or care paths. These can be very helpful in guiding staff to attend to common areas, such as pain and other symptom management. Unfortunately, because dying patients do not fit neatly into single diagnostic categories, use of such standardized tools may result in more variances than compliance. If care paths are to be used, they must be written broadly enough to encompass the many different kinds of issues that come up.

A slightly different approach that has a rationale from the care path literature is to add standards to already existing care paths. For example, in the ICU, dying patients experience some specific, common trajectories and syndromes, including long-term mechanical ventilation, end-stage congestive heart failure, multi-organ system failure, and liver failure. It is therefore reasonable to add palliative care elements to any care paths used for these populations. These elements can be written with some flexibility, using such standards as holding a discussion of treatment limitation by the patient's fifth day in the ICU and repeating this discussion at least every 3 days therafter, involving the patient's clergy if desired by the patient and/or family by the third day of ICU stay; consulting with a social worker by day 3; and providing appropriate support resources to the family (e.g., grief counseling, support group name and number) by the day of the patient's death. This serves multiple purposes: it guides staff in knowing what behaviors are expected, it sets a standard for monitoring care as the patient is dying, and, perhaps most importantly, it works against the tendency to avoid thoughts of death.

Continuous Quality Improvement

Regardless of whether the issue of palliative care is addressed through major changes in the environment or minor modifications in procedure, attention to effectiveness must be ongoing, or else the strong technological and interventionist biases of the critical care environment are likely to overcome positive changes. The principles of continuous quality improvement (CQI) can be very useful in ensuring that ongoing needs are monitored and addressed.

Much has been written about this management technique.[35,36] Briefly, CQI is best understood as a framework for ensuring that there are continual improvements in the work of an organization.[37] The assumptions underlying the framework include, first and foremost, recognition that work production occurs within a system of interdependent parts and that improvements are a function of the application of values, professional knowledge, and knowledge of how to make improvements. Analysis of opportunities for improvement requires a thorough understanding of the processes of work that occur between the parts, as well as the identification of what constitutes quality, from both the consumer and professional standpoints.

The CQI approach to management departs from traditional management approaches in assuming, as in sociotechnical theory, that workers are creative and invested in their work, that identifying and removing barriers to productive work will enable them to achieve desired goals, and that learning and mastery are fundamental needs of all humans. Thus, motivating individuals to perform better does not require more rigid structures and rules but may instead require providing opportunities for employees to take part in the analysis of such barriers and to redesign more effective processes. Variations are not assumed to reflect poor performance of individuals but are instead analyzed to determine if the variation is assignable to system problems or if it is merely a common, random variation that cannot be reduced without altering the input or characteristics of the task.

This process can be illustrated through the following simplified analysis of a common problem in critical care units. Because of the complexity of illness in most patients, consultants are used quite routinely. Ideally, input from the consultants is transmitted through the primary team. That is, decision making remains with the primary team, and communication with patients and families should be made with the agreement of the team, through the team, or in the presence of someone from the primary team. In all cases, the consultant must be aware of the goals already established between patient and providers and of the plan of care. If several of the consultants frequently talk directly to patients' families without talking first with the primary team, this results in inconsistent messages to family members, confusion, and the need to reassess and regroup. One approach to addressing this problem might be to assume that the individual consultants are at fault. This might be followed by either ceasing to use these experts or by establishing a policy that no consultant may talk with the patient's family without first talking with the patient's primary physician. In this approach, it is assumed that the source of variance in question (inconsistent communication) can be traced to individuals not performing appropriately, without further analysis of any system factors that might generate this behavior.

A CQI analyst would instead first investigate the processes surrounding this aspect of work. Figure 20–1 is a simplified schema of the processes of communication regarding patient condition. The lines represent processes occurring between parts of the system, in this case, communication between different sets of people. The black circles represent points of analysis, indicating that every process surrounding the identified variance in procedure must be under-

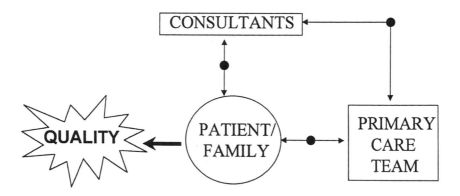

Figure 20–1. Continuous quality improvement process map of communication links related to contribution of consultant communication to quality of care. Arrows indicate two-way communication processes; black circles (nodes) indicate possible sources of variance.

stood and assessed as an opportunity for improvement. In our hypothetical situation, a discussion among all involved might reveal that first, there is some common variance in their behavior, simply because of unique, uncontrollable features of the clinical situation. Patients and their families, for example, may ask consultants to explain their findings as they are examining the patient; thus it is not reasonable to expect that no communication take place. In addition, there is often no one from the primary team available when the consultant examines the patient. Given this, it is imperative that the consultant have at least a basic understanding of the plan of care and current goals, knowledge of what further decisions are contingent on the consultant's recommendations, and a clear agreement with the primary team about communication with the patient and family. Thus, the process to target for improvement is not communication between consultant and family but rather the communication process that takes place between primary team and consultant prior to the consultation.

As can be seen from this example, CQI differs from isolated quality assurance projects in that it requires a philosophical commitment to both principles of improvement and human relations. It is founded on a deep appreciation of organizations as systems of interconnected and interdependent processes. A considerable body of literature has been developed on this topic and the reader is referred to these references for a more complete discussion.[35,37–39]

Conclusion

This chapter is intended to complement the more specific discussions of discrete areas for improving the care of dying patients in critical care units. Discussions in other chapters address the essential components of this care, such as pain management, communication techniques, and treatment withdrawal methods. This chapter has argued that in order to facilitate changes in one area and incorporate these changes into stable components, attention must be paid to the overall environment in which care takes place.

Features of the organizational environment that are most readily addressed are the physical location and the knowledge and skills of personnel. While these are always appropriate to target for improvement, a comprehensive understanding of the environment as a system of both parts and processes is required if we are to design and redesign ICUs that are not overwhelmingly characterized by the rule of rescue.

References

1. Wilson-Barnett J, Richardson A. Nursing research and palliative care. In: Oxford Textbook of Palliative Medicine (Doyle D, Hanks GWC, MacDonald N, eds.). New York: Oxford University Press, 1993, pp. 97–102.
2. Institute of Medicine, Committee on Care at the End of Life. Approaching Death. Washington, DC: National Academy Press, 1997.
3. Jastremski CA, Harvey M. Making changes to improve the intensive care unit experience for patients and their families. New Horizons. 1998;6:99–109.
4. Solomon MZ, O'Donnell L, Jennings B, Guilfoy V, Wolf SM, Nolan K, Jackson R, Koch-Wesner D, Donnelley S. Decisions near the end-of-life: professional views on life-sustaining treatments. Am J Public Health. 1993;83:14–23.
5. Puntillo K. Pain experiences of intensive care patients. Heart Lung. 1990;19:526–533.
6. Tittle M, McMillan SC. Pain and pain-related side-effects in an ICU and on a surgical unit: nurses' management. Am J Crit Care 1994;3:25–30.
7. SUPPORT Principle Investigators. A controlled trial to improve care for seriously ill hospitalized patients: the Study to Understand Prognoses and Preferences for Outcomes and Risks of Treatments (SUPPORT). JAMA. 1995;274:1591–1598.
8. Buckman R. Communication in palliative care: a practical guide. In: Oxford Textbook of Palliative Medicine (Doyle D, Hanks GWC, MacDonald N, eds.). New York: Oxford University Press, 1993, pp. 47–60.
9. Jacob D. Family decision making for incompetent patients in the ICU. Crit Care Nurs Clin North Am 1997;9:107–114.
10. Weir RF. Abating Treatment with Critically Ill Patients. New York: Oxford University Press, 1989.
11. U.S. Congress, Office of Technology Assessment. Institutional Protocols for Decisions about Life-Sustaining Treatments. Washington, DC: U.S. Government Printing Office, OTA-BA-389, 1988.
12. O'Toole EE, Youngner SJ, Juknialis BW, Daly BJ, Bartlett ET, Landefeld CS. Evaluation of a treatment limitation policy with a specific treatment-limiting order page. Arch Intern Med 1994;154:425–432.
13. Meisel A. The legal consensus about forgoing life-sustaining treatment: its status and its prospects. Kennedy Inst Ethics J 1993;2:309–343.

14. Seamark DA, Williams S, Hall M, Lawrence CJ, Gilbert J. Palliative terminal cancer care in community hospitals and a hospice: a comparative study. *Br J Gen Pract* 1998;June:1312–1316.
15. Morris JN, Mor V, Goldberg RJ, Sherwood S, Greer DS, Hiris J. The effect of treatment setting and patient characteristics on pain in terminal cancer patients: a report from the National Hospice Study. *J Chron Dis* 1986;39:27–35.
16. Elpern EH, Silver MR, Rosen RI, Bone RC. The noninvasive respiratory care unit. *Chest* 1991;99:205–208.
17. Gracey DR, Naessens JM, Viggiano RW. Outcomes of patients cared for in a ventilator-dependent unit in a general hospital. *Chest* 1995;107:494–99.
18. Becker FD. Workspace: Creating Environments in Organizations. New York: Praeger, 1981.
19. Passmore, WA. Designing Effective Organizations: The Sociotechnical Systems Perspective. New York: John Wiley & Sons, 1988.
20. Happ MB.Sociotechnical systems theory. *J Nurs Admin* 1993;23(6):47–54.
21. Mount BM. The problem of caring for the dying in a general hospital; the palliative care unit as a possible solution. *Can Med Assoc J* 1976;115:119–121.
22. Fisher RH, Nadon GW, Shedletsky R. Management of the dying elderly patient. *J Am Geriatr Soc* 1983;31:563–564.
23. Ford G. The development of palliative care services. In: Oxford Textbook of Palliative Medicine (Doyle D, Hanks GWC, MacDonald N, eds.). New York: Oxford University Press, 1993, pp. 36–47.
24. Asch DA, Shea,JA, Jedrziewski MK, Bosk CL. The limits of suffering: critical care nurses views of hospital care at the end of life. *Soc Sci Med* 1997;45:1661–1668.
25. Samarel N. Nursing in a hospital-based hospice unit. *Image* 1989;21:132–136.
26. Mathew LM, Jahnigen DW, Scully JH, Rempel P, Meyer TJ, LaForce FM. Attitudes of house officers toward a hospice on a medical service. *J Med Ed* 1983;58:772–777.
27. Campbell ML, Field BE. Management of the patient with do-not-resuscitate status: compassion and cost containment. *Heart Lung.* 1991;20:345–348.
28. Campbell ML, Frank RR. Experience with an end-of-life practice at a university hospital. *Crit Care Med* 1997;25:197–202.
29. Woodruff RK, Jordan L, Eicke JP, Chan A. Palliative care in a general teaching hospital. *Med J Aust* 1991;155:662–665.
30. Frommelt KHM. The effects of death education on nurses' attitudes toward caring for terminally ill persons and their families. *Am J Hospice Palliat Care* 1991; 8(5):37–43.
31. Hamilton J, Edgar L. A survey examining nurses' knowledge of pain control. *J Pain Symptom Manage* 1992;7(1):18–26.
32. McCaffery M, Pasero C. Pain Clinical Manual, 2nd ed. St. Louis: Mosby, 1999.
33. Meier DE, Morrison S, Cassel CK. Improving palliative care. *Arch Intern Med* 1997;127:225–230.
34. Voigt L, Paice JA, Pouliot JA. Standardized pain flowsheet: impact on patient-reported pain experiences after cardiovascular surgery. *Am J Crit Care* 1995;4:308–313.
35. Deming W. Out of the Crisis. Cambridge, MA: Massachusetts Institute of Technology; 1986.
36. Berwick DM. Continuous improvement as an ideal in health care. *N Engl J Med* 1989;320:55–56.

37. Batalden PB, Stoltz PK. A framework for the continual improvement of health care. *J Qual Improv* 1995;19:424–452.
38. Laffel G, Blumenthal D. The case for using industrial quality management science in healthcare organizations. *JAMA* 1989;262:2869–2873.
39. Cesta TG. The link between continuous quality improvement and case management. *J Nurs Admin* 1993;23(6):55–61.

Chapter 21

An International Perspective on Death in the ICU

MALCOLM FISHER

*T*he complex rituals and practices associated with death and dying vary among countries. Over the last 15 years, developed countries have shown a major interest in the period of dying, particularly as to the appropriate application and withdrawal of artificial forms of life support. The provision of a comfortable, dignified death was once a priority for the medical and nursing professions. In learning to use life support technology, medicine in developed countries focused on prolonging life, which, for some patients, led to a prolongation of suffering. This focus on life preservation led to the loss of the traditional skills of the healing professions in dealing with the dying patient. Much of the current literature on appropriate care of the dying stems from a desire to recapture those skills. Many factors, from both within the health professions and society at large, influence the international variability in end-of-life care in the ICU. Unfortunately, there is relatively little data on which to base formal comparisons between countries. Five factors that influence the variability in practice across countries are economic, cultural and religious, and legal issues and medical training.

Economic Factors

There is a close correlation between a country's gross domestic product and the life expectancy of its inhabitants. Of the 30,000,000 people who die annually, one-third die from infectious diseases. Three million people die of gastroenteritis and tuberculosis (TB). Four million children die of lung infections. AIDS-related disease is the most common cause of death in some African countries.[1] In contrast, in Western societies the "diseases of affluence" play a major role. In the least developed countries life expectancy is 52 years, in developing countries it is 64 years, and in the most developed countries it is 77 years.[1]

Even in affluent societies personal wealth plays a major role in the incidence of and outcome from disease. The complex issues that surround the prolongation of life by artificial means are of little relevance in many countries where intensive care is nonexistent or not regarded as a priority. In poor countries, health care needs related to sanitation, particularly water management, and vaccination take precedence over aggressive intensive care. The problems associated with survival so far outweigh the problems related to dying that the dilemmas faced by developed countries related to end-of-life care are inconsequential or nonexistent. Kavalier[2] wrote that in a hospital in Northern Uganda, medical practice was based on an expectation (shared with the patient) that the hospital is a place one goes to die, although his article produced strong reactions from others who had worked in the hospital.[3,4] In countries where the majority of the population have access only to rudimentary health care, the rich may have access to the best of technology and the latest treatment.[5] Those who practice in such environments justify this on the basis that quality health care must develop down as well as up. In developed countries, the poor and those of fringe religious and cultural beliefs may have greater ability to determine their medical care because of a greater access to medical care and a greater emphasis on human rights and equality. The availability of intensive care beds has an impact on the use of critical care for dying patients. Studies have shown that shortages of intensive care beds have a major influence on whether treatment is instituted or withheld and that even in counties where there are major bed shortages, patients are admitted to ICUs when there is little chance of survival.[6,7]

Cultural and Religious Factors

Lynn Payer, in her landmark book *Medicine and Culture*,[8] argues that cultural beliefs play a major role in the variability of health care in different countries, and that cultural beliefs may play a greater role than science in determining how medicine is practiced. The undesirable effects of the medicalization of dying are phenomena of affluent societies. People no longer die at home but in hospitals. Old age is not recognized in disease classification systems as a cause of death. Death is equated with medical failure. Magisterial processes investigate "unnatural death." Literature such as the Study to Understand Prognoses and Preferences for Outcomes and Risks of Treatments (SUPPORT) in the United States have identified a number of patients who die in pain or after treatment they do not wish to have, in spite of interventions to reduce this.[9]

Western ethical and cultural values have little meaning in other countries.[10] The basic ethical values of truth, beneficence, justice, and autonomy are assigned different relative values by different cultures. What is seen as appropriate by some is seen as paternalism and rejection of basic rights by others. Conflict due to differing values can be a major problem in cultures transplanted into other environments where the traditional beliefs of immigrant ethnic groups are not shared by the majority population. In Australia, for example, many Chinese and some Middle Eastern immigrants believe it is wrong to inform a patient of their impending death, whereas the Australian ethical standard is that the patient has the right not only to that information but also to determine who else receives the information. The advent of vocal advocacy groups, for example, ACT UP, which speaks for patients with AIDS, have forced discussions on improving the quality of terminal care and legalizing euthanasia.

Religion plays a major role in the shaping of a society's views on sanctity of life, the hereafter, and the right to die. Where religion plays a major role in government, lawmaking, and punishment, as in the Middle East, religion becomes the major driving force behind customs and laws relating to end-of-life decision making. In countries where prolonged life support is not available, religious views are characteristically more fatalistic and their role is restricted to the rituals surrounding death. Even for individuals from within a single religion, heterogeneity occurs. For this reason, it is important that the views of the patient and family be obtained, rather than assuming ideals based on perceived or attributed beliefs. At times, religious beliefs may conflict with requirements of civil law. For example, in Australia the Muslim belief that postmortem examination is wrong places them in conflict with the laws regarding magisterial referral and postmortem. At times the laws may be waived by the coroner on receipt of a statement asserting the family is without complaint or question with respect to the final illness and post mortem examinations are contrary to their beliefs.

The religious beliefs of health professionals have also been shown to have an impact on end-of-life decisions. Vincent[6] found that Roman Catholic doctors in Europe were more likely to treat a patient fully even if this was not the patient's wish. Withdrawal of care is unusual in Israel, but withholding care is permitted. Surprisingly, a U.S. study showed that Jewish doctors were more likely to withhold or withdraw life support than their Roman Catholic colleagues.[11]

Legal Factors

The appropriate role of the law and the courts in end-of-life decision making in terms of both legislation and medical care for individuals, is controversial. This controversy is expected in societies that have marked variation in the numbers of lawyers, the perceived role of lawyers, and access of the population to the legal system. Just as access to health care has a profound effect on the medicalization of death in a given society, access to and reliance on judicial relief has a similar effect on the role of the legal system in death.

The law can have an impact on end-of-life decision making in several ways. Formally, legislatures can pass laws related to the care of dying patients. For example, in the United States, a National Death Act was passed that established a national definition of death, including brain death criteria. In addition, highly publicized, precedent-setting cases ruled on by judges (for example, the *Cruzan* or *Quinlan* cases) affect future rulings and clinical practice. Finally, clinical practice may be subject to either criminal prosecution (which is extraordinarily rare for end-of-life care) or civil action. Physicians' perceptions of their risk for legal review in different countries are likely to influence their care of dying patients in the ICU, just as these perceptions influence their care in other areas of medicine.

Teaching

A further influence on practices at the end of life is medical training. Critical care fellows who train in other countries are able to witness end-of-life processes and adapt those they find of value and use to their own culture. Tai and Lew[12] noted that the practice of intensivists from Singapore with respect to management of the dying patient in ICU was substantially influenced by the intensivists trainingin Australia and the USA.

Consistent Findings in Developed and Developing Countries

Although there is considerable variation in the care of patients dying in ICUs, there are some broad features that distinguish this kind of care in developed countries from that in developing countries (Table 21–1). Evidence from several studies indicates that limitation of life-sustaining treatment from dying, critically ill patients is occurring more frequently in developed nations. Sprung and Eidleman[13] suggest that 25 years ago, most ICU patients died with aggressive resuscitative attempts, while in 1996, 35%–87% of deaths occurred after limitation of life support. Euthanasia, or the provision of treatments by clinicians to hasten death, is illegal in all countries. Nevertheless, there is evidence of the practice of euthanasia in some countries and it is likely that it is practiced covertly in most countries.[14,15]

While these features hold as generalities, there are considerable differences among countries. For example, the relative role of family, patient, and surrogates versus the role of physicians in making decisions for patients varies among countries. Differences in the availability of hospice and palliative care services as well as in the role of ethicists in bedside decision making also occur. There are major differences in the availability, usage, validity, and perceived

Table 21–1. Features distinguishing care of patients dying in ICUs of developed countries from that in developing countries

Developed Countries	Developing Countries
A desire to improve the quality of care of the dying patient	Restricted access
Value of autonomy, including respect for the rights of patients to refuse treatment and to a peaceful death	High-technology medicine has a relatively poor cost-benefit ratio compared to that of preventive medicine
Acceptance of an ethical and legal difference between killing and letting a patient die	Greater gaps between rich and poor for access and, in some cases, an apparent disregard by the rich and powerful for the fair distribution of resources
A desire to apply life-supporting technology appropriately	
Acknowledgment of the difficulty of outcome prediction	Death due to infectious diseases is more prominent
Acceptance that health professionals, patients, and families should be involved in end-of-life decisions, and patients and families should be treated in the context of their spiritual and cultural beliefs	End-of-life decision making is not a major social issue
Acceptance that use of "double-effect" drugs and withdrawal of artificial life support do not constitute criminal acts	
Illegality of assisted suicide and euthanasia	
Belief that society condones health professionals and families endeavouring to determine what an incompetent patient would want	
Health professionals' fear of decision making is based on financial incentives or bed shortages	
Increase in the rate of withholding or withdrawal of life-sustaining treatments in patients who die in the ICU.	

value of advance directives among countries. Following is a geographic outline of some of the variations that have been observed in end-of-life care of critically ill patients.

End-of-Life Care in Europe and Individual Countries

Europe

Two comprehensive studies of European attitudes and practices have been undertaken by Vincent.[6,7] In the first study, admissions were limited by bed availability but most units admitted patients little hope of survival. There was less information given to families than in the United States. Vincent noted that critically ill patients in Europe are rarely informed about their condition. Only 16% of respondents, for example, would inform the patient or relatives of an adverse incident although 50% felt they should. Only 10% of respondents believed they delivered complete information to their patients and only 13% felt they should do so. There was marked variation in the use of do-not-resuscitate (DNR) orders (used by 83% of respondents), withholding and withdrawing life support (used by 63% of respondents), and practicing euthanasia (used by 36% of respondents). In the second study it was noted that the withholding and withdrawal of treatment had increased since the previous study (93% vs. 83% for withholding, and 77% vs. 63% for withdrawal), and it was suggested that these practices had become more generally accepted by the medical profession in Europe. Most deaths in European ICUs occur following the withdrawal of life-sustaining therapies. The deliberate administration of drugs until death ensues did not markedly increase. In contrast to the United States, most decisions were made by doctors; families' requests to limit life-sustaining treatment had little influence on decision making.

There is a heterogeneity of attitudes and practice in Europe, regarding care for the dying. Eighty percent of respondents felt that written DNR orders should be applied, but only 58% did so, with a wide variation occurring according to country (from 8% in Italy to 91% in The Netherlands). The countries of southern Europe apply DNR orders less than those of the north. Important differences in attitudes also exist among European countries. Written DNR orders were applied by 58% of respondents, with considerable variation occurring among countries, ranging from 8% in Italy to 91% in The Netherlands. In northern European countries, The Netherlands, Switzerland, and the United Kingdom, DNR orders were more frequently discussed with the patient than in Spain, Greece, and Portugal.

Bed availability was a major factor in the use of intensive care in Spain, Portugal, and the United Kingdom. Fifty-two percent of respondents involved the entire ICU staff in decisions to withdraw life support and 45% limited participation in decision making to medical staff. Decisions were more commonly made by physicians in Italy, Greece, and Portugal and by the ICU staff as a whole in the United Kingdom and Switzerland. Doctors with a Catholic background were less likely to withhold ($p < 0.05$) and withdraw ($p < 0.01$) therapy than their protestant or agnostic counterparts. Physicians from Switzerland, the United Kingdom, Belgium, and the Netherlands withdrew therapy more commonly than doctors from Greece, Italy, and Portugal ($p < 0.01$). Deliberate drug administration to hasten death was more common in France, The Netherlands, and Belgium, and less common in Portugal and Italy. Ninety-three percent of doctors sometimes withheld treatment from patients with no hope of a meaningful life, but withdrawal of treatment was less common.

United Kingdom

Intensive care in the United Kingdom is characterized by a smaller number of beds per person and less funding than in other developed countries and, consequently, greater acuity of illness.[16] In a study from one unit, 81.5% of 65 patients who died had some limitation of therapy.[17] The mean time from decision not to continue active treatment to death was 13.2 hours. Granger and colleagues[18] noted major inadequacies in ICUs in the United Kingdom in both facilities for and training in management of the bereaved. As in the United States and Australia, there is support for euthanasia and physician-assisted suicide among members of the public and patients. In a small study, Emanual and colleagues found that two-thirds of oncology patients and the public viewed euthanasia and physician-assisted suicide as acceptable. There was a lower acceptance among oncologists.[19] Urwin[20] noted that guidelines for withdrawing life support were less readily available than in the United States and that such issues tend to be treated in a secretive manner.

The House of Lords condemned euthanasia and suggested that a code of practice rather than legislation dictate care for competent patients.[21] United Kingdom case law has established a legal difference between killing and relieving of suffering that shortens life. The law has endorsed the rights of competent patients to refuse treatment and that disconnection of artificial ventilation on request does not constitute assisted suicide.[20] A recent U.K. case that received considerable attention was the decision that it was not unlawful to withdraw feeding from Tony Bland, a young man in a persistent vegetative state. This led to a process by which appeals to the High Court for a decision to withdraw treatment may be made by families having two supporting medical specialists.[22] The Roman Catholic Church expressed strong dissenting views based on the Vatican Statement of 1990 and a consensus statement of Bishops equating withdrawal of feeding with lethal injection.[23] One interesting U.K. development was that the Exeter Health Region introduced resuscitation of dead patients to provide organs for transplantation. This was declared illegal some time after introduction of this practice.

Japan

Fukara et al.[24] (1995) found that DNR orders were written for most (72%) patients who died in a Japanese teaching hospital but that only 5% of patients were involved in decisions about their own DNR orders. A 1995 court case in Yokohama found that life support could be withdrawn if a terminally ill patient or the patient's family, acting on their understanding of the patient's wishes, requested it. One of the unique aspects of Japanese medicine is the absence of transplantation from beating heart donors. In Japan, it is illegal to take organs under these circumstances even if the patient is brain dead.

Israel

Israel religion, politics, and law are more interrelated than in many other societies. According to Jewish law, one is prohibited from hastening death in the terminally ill by withdrawing care, although withholding care is permitted.[25] Where the practice of intensive care occurs in institutions with a strong Orthodox view, therapy is only withdrawn in patients who are brain dead or in whom the therapy is shown to have no effect. Two studies have shown that withholding treatment leads to death within 48 hours in most critically ill patients[25] and Eidleman and colleagues suggest that the withholding of treatment should often be considered an alternative to withdrawal.[25] In contrast, most doctors who responded to a questionnaire in the United States regarded withholding and withdrawal of life support as the same, although 26% were "more disturbed" by withdrawing it than by withholding it.[26] It is interesting to note that in a small questionnaire study of nurses who care for cancer and dementia patients, 50% of Israeli nurses favored including euthanasia as a treatment option.[27]

Ireland

The Irish Supreme Court recently judged that it would be an inequitable denial of a constitutional human right if a patient unable to express his or her wishes were not permitted a mechanism of terminating a medical intervention through a surrogate decisionmaker.[28]

New Zealand

Streat and Judson[29] have described a gatekeeping role for intensivists who "do not admit patients who are very unlikely to benefit." They note that there is little constraint generated by concerns about autonomy in situations where therapy is not indicated on medical grounds. They further state that withdrawal of therapy involves medical consensus followed by family discussion. In general, "families are not asked to make life-and-death decisions, or even to participate in these decisions, because clinicians consider these decisions our medical responsibility. Consensus rather than permission is sought but families are asked to for their agreement to withdraw care." This is similar to the process in Australia. In a landmark case in New Zealand it was ruled that disconnecting a patient (who could not participate in decision making) with severe Guilliane Barre syndrome from a ventilator did not constitute an offence. The ventilator was disconnected.[29]

Hong Kong

Ip et al.[30] have noted that there are competitive cultural and ethical values in Hong Kong because of the coexistence of Chinese and Western medicine and a predominantly Chinese population practicing many Chinese cultural traditions.

The Chinese think harmony, responsibility, and respect for patients and ancestors are more important than the Western values of autonomy, individual rights, and self-determination. Do-not-resuscitate orders are rarely used. It is very unusual for doctors to discuss advance directives or suitability of resuscitation. To tell someone that they are dying is considered rude and dangerous. Decisions to withdraw life support are usually initiated by doctors and made with the consent of the family. Euthanasia is prohibited by law, but there is no legislation regarding autonomy, advance directives, or withdrawal of life support. Medical litigation is rare.

United States

Although most medical, legal, and ethical writing about end-of-life care comes from the United States, to the outsider, the situation there can be confusing. The conflicts are related to the cosmopolitan and multicultural nature of the population, the contractual relationship between doctor and patient, and the U.S. propensity to invoke the legal system in end-of-life decisions. It further appears that in the United States, the wishes of families, irrespective of the possibility of survival, play a major part in continuing inappropriate therapy. The SUPPORT studies[9] in particular are very disturbing, as they report an unacceptable incidence of patients dying in pain, receiving treatment they do not wish, and not understanding what is going on. The provision of a team of support workers and detailed prognostic information to attempt to rectify the situation made no difference. It is therefore not surprising that Asch[15] found a significant incidence of nurse-assisted suicide or euthanasia in ICUs. He suggested that of 852 nurses in U.S. ICUs, 17% had received requests for active euthanasia and 16% had complied with the requests and an additional 4% reported they had hastened death by "pretending" to provide life-sustaining treatment.[15] While the validity of the survey has been challenged, these results are though provoking.

In many hospitals, doctors avoid determining or simply override the wishes of patients.[9] Nonetheless, there is evidence that the withdrawal of life support is increasing.[31] A study of the rate of DNR decisions showed that this rate doubled between 1984 and 1988[32] and a second regional study found recommendations to withdraw or withhold therapy from ICU patients had increased from 51% in 1987/1988 to 91% in 1992/1993.[33] A more comprehensive study showed a reduction in attempts at carciopulmonary resuscitation (CPR) prior to death and an increase in withdrawal of life support. Of 5910 patients who died, 23% received full ICU care including failed CPR, 22% received full ICU care without CPR, 10% had life support withheld, and 38% had life support withdrawn. There was a wide variation among different units.[34] The intriguing possibility that the method of remuneration of the attending physician may be important determinants of end-of-life management has been raised by Cher and Levert.[35] Their data suggested that expensive and futile interventions were less common in patients receiving managed care than in fee-for-service patients. Curtis and Rubenfeld have criticized the study and suggest that a death which appears economically sound may not be what the patients would wish and that limitation of technology may be associated with limitation of opportunity for a good outcome.[36] Attending physician behavior seems to have an important affect on care at the end of life. Kollef[37] reviewed 159 patients' deaths in an academic tertiary care MICU. Withdrawal of treatment was 2.5 times more likely if the patient received care from the ICU attending rather than their private non-ICU attending physician.

In the United States, most of the public and many physicians favor legalization of physician-assisted suicide.[38] An active political and legal debate is occuring including patient-sponsored referenda and new legislation. Critics have commented on the efforts to change euthanasia laws by observing that the costs of advertising campaigns to retain or eliminate Oregon's assisted suicide laws would fund hospice care for uninsured Oregonians for 3 years.[39]

It is certainly possible that we have a better idea of what is wrong with end-of-life care in the United States because of the considerable amount of information about practices and attitudes that is available from this country. However, there is an apparent dichotomy between the practice guidelines produced by experts and medical societies and the actual practice in the United States. It is likely that similar problems occur in other countries.

Australia

Although a cosmopolitan and multiracial society as diverse as the United States, Australia has a much smaller population and the attitudes to withdrawal of treatment seem to lie between those of Europe and the United States. Raper and Fisher[40,41] noted that 80% of their patients who died did so after withdrawal of life support and suggested that in Australia, the families of the critically ill, irrespective of ethnic and social background, preferred to acquiesce to the decisions of doctors rather than make decisions themselves regarding withdrawal of care. These authors advocated a system in which all the involved health care workers should reach consensus about appropriateness before seeking agreement with patient and/or family. Daffurn and colleagues[42] described a policy that excluded family from the clinical decision and the family were simply told the patient was dying. When this decision had been reached, all observations, monitoring, drugs (except narcotics), procedures, and routine care (including feeds and fluids) were ceased. If mechanical ventilation was continued, the oxygen concentration was reduced to room air.

Surveys of doctors and lay people in Australia usually show attitudes supportive of euthanasia and assisted suicide, but medical organizations oppose the introduction of both practices. In a 1993 study of 943 nurses in Victoria, 759 supported active euthanasia, 93% had been asked by patients to hasten death, and 1 out of 10 had complied with this request without medical consultation.[43] Kuhse and colleagues showed in 1997 that of all Australian deaths that involved a medical end-of-life decision, 1.8% involved euthanasia or assisted suicide, the ending of life without specific patient request in 3.5%, withholding or withdrawal of potentially life-prolonging treatment in 28.6%, and use of opioids in doses large enough to shorten life in 30.9%. They suggested that in 30% of all Australian deaths, a medical decision was made with the explicit intent of shortening life and 4% of these decisions were made at the request of the patient. These authors conclude that Australian law does not prevent such practices among doctors.[14]

Australia shares with the United States a diversity of state laws regarding brain death, surrogacy, and living wills. There is also diversity among states as to making decisions regarding end of life. In South Australia, The Living Will has legal status, although few patients have obtained the document. In Victoria a nominated spokesperson has legal status and in New South Wales, a Guardianship Board is the legal representative of the incompetent patient both for end-of-life decisions and consent for procedures and to participate in clinical trials. In spite of the legality of the situation in New South Wales, end-of-life decisions are invariably made by health workers and families. Proposed Right to Die legislation in New South Wales was rejected by all groups at a public meeting. As a result of this process, Health Department "Interim Guidelines For Withdrawal of Care" were established, leaving such matters to doctors, patients, and families.[44] Withdrawal of life support, and for a brief period, euthanasia were legal in the Northern Territory but the legislation was overturned by Federal parliament. Kissane and colleagues[45] reviewed the seven patients who made use of the Terminally Ill Act. Four patients died and the process in the deaths was assisted suicide using a computer to control self-administration of a lethal intravenous cocktail, rather than euthanasia. Kissane and colleagues noted differing medical opinions regarding the terminal nature of the illnesses and the common symptoms of depression, and commented on the social isolation of three patients. Thirteen Victorian doctors in Australia have publicly announced that they have taken patient's lives and no prosecutions have followed. In another case, a lay person was found guilty of assisting in a suicide but given a suspended sentence. In general, the Australian legal system appears reluctant to be involved in end-of-life decision making.

Saudi Arabia

Chang[46] has noted the concern of Saudi doctors over whether transplantation contravened the dictates of the Prophet Mohammed. A fatwa (Muslim religious decision) permitting organ retrieval from cadavers was passed in 1982 and subsequently brainstem death was deemed equatable with cardiorespiratory death. Religious considerations and a need for unanimity dominate medical decision making in this country. Relatives involved in organ donation decision making usually require a unanimous decision by family and it is likely that a religious representative will be present to explain both the fatwa and the Prophet's teaching.

South Africa

South African medicine is a unique balance of first- and third-world medicine and disease. In a study of one unit, 86% of 45 patients who died had had treatment limited.[17] Recently, the South African government has openly endorsed rationing by effectively restricting the artificial ventilation of neonates of less than 1000 g weight with the limitation of supplies of surfactant. In addition, the cardiac transplant program at Groote Schur Hospital (where the first heart transplant was performed) has been stopped for economic reasons.

Switzerland

Thirty percent of families of patients who died in the ICU reported that they were dissatisfied with the standard of communication and that this was more likely to be so if the news of death was received by telephone rather than in person.[47]

India

Udwadia and colleagues[5] note that that although the major health problems remain malnutrition and infection, there are ICUs, particularly in the private sector. In spite of religious, cultural, and philosophical diversity, the fundamental ethical values of good and evil, right and wrong, and the sanctity of life are similar. There are no living wills with legal validity. Withholding of life support is practiced in almost all ICUs, and although withdrawal of life support in the absence of brain death has no legal sanction, it is increasingly practiced. Brain death is legally recognized for purposes of transplantation.

Canada

Wood and Martin[48] showed a 64.5% incidence of withdrawal of treatment in 110 deaths in one unit over 12 months. The Canadian Clinical Trials Group[49] used a questionnaire with hypothetical cases to examine the attitudes of health care workers about withdrawal of life support and found that likelihood of long-term survival, survival of the acute episode, premortem cognitive function, and age were major factors leading doctors to consider termination of life support, and that in only 1 of 12 scenarios was the same action chosen by more than 505 of 1361 respondents. Opposite extremes of care were chosen by greater than 20% in 8 of 12 scenarios, and identifiable factors affecting choice were the number of years from graduation from medical school, ICU size, and location. The authors concluded that most patients' care is determined in large part by provider attitudes and that many patients would find this unsatisfactory.

Keenan and colleagues[50] found that more intensive care patients had life support withheld in community hospitals than in teaching hospitals and more teaching hospital patients had life support withdrawn.

In Canada, a government inquiry has outlawed euthanasia and two court cases have occurred over assisted death, one leading to the conviction and disbarring of the doctor and a second in which the doctor was exonerated by a lower court. In 1998 a Manitoba court gave a Winnipeg hospital the right to impose a DNR order on a comatose child over the wishes of the child's parents. In 1999 the court ordered physicians to rescind a DNR order on a 79-year-old man whom doctors said would degenerate into a vegetative state if he received CPR. Madam Justice Beard rejected the doctors' argument that doctors are the best qualified to make medical decisions on DNR orders, as "doctors can and do make mistakes."[51] Maurice Generaux, a Canadian doctor, was recently sentenced to years imprisonment with 3 years probation after he pleaded guilty to assisting suicide.

The Netherlands

In a recent study of European countries, Vincent[7] found that intensive care doctors from The Netherlands were most likely to involve the patient and family in end-of-life decisions and to write DNR orders. The Netherlands is unique in its adoption of voluntary euthanasia as a condoned rather than legal practice while still officially illegal. Nevertheless, this practice is still quite rare. Van der Wal and colleagues[52] showed that 2.4% of deaths studied resulted from euthanasia and 0.2%–0.4% from physician-assisted suicide. In 0.7% of cases, the decision was made without the explicit consent of the patient. Pain and symptoms were alleviated with doses of opioids that may have shortened life. In 20.2% of patients, decisions to withdraw or withhold life support were made.

The Dutch legal basis for the practice of euthanasia, discussed by Brahams,[53] is as follows. A doctor who acts with due care and within generally accepted medical standards should not be convicted under the penal code, and a physician's duty to abide by the law and respect the life of the patient may be outweighed "by his other duty to help a patient who is suffering unbearably, who depends on him and for whom, to end his suffering, there is no alternative but death." Brahams[53] notes two successful defenses of doctors who injected lethal doses of d-tubocurarine in terminally ill patients. The Court's response to a request by a patient's husband for cessation of tube feeding was to rule that the decision was a medical one and must be made by the doctors.

Conclusion

The literature on international variations in the management of the dying, critically ill patient reflects the diverse economic, cultural, legal, and religious beliefs of countries and societies. The literature also shows that efforts are being made to improve the appropriateness and compassion with which intensive care patients are managed, but there appears to be a greater ability to document the principles of care than to deliver this care at the bedside. There is an apparent desire to improve the quality of care and to fulfill the goals expressed by Dunstan in 1985: "The success of intensive care is not to be measured only by the statistics of survival, as though each death were a medical failure. It is to be measured by the quality of lives preserved or restored, the quality of the dying of those in whose interest it is to die, and by the quality of relationships involved in each death."[54]

References

1. McGregor A. "Fatal complacency" over health says WHO. *Lancet* 1996;347:1478.
2. Kavalier F. Uganda: death is always just around the corner. *Lancet* 1998;352:141–142.
3. Murphy O. Support for Mbarara Hospital. *Lancet* 1998;352:735–736.
4. Mutakooha, EK Support for Mbarara Hospital. *Lancet* 1998:352;735
5. Udwadia FE, Guntupalli KK, Vidyasagar D. Critical care in India. *Int Perspect Crit Care* 1997;13:317–329.
6. Vincent JL. European attitudes towards ethical problems in intensive care medicine: results of an ethical questionnaire. *Intensive Care Med* 1990;16:256–264.
7. Vincent JL. Foregoing life support in Western European intensive care units: The results of an ethical questionnaire. *Crit Care Med* 1999;27:1626–1633.
8. Payer L. Medicine and Culture: Notions of Health and Sickness. London: Victor Gollancz, 1990.
9. Support Principal Investigators. A controlled trial to improve care for seriously ill patients: the Study to Understand Prognoses and Preferences for Outcomes and Risks of Treatments (SUPPORT) *JAMA* 1995;274;1591–1636.
10. Nyman DJ, Sprung CL. International perspectives on ethics in critical care. *Int Perspect Crit Care* 1997;13:409–416.
11. Society for Critical Care Medicine Ethics Committee. Attitudes of critical care medicine professionals concerning forgoing life-sustaining treatments. *Crit Care Med* 1992;20:320–326.
12. Tai, DYH, Lew TWK. Foregoing life support in medically futile patients. *Ann Acad Med Singapore* 1998;27:430–436.
13. Sprung CL, Eidelman LA. Worldwide similarities and differences in the forgoing of life-sustaining treatments. *Intensive Care Med* 1996;22:1003–1005.
14. Kuhse H, Singer P, Baume P, Clark M, Rickard M. End-of-life decisions in Australian medical practice. *Med J Aust* 1997;166:191–196.
15. Asch DA. The role of critical care nurses in euthanasia and assisted suicide. *N Engl J Med* 1996;334:1734–1739.
16. Bion J. Europe. *New Horizons* 1994;2:341–344.
17. Turner JS, Michell WL, Morgan CJ, Benetar SR. Withdrawal of life support. Frequency and practice in a London and a Cape Town intensive care unit. *Intensive Care Med* 1996;22:1020–1025.

18. Granger, CE, George C, Shelley MP. The management of bereavement on intensive care units. *Intensive Care Med* 1995;21:429–436.

19. Emanual GJ, Fairclough DL, Daniels ER, Claridge BR. Euthanasia and physician-assisted suicide attitudes and experiences of oncology patients, oncologists, and the public. *Lancet* 1996;347:1805–1810.

20. Urwin JL. United Kingdom. In: Critical Care: Standards, Audit and Ethics. (Tinker J, Browne DRG, Sibbald WJ, eds.). London: Hodder Healing, 1996, pp. 367–372.

21. Editorial: Their Lordships on euthanasia. *Lancet* 1994:343:430–431.

22. Brahams P. Persistent vegetative state. *Lancet* 1993;XX:341–428.

23. Cole AP. Letting vegetative patients die. *BMJ* 1993;306:142–143.

24. Fukaura A, Tazawa H, Nakajima H, Adachi M. Do-not-resuscitate orders at a teaching hospital in Japan. *New Engl J Med* 1995;333:805–808.

25. Eidelman LA, Jakobson DJ, Pizov R, Geber D, Leibovitz L, Sprung CL. Forgoing life-sustaining treatment in an Israeli ICU. *Intensive Care Med* 1998;24:162–166.

26. Society of Critical Care Medicine. The Society of Critical Care Medicine Ethics Committee consensus statement on the triage of critically ill patients. *JAMA* 1994;271:1200–1203.

27. Davis AJ, Davidson B, Hirschfield M, Lauri S, Ying Lin J, Norberg A, Phillips L, Pitman E, Hui Shen C, Vaander Laan R, Zhang HL, Ziv I. An international perspective of active euthanasia: attitudes of nurses in seven countries. *Int J Nurs Stud* 1993;30:301–310.

28. Phelan D. hopeless cases in intensive care. *Care Crit Ill* 1995;11:196–197.

29. Streat S, Judson JA. New Zealand. *New Horizons* 1994;2:392–403.

30. Ip M, Gilligan T, Koenig B, Raffin TA. Ethical decision making in critical care in Hong Kong. *Crit Care Med* 1998;26:447–451.

31. Koch KA, Rodeffer HD, Wears RL. Changing patterns of terminal care management in an intensive care unit. *Crit Care Med* 1994;22:233–243.

32. Prendergast TJ, Luce JM. Increasing incidence of withholding and withdrawal of life support from the critically ill. *Am J Respir Crit Care Med* 1997;155:15–20.

33. Prendergast TJ, Claessens MT, Luce JM. A national survey of end-of-life care for critically ill patients. *Am J Respir Crit Care Med* 1998;158:1163–1167.

34. Cher DL, Levert LA. Method of Medicare reimbursement and the rate of potentially ineffective care of critically ill patients. 1997;278:1001–1007.

35. Curtis JR, Rubenfeld GD. Aggressive medical care at the end of life: does capitated reimbursement encourage the right care for the wrong reasons. *JAMA* 1997;275:1001–1007.

36. Kollef M. Private attending physician status and withdrawal of life-sustaining interventions in the medical intensive care population. *Crit Care Med* 1996;24:968–273.

37. Sprung C, Oppenheim A. End-of-life decisions in critical care medicine—where are we headed. *Crit Care Med* 1992;26:200–202.

38. Tolle SW. Care of the dying: clinical and financial lessons from the Oregon experience. *Am Intern Med* 1998;128:567–568.

39. Fisher MM, Raper RF. Withdrawing and withholding treatment in intensive care. Part 1. Social and ethical dimensions. *Med J Aust* 1990;153:217–220.

40. Fisher MM, Raper RF. Withdrawing and withholding treatment in intensive care. Part 1. Social and ethical dimensions. *Med J Aust* 1990;153:217–220.

41. Fisher MM, Raper RF. Withdrawing and withholding treatment in intensive care. Part 3. Practical aspects. *Med J Aust* 1990;153:222–225.

42. Daffurn K, Kerridge R, Hillman KM. Active management of the dying patient. *Med J Aust* 1992;157:701–704.

43. Kuhse H, Singer P. Voluntary euthanasia and the nurse. An Australian survey. *Int J Nurs Stud* 1993;30:311–322.

44. New South Wales Health Dying With Dignity. Interim Guidelines on Management. State Health Publication No. (HPA) 93–93. 1993.

45. Kissane DW, Street A, Nitschke P. Seven deaths in Darwin: case studies under the Rights of the Terminally Ill Act, Northern Territory, Australia. *Lancet* 1998; 352:1097–1102.

46. Chang RW. Saudi Arabia. *New Horizons* 1994;2375–2380.

47. Malacrida R, Bettilini CM, Degrate A, Martinez M, Badia A, Piazza J, Vizzardi N, Wullschleger R, Rapin CH. Reasons for dissactisfaction: a survey of relatives of intensive patients who died. *Crit Care Med* 1998;26:1187–1193.

48. Wood GG, Martin E. Withholding and withdrawing life-sustaining treatment in a Canadian intensive care unit. *Can J Anesth* 1995;42:186–191.

49. Cook D, Guyatt GH, Jaeschke R, Reeve J, Spanier A, King D, Molloy DW, Willan A, Streiner DL. Determinants in Canadian healthcare workers of the decisions to withdraw life support from the critically ill. *JAMA* 1995;273:703.

50. Keenan SP, Busche KD, Liddy MC, Rosmin E, Inman KJ, Sibbald WJ. Withdrawal and witholding of life support in the intensive care unit: a comparison of teaching and community hospitals. *Crit Care Med* 1998;26:245–251.

51. Kondro W. Do-not-resuscitate order lifted in Canada. *Lancet* 1998;352:1689.

52. van der Wal G, Haverkate I, Van Der De Graff CLM, Kester JCG, Onwuteaka-Philipsen DB, van der Heide A, Bosma JM, Willems DLL. Euthanasia, physician-assisted suicide, and other medical practices involving the end of life in The Netherlands, 1990–1995. *N Engl J Med* 1996;335:1699–1705.

53. Brahams D. Euthanasia in The Netherlands. *Lancet* 1990;335:591–592.

54. Dunstan GR. Hard questions in intensive care. *Anaesthesia* 1985;40:479–482.

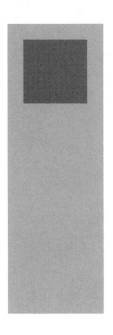

Part V

*Specific
Diseases and
Special
Populations*

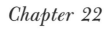

Chapter 22

AIDS

MARK J. ROSEN

Since the start of the human immunodeficiency virus (HIV) epidemic almost two decades ago, the demographics of acquired immunodeficiency syndrome (AIDS) and the treatment of HIV-related disorders has seen more rapid and dramatic changes than perhaps any other illness in recent history. New preventive and therapeutic strategies changed the incidence of life-threatening diseases and their outcomes. Even though the number of patients with AIDS admitted to ICUs is far smaller than those with heart disease, lung disease, and cancer, our experience with AIDS shows clearly how new treatments change outcomes, which in turn influence medical practice and the attitudes of patients and providers about life-sustaining treatments and end-of-life care. Also, political and social advocacy efforts engendered by the AIDS epidemic surely helped to catalyze progress in palliative care.

By July 1998, over 665,000 cases of AIDS were reported in the United States, and over 400,000 died.[1] The worldwide impact is far more devastating, as the vast majority of all HIV-infected persons live in the underdeveloped nations of Africa and Asia. In these parts of the world, intensive care is usually not available, and end-of-life issues are not as complex. Therefore, this section will deal with intensive care in patients with HIV in developed nations.

Epidemiology

In the 12 months before July 1, 1998, 54,407 new cases of AIDS were reported to the Centers for Disease Control, a 15% decline from the previous 12 months. New cases are increasingly likely to be injection drug users and heterosexual partners of HIV-infected persons, and less likely to be gay men. The

U.S. death rate associated with AIDS also declined dramatically since 1995. Rates of opportunistic infections are declining in all transmission categories and racial/ethnic groups. As a result, more people in the United States are living with AIDS; as of July 1998, over 258,000 are living with HIV infection without an AIDS-defining disorder. These people are also increasing likely to be African-American or Latino, groups who may have difficulty accessing good health care, and who may have special issues about communication with providers and about end-of-life care.

The dramatic decline in AIDS mortality since 1996 is attributed primarily to the use of potent antiretroviral therapy (PAT).[2] This form of treatment uses combination therapy, usually including a protease inhibitor, with the goal of inhibiting HIV replication and enhancing immune function.[3] The success of this strategy changed the perception of AIDS as a progressive and fatal disease to a chronic controllable illness. The effects of PAT on admissions to ICUs and ICU mortality by persons with HIV infection are not known, as specific data on this question are not yet available. It is reasonable to infer that the overall reductions in AIDS-related mortality are probably reflected in fewer ICU admissions and deaths, but one could also speculate that increased hope for prolonged survival would encourage patients to choose aggressive support that they may otherwise forego. More research is needed to determine the effects of these treatments on ICU utilization and patients' and providers' attitudes on the use of mechanical ventilation and other invasive interventions in patients with AIDS.

Patient Preferences

A few surveys have examined HIV-infected persons' preferences about life-sustaining treatments, but they are limited by the small numbers and cross section of subjects, who are predominantly gay men. In 1985, 118 gay men were interviewed about their attitudes concerning life-sustaining treatment.[4] In the hypothetical scenario of severe *Pneumocystis carinii* pneumonia (PCP), 55% wanted admission to an ICU and mechanical ventilation, and 46% wanted cardiopulmonary resuscitation (CPR); these results demonstrate considerable variability in patients' preferences. More recently, Singer and colleagues showed that of 101 patients with HIV infection, over 60% preferred mechanical ventilation and CPR in the event of a potentially reversible illness.[5] Another study showed that patients' preferences were associated with ethnicity, as white patients were twice as likely to prefer the primary goal of relieving pain to that of extending life. This association persisted after controlling for education, income, and HIV risk behavior.[6]

Although patients with HIV infection may have preferences about end-of-life care, and communication with their providers increases the likelihood that they will receive the care they desire, these discussions do not always occur.[7] In a 1985 survey, 73% of patients wanted to discuss life-sustaining treatment with their physicians, but only a third reported having done so. In another study, 68% of over a thousand persons with AIDS knew about advance directives, but only 11% ever talked with their providers about them; gay men were more likely to have been counseled and to have executed an advance directive than drug users or women.[8] Another study showed that even though whites and nonwhites wanted to discuss end-of-life care with their doctors in equal proportions, white patients were more likely to have had that discussion.[9]

ICU Utilization

Patients with AIDS are admitted to ICUs because of critical illnesses that are usually related to HIV infection. In most studies, the most common cause for ICU admission is PCP, which is also the most common AIDS-indicator disorder.[10] However, patients are admitted with a wide range of critical illnesses that may or may not be related to HIV infection, including other opportunistic infections, sepsis, hypotension, gastrointestinal hemorrhage, seizures, trauma, and drug overdose.

Data on how often patients with AIDS are admitted to ICUs are scarce, but it seems that the great majority of deaths of patients with AIDS do not involve an ICU admission. In the Pulmonary Complications of HIV Infection Study, 1130 HIV-infected adults who did not have AIDS at the time of enrollment were followed prospectively for a mean of 3.8 years in six U.S. centers.[11] By the end of the study, 354 (31%) of the original cohort died, but only 209, or 59% of all deaths, occurred in the hospital. Of the 1320 total hospital admissions, only 68 (5%) included admission to an ICU, and only 25 deaths (7% of all deaths) occurred during a hospitalization with an ICU admission. Therefore, ICUs were involved in a very small proportion of hospital admissions and deaths. The reasons for the low ICU utilization could not be determined because these data were not collected systematically. In many cases, physicians did not recommend invasive interventions in patients with advanced HIV disease, and patients often declined hospitalization and ICU care.[4,12] These data should not be extrapolated to current patients with AIDS for several reasons. First, this study took place before PAT was widely used; admission rates are now probably lower, but patients and caregivers may be more likely to choose intensive care. The cohort also had ongoing access to providers who were available to counsel them on hospitalization and ICU care, a resource not available to many patients. Finally, 72% of the cohort were gay men, who may be more likely than others with AIDS to choose comfort measures if they develop a critical illness.

Outcomes of Respiratory Failure Due to PCP

Most investigations of intensive care for patients with AIDS focused on patients with respiratory failure due to PCP. Respiratory failure is usually defined as the need for intubation and mechanical ventilation, and survival is defined as discharge from the hospital. As changes in therapy modified the prognosis, three "eras" of critical care for patients with PCP and respiratory failure were identified.[13] The first comprised the experience through 1986, when outcomes were uniformly dismal. From 1986 through 1993, the prognosis seemed to improve, but after 1993, survival of patients with PCP and respiratory failure was again reported to be unlikely. Although not extensively documented, each of these three periods probably saw changes in attitudes of providers and patients about whether mechanical ventilation should be offered or chosen, and ICU utilization probably changed as well. Table 22.1 summarizes the results of several studies on outcomes of mechanical ventilation for PCP.

Early in the epidemic, the likelihood of survival after mechanical ventilation for PCP was only around 15%. In the 1984 National Institutes of Health Workshop on the Pulmonary Complications of AIDS, 88 of the 102 patients with AIDS who received mechanical ventilation died and "nearly all" had PCP.[14] These data were confirmed and expanded in several centers. By mid-1985, only 4 of 25 patients (14%) with PCP who required mechanical ventilation at Mount Sinai Hospital in New York survived to hospital discharge, and each survivor had a prolonged and complicated hospital course.[15] By the end of 1985, 82 patients with AIDS were admitted to the ICU at San Francisco General Hospital, 45 of whom had PCP and respiratory failure requiring mechanical ventilation.[6] Only six survived (13%), and five of them died within a year of hospital discharge. Other studies from individual centers confirmed that survival after respiratory failure was around 15%.[16-18] In centers with a large experience treating patients with AIDS, it was widely accepted that endotracheal intubation and mechanical ventilation were unlikely to meaningfully improve survival in patients with PCP. In some centers, ICU utilization declined despite increasing numbers of hospital admissions for PCP, because physicians did not recommend aggressive interventions and patients were more likely to decline ICU care.[12,19]

After 1986, survival rates seemed to improve to around 50%, which was attributed to selection of patients with a better prognosis and to the benefits of adjunctive corticosteroid therapy.[20-23] At San Francisco General Hospital, Wachter et al. compared the outcomes of patients with PCP and respiratory failure from 1986 to 1988 with those hospitalized before 1986.[23] Mortality was 87% before 1986 and 60% after 1986. Only 5% of the earlier patients were treated with corticosteroids, compared with 74% of the later patients. Overall, the mortality rate was 78% among those who did not receive corticosteroids, and 54% among those who did. Other centers reported survival that varied from 12% to 47%.[24-28] The improving survival rates during these years show that the possi-

Table 22–1. Studies of outcomes of mechanical ventilation in patients with AIDS and *pneumocystis carinii* pneumonia

Reference	Study period	Patients (n)	In-hospital survival rate (%)
Era I			
Murray et al., 1984[14]	10/80–7/83	102	14
Schein et al., 1986[16]	5/81–10/83	13	8
Rosen et al., 1986[15]	1/82–6/85	25	16
Wachter et al., 1986[12]	3/81–12/85	45	13
Deam et al., 1988[17]	Pre–1986	22	18
Baggot and Baggot, 1987[18]	1/85–6/86	45	9
Era II			
El-Sadr and Simberkoff, 1988[20]	1/82–12/86	19	42
Montaner et al., 1989[21]	1/81–3/87	24	50
Rogers et al., 1989[28]	7/81–3/87	24	37
Efferen et al., 1989[22]	12/84–6/88	32	54
Wachter et al., 1991[23]	1/86–12/88	35	40
Smith et al., 1989[25]	1/84–9/88	37	13
Friedman and Franklin, 1990[26]	1/87–12/90	75	47
Peruzzi et al., 1991[287]	1/85–4/89	17	12
Benson et al., 1991[28]	4/85–12/87	12	42
Era III			
Hawley et al., 1994[29]	4/87–3/91	27	11
Wachter et al., 1995[30]	1/89–12/91	37	24
Staikowsky et al., 1993[31]	1/87–1/92	33	18
Lazard et al., 1996[32]	10/90–10/92	84	31
De Palo et al., 1995[33]	11/91–11/92	16	19
Rosen et al.,1997[11]	11/88–3/94	7	29
El-Solh et al., 1996[34]	1/90–9/94	41	12

bility of new and effective treatments should always be considered when counseling patients on whether to undergo intensive care.

We are now in a third era of outcomes: since 1993, respiratory failure due to PCP is again associated with higher mortality rates, thus clinicians' optimism that patients with PCP have a good chance of surviving mechanical ventilation has been tempered.[5,29–34] Since the treatment of severe PCP has not changed significantly in the last 10 years, the apparent decline in survival is best explained by patient characteristics. At San Francisco General Hospital, mortality increased from 61% in the period from 1986 through 1988 to 76% over the next 2 years.[3] In the latter period, more patients were injection drug users, and there were more episodes of recurrent PCP. Mortality was strongly associated with a CD4 lymphocyte count $< 50/mm^3$ (94%) and with the development of pneumothorax (no survivors).

Recent patients who required mechanical ventilation were also more likely to be "treatment failures" who would be expected to have a poor prognosis. Staikowsky et al. found an overall mortality rate of 82% among patients who required mechanical ventilation for the treatment of PCP between 1987 and 1992.[31] Only 1 of the 22 patients (5%) who started mechanical ventilation after 5 days of treatment with trimethoprim-sulfamethoxazole and corticosteroids survived, compared with 5 of the 14 (36%) who received a shorter course of therapy before mechanical ventilation. At Beth Israel Hospital, New York, 13 of 16 (81%) patients who required mechanical ventilation for PCP from July 1991 to June 1992 died, despite the routine use of adjunctive corticosteroids.[33] In Vancouver, the proportion of patients who received mechanical ventilation for PCP decreased from 1981 through 1991, but mortality rates increased from 50% in 1981–1987 to 89% in 1987–1991.[29] During the same periods, corticosteroid use before intubation increased from "almost never" to 50%. Taken together, these and other studies show that when respiratory failure follows several days of appropriate therapy for PCP, the probability of survival is only 10%–20%. Patients who require intubation before receiving antipneumocystis treatment have a better prognosis.

There is little evidence of a threshold duration of mechanical ventilation for PCP that is associated with a zero survival rate, denoting "futility" that would justify prompt withdrawal of ventilatory support. In a multicenter trial of corticosteroids for PCP, survival after 2 weeks of mechanical ventilation was unprecedented.[35] However, the number of patients in this analysis was too small to support a conclusion that ventilatory support for more than 2 weeks is futile, and other centers have contradictory experience.[35a]

The prospects for prolonged survival following PCP and respiratory failure are surely more hopeful than earlier in the epidemic, when patients who survived to be discharged from the hospital rarely lived longer than 1 year.[6,10] Friedman et al. studied 73 patients with 75 episodes of PCP who received positive pressure ventilation in the ICU from 1987 through 1990; of the 34 survivors, 20 (74%) survived for 1 year.[36] In a follow-up study from the same center that included more patients, the survival rate was 80% at 1 year, 49% at 2 years, 18% at 3 years, and 6% at 4 years.[37] Prolonged survival may have been related to selection of patients for mechanical ventilation who have a better prognosis and to improvements in prophylaxis and treatment of subsequent infections. Although the data are not yet available, it is very likely that survivors of a life-threatening illness who never received PAT should enjoy a far better prognosis than before. Also, patients and providers may be more likely to pursue aggressive interventions than previously.

Special Concerns

Since the population of HIV-infected persons increasingly consists of injection drug users and racial/ethnic minorities, providers face special challenges in communicating with patients and their families, especially regarding advance directives and end-of-life care (see Chapter 8). In a study of barriers to communication between caregivers and patients with AIDS, fears of discrimination and concerns about inadequate pain control at the end of life were identified by some.[38] Also, there are often sensitive issues regarding confidentiality in patients with life-threatening illness in the ICU. Most providers who care for patients with AIDS in the ICU have faced the difficult situation of communicating with family and friends who do not know that their loved one has HIV infection. The basic ethical and legal principles for providers are that caregivers must not divulge confidential information against the patient's implied or overt request, *except* when there is a high likelihood that great harm would come to a party if the information remains confidential. In the case of HIV, the laws vary by state, but some encourage and others require that sexual and/or needle-sharing partners of HIV-infected persons be informed of possible risks to them.

Conclusions

The history of the AIDS epidemic in the United States illustrates several principles in end-of-life care. In AIDS, as in other diseases, new treatments have changed outcomes, which in turn strongly influence patient and physician preferences. With HIV, the use of corticosteroids as adjunctive therapy for PCP has been associated with improved survival and, with it, changes in ICU utilization. Potent antiretroviral therapy has dramatically reduced mortality due to AIDS in the United States. The effects of these therapies on ICU utilization, outcomes, and patient and provider preferences are unknown, and more research is clearly needed in this area.

References

1. Centers for Disease Control and Prevention. HIV/AIDS Surveillance Report. 1998; 10(1):1–40.
2. Palella FJ, Delaney KM, Moorman AC, Loveless MO, Fuhrer J, Satten GA, Aschman DJ, Holmberg SD, and the HIV Outpatient Study Investigators. Declining morbidity and mortality among patients with advanced human immunodeficiency virus infection. *N Engl J Med* 1998;338:853–860.
3. Centers for Disease Control and Prevention. Report of the NIH Panel to Define Principles of Therapy of HIV Infection, and Guidelines for the Use of Antiretroviral Agents in HIV-Infected Adults and Adolescents. *MMWR Morb Moral Wkly Rep* 1998;47(RR-5).
4. Steinbrook R, Lo B, Moulton J, Saika G, Hollander H, Volberding PA. Preferences of homosexual men with AIDS for life-sustaining treatment. *New Engl J Med* 1986; 314:457–460.

5. Singer PA, Thiel EC, Flanagan W, Naylor CD. The HIV-specific advance directive. *J Gen Intern Med* 1997;12:729–735.

6. Mouton C, Teno JM, Mor V, Piette J. Communication of preferences for care among human immunodeficiency virus–infected patients. *Arch Fam Med* 1997; 6:342–347.

7. Teno JM, Mor V, Fleishman J. Preferences of HIV-infected patients for aggressive versus palliative care [letter]. *N Engl J Med* 1991;324:1140.

8. Teno J, Fleishman J, Bork DW, Mor V. The use of formal prior directives among patients with HIV-related diseases. *J Gen Intern Med* 1990;5:490–494.

9. Haas JS, Weissman JS, Cleary PD, Goldberg J, Gatsonis C, Seage GR 3d, Fowler JF, Massagli MP, Makadon HJ, Epstein AM. Discussion of preferences for life-sustaining care by persons with AIDS. *Arch Intern Med* 1991;153:1241–1248.

10. Rosen MJ, De Palo VA. Outcome of intensive care for patients with AIDS. *Crit Care Clin North Am* 1993;9:107–114.

11. Rosen MJ, Clayton K, Schneider RF, Fulkerson W, Rao AV, Stansell J, Kvale PA, Glassroth J, Reichman LB, Wallace JM, Hopewell PC, and the Pulmonary Complications of HIV Infection Study Group. Intensive care of patients with HIV infection: utilization, critical illnesses and outcomes. *Am J Respir Crit Care Med* 1997;155:67–71.

12. Wachter RM, Luce JM, Turner J, Volberding P, Hopewell PC. Intensive care of patients with the acquired immunodeficiency syndrome. Outcome and changing patterns of utilization. *Am Rev Respir Dis* 1986;134:891–896.

13. Wachter RM, Luce JM. Respiratory failure from severe *Pneumocystis carinii* pneumonia: entering the third era. *Chest* 1994;106:1313–1315.

14. Murray J, Felton CP, Garay SM, Gottlieb MS, Hopewell PC, Stover DE, Teirstein AS. Pulmonary complications of the acquired immunodeficiency syndrome: report of National Heart, Lung and Blood Institute Workshop. *N Engl J Med* 1984; 310:1682–1688.

15. Rosen MJ, Cucco RA, Teirstein AS. Outcome of intensive care in patients with the acquired immunodeficiency syndrome. *J Intensive Care Med* 1986;1:55.

16. Schein RMH, Fischl MA, Pitchenik AE, Sprung CL. ICU survival of patients with the acquired immunodeficiency syndrome. *Crit Care Med* 1986;14:1026–1027.

17. Deam R, Kimberley APS, Anderson M, Soni N. AIDS in ICU's: outcome. *Anaesthesia* 1988;45:150–151.

18. Baggot LA, Baggot BB. *Pneumocystis carinii* pneumonia (PCP) in AIDS patients in intensive care. *Chest* 1987;92:132S.

19. Curtis JR, Greenberg DL, Hudson LD, Fisher LD, Krone MR, Collier AC. Changing use of intensive care for HIV-infected patients with *Pneumocystis carinii* pneumonia. *Am J Respir Crit Care Med* 1994;150:1305–1310.

20. El-Sadr W, Simberkoff MS. Survival and prognostic factors in severe *Pneumocystis carinii* pneumonia following mechanical ventilation. *Am Rev Respir Dis* 1988; 137:1264–1267.

21. Montaner JSG, Russel JA, Lawson L, Ruedy J. Acute respiratory failure secondary to *Pneumocystis carinii* pneumonia in the acquired immunodeficiency syndrome. A potential role for systemic corticosteroids. *Chest* 1989;95:881–884.

22. Efferen LS, Nadarajah D, Palat DS. Survival following mechanical ventilation of *Pneumocystis carinii* pneumonia in patients with the acquired immunodeficiency syndrome: a different perspective. *Am J Med* 1989;87:401–404.

23. Wachter RM, Russi MB, Bloch DA, Hopewell PC, Luce JM. *Pneumocystis carinii*

pneumonia and respiratory failure in AIDS. Improved outcomes and increased used of intensive care units. *Am Rev Respir Dis* 1991;143:251–256.

24. Rogers PL, Lane HC, Henderson DK, Parillo J, Masur H. Admission of AIDS patients to a medical intensive care unit: causes and outcome. *Crit Care Med* 1989;17:113–117.

25. Smith RL, Levine SM, Lewis ML. Prognosis of patients with AIDS requiring intensive care. *Chest* 1989;96:857–861

26. Friedman Y, Franklin C. Admission of AIDS patients to a medical intensive care unit: causes and outcome. *Crit Care Med* 1990;18:346–347.

27. Peruzzi WT, Skoutelis A, Shapiro BA, Murphy RM, Currie DL, Cane RD, Noskin GA, Phair JP. Intensive care unit patients with acquired immunodeficiency syndrome and *Pneumocystis carinii* pneumonia: suggestive predcictors of hospital outcome. *Crit Care Med* 1991;19:892–900.

28. Benson CA, Spear J, Hines D, Pottage JC, Kessler HA, Trenholme GM. Combined APACHE II score and serum lactate dehydrogenase as predictors of in-hospital mortality caused by first episode *Pneumocystis carinii* pneumonia in patients with acquired immunodeficiency syndrome. *Am Rev Respir Dis* 1991;144:319–323.

29. Hawley, PH, Ronco JJ, Guilleni SA, Quieffin J, Russell JA, Lawson LM, Schechter MT, Montaner JS. Decreasing frequency but worsening mortality of acute respiratory failure secondary to AIDS-related *Pneumocystis carinii* pneumonia. *Chest* 1994;106:1456–1459.

30. Wachter RM, Luce JM, Safrin S, Berrios DC, Charlebois E, Scitovsky AA. Cost and outcome of intensive care for patients with AIDS, *Pneumocystis carinii* pneumonia, and severe respiratory failure. *JAMA* 1995;273:230–235.

31. Staikowsky F, Lafon B, Guidet B, Denis M, Mayaud C, Offenstadt G. Mechanical ventilation for *Pneumocystis carinii* pneumonia in patients with the acquired immunodeficiency syndrome: is the prognosis really improved? *Chest* 1993;104:756–762.

32. Lazard T, Retel O, Guidet B, Maury E, Valleron A-J, Offenstadt G. AIDS in a medical intensive care unit. Immediate prognosis and long-term survival. *JAMA* 1996;276:1240–1245.

33. De Palo VA, Millstein BH, Mayo PH, Salzman SS, Rosen MJ. Outcome of intensive care in patients with HIV infection. *Chest* 1995;107:506–510.

34. El-Solh AA, Stubeusz DL, Grant GB, Grant BJB. Outcome of AIDS patients requiring mechanical ventilation predicted by recursive partitioning. *Chest* 1996;109:1584–1590.

35. Bozzette SA, Feigal D, Chiu J, Gluckstein D, Kemper C, Sattler F. Length of stay and survival after intensive care for severe *Pneumocystis carinii* pneumonia; a prospective study. *Chest* 1992;101:1404–1407.

35a. Curtis JR, Yarnold P, Schwartz D, Weinstein RA, Bennett CL. ICU use and outcomes of acute respiratory failure for patients with HIV-related *Pneumocystis carinii* pneumonia. *Am J Respir Crit Care Med*, 2000, in press.

36. Friedman Y, Franklin C, Freels S, Weil MH. Long-term survival of patients with AIDS, *Pneumocystis carinii* pneumonia, and respiratory failure. *JAMA* 1991;266:89–92.

37. Franklin C, Friedman Y, Wong T, Tzyy-Chyn H. Improving long-term prognosis for survivors of mechanical ventilation in patients with AIDS with PCP and acute respiratory failure. *Arch Intern Med* 1995;155:91–95.

38. Curtis JR, Patrick DL. Barriers to communication about end-of-life care in AIDS patients. *J Gen Intern Med* 1997;12:736–741.

Chapter 23

Cancer

ANTHONY BACK

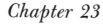

*P*atients with cancer are most commonly admitted to an ICU for postoperative recovery, respiratory failure, sepsis, or multiorgan system failure. Less commonly, the indication for admission is a complication of progressive cancer (such as pericardial tamponade) or a complication of anticancer therapy (such as neutropenic sepsis). Overall, the most common cause of death for patients with cancer in ICUs is infection, rather than progressive cancer. However, the exact cause of death may be difficult to identify clinically, and in one autopsy study that included 69% of the deaths in a medical oncology ICU, the clinically identified cause of death was correct in only 41% of cases.[1]

The high cost of ICU care and poor prognosis for many patients with cancer admitted to ICUs has resulted in a number of studies evaluating outcomes.[2] However, the studies that are relevant to ICU outcomes for patients with cancer do not necessarily have study populations defined by ICU admission. Because many inpatient cancer units have the capacity to provide some level of critical care, criteria for ICU admission are highly institution-specific. For example, in some stem cell transplantation units, patients do not require transfer to an ICU for mechanical ventilation. Thus a study population may be defined by use of a specific intervention such as mechanical ventilation, rather than by ICU admission. Table 23–1 summarizes a number of outcomes studies for mechanically ventilated cancer patients. In addition, the complex trajectory of a cancer patient's illness has not been well captured in some prognostic models developed for ICUs: the implications of admission for sepsis in the setting of progressive metastatic cancer are quite different from those for sepsis with cancer that has responded to anticancer therapy. Consequently, some prognostic models perform poorly on patients with

Table 23–1. Outcome for mechanically ventilated patients with cancer[a]

Reference	Ventilated (N)	Solid malignancy (N)	Hematologic malignancy (N)	BMT (N)	In-hospital mortality (%)	6-month mortality[b] (%)	Factors associated with increased mortality
Snow et al., 1979[13]	180	100	80	0	—	93%	AML, ALL, lung CA
Peters et al., 1988[14]	116	0	110	0	82%	—	—
Crawford et al., 1988[15]	232	0	232	232	—	93%	Age
Brunet et al., 1990[16]	111	0	111	0	83%	—	Dialysis, >1 organ failure, SAPS >15
Crawford et al., 1992[15]	348	0	348	0	96%	—	Age, relapse, HLA mismatch
Faber-Langendoen et al., 1993[17]	191	0	191	191	—	97%	Age >40, MV within 90, Days of BMT
Epneret al., 1996[18]	157	0	157	71	75% no BMT 90% BMT	—	Age >20 years, >first complete remission, neutropenia >30d, BMT, Apache III
Groeger et al., 1999[7]	782	305	477	208	76%	—	Ventilation initiated after first hospital day, Leukemia progression or recurrence, Allogeneic BMT, Arrhythmias, DIC, Vasopressors

ALL, acute lymphatic leukemia; AML, acute myeloid leukemia; BMT, bone marrow or stem cell transplant; DIC, ; HLA, ; SAPS, .

[a]Data are from reports with >100 patients.

[b]Mortality at 6 months from study entry.

cancer.[3] Future prognostic studies are likely to be increasingly sensitive to these issues of disease trajectory.

In addition to the difficulty of accurate prognostication, communication between physician and patient and differing thresholds for pursuing life-sustaining therapy have been empirically demonstrated to be significant factors in ICU utilization for patients with cancer. First, the accuracy of a cancer patient's understanding of their own prognosis correlates strongly with the patient's preference for life-sustaining treatment. Patients whose estimate of survival corresponds with their physician's estimate are less likely to prefer life-sustaining therapy than patients whose estimates of survival are more optimistic than their physicians' estimates.[4] Second, any survival probability statistic is subject to variable interpretations. Intensivists who see their task as selecting those patients who have a high chance of benefit from an ICU stay may interpret a 10% chance of survival quite differently from that of a patient with cancer who has been actively pursuing treatment because it promises a survival of 10%.

A final issue in caring for patients with cancer in the ICU involves the culture of high-tech cancer care. Many cancer patients enter anticancer treatment expecting toxicity that may be life threatening; they expect that their treatment will either kill them or cure them. These patients are often highly knowledgeable about their treatment regimens, and may have great faith in medical technology based on extensive personal experience. In general, cancer caregivers have not yet learned how to incorporate an idea about a good death into the mainstream conception of what constitutes good cancer treatment. Our society's dominant imagery of cancer treatment engages patients in a battle with their cancer, in which an ICU admission may be seen as "fighting the good fight."[5,6] Reorienting patients, or more often, family members toward a good death requires that intensivists build trust and communicate well, in addition to understanding prognostication and both the patient's and family's values.

Issues in the Decision to Limit ICU Care

Prognostication of outcome

The general prognosis for cancer patients admitted to an ICU because of critical illness is poor, with mortality rates ranging from 50% to 80%. The prognosis for those who leave the hospital after an ICU stay is also poor. In one study, approximately 75% of cancer patients admitted to an ICU who survived to hospital discharge lived less than 3 months.[3]

The best known prognostic models of ICU mortality developed for the adult medical population, such as the Acute Physiology and Chronic Health Evaluation (APACHE), do not include cancer-specific variables and have not been extensively validated in cancer patients. These ICU prognostic scoring systems generally underestimate the chance of hospital mortality for cancer patients admitted to an ICU.[3] In particular, APACHE appears to underestimate survival in both patients with hematologic malignancies and those undergoing a marrow transplant.

In the most comprehensive mortality prediction model that has been developed specifically for cancer patients admitted to an ICU, Groeger and colleagues identified three cancer-specific variables as significant: allogeneic bone marrow transplantation, disease progression, and poor performance status (all correlate with increased mortality).[3] The other 13 variables include laboratory values (such as PaO_2/FiO_2) and clinical variables (such as days of hospitalization before ICU admission). This model was developed in four tertiary cancer centers and has not been validated in other settings.

In a different multicenter observational study specifically examining outcome for cancer patients requiring mechanical ventilation, Groeger et al. found that overall hospital mortality was 76%.[7] Seven variables were associated with an increased risk of death: intubation after 24 hours of hospitalization, leukemia, progression or recurrence of cancer, allogeneic bone marrow transplantation, cardiac arrhythmias, presence of disseminated intravascular coagulation, and need for vasopressor therapy. In particular, patients who were admitted with respiratory failure had a better prognosis than patients who developed respiratory failure after 24 hours of hospital therapy. Also, patients who were mechanically ventilated because of prior surgery had a decreased risk of death, probably because these are largely patients who underwent anticancer surgery with curative intent.

Specifically for neutropenic cancer patients, single institution studies have indicated that patients with a hematological malignancy (leukemia or lymphoma) are more likely to be admitted for respiratory failure than patients with solid tumors, and that, like other critically ill patients, the number of organ system failures correlates with ICU mortality.[8]

For patients who have undergone marrow or stem cell transplantation, Rubenfeld and Crawford developed a prognostic system aimed at identifying a group of patients with respiratory failure for whom survival was unprecedented.[9] There were no survivors among an estimated 398 post-transplant patients who had lung injury and either required more than 4 hours of vasopressor support or had sustained hepatic and renal failure. Survival after respiratory failure for patients undergoing marrow or stem cell transplantation is poor; however, these authors note that during the past 5 years, the survival rate for post-transplant patients at the Fred Hutchinson Cancer Research Center has improved from 5% to 16% ($P = 0.008$). This increased survival is not explained by changes in the age of the patients, the rate or timing of intubation, or the percentage of allogeneic transplants that were not HLA-identical. A possible explanation for this improved survival is that physicians have become more experienced in selecting patients for mechanical ventilation and do not provide mechanical ventilation to patients they judge to have a very low chance of survival.

The only ICU prognosis study that has been specifically designed to identify situations in which ongoing ICU therapy is futile for patients with cancer is the Rubenfeld and Crawford study. In this study, the authors conclude that mechanical ventilation is futile for patients who have undergone a marrow or stem cell transplant and have severe lung injury, more than 4 hours vasopressor support, and sustained hepatic or renal failure, because the predicted survival rate is zero. There are no other studies specifically designed to identify situations in which ICU therapy would be futile.

Finally, a common issue arising for patients with metastatic cancer who are considering advance care plans is the likelihood of surviving in-hospital cardiopulmonary resuscitation (CPR). A review of studies, summarized by Faber-Langendoen,[10] revealed that zero patients with metastatic cancer survived to hospital discharge after in-hospital CPR, even though some patients initially responded. Thus patients with metastatic cancer should be counseled about the medical futility of in-hospital CPR and subsequent ICU admission.

Issues in communication with patients and families

Uncertainty about using prognostic models to predict outcome for an individual patient
In the Study to Understand Prognoses and Preferences for Outcomes and Risks of Treatment (SUPPORT), an analysis was specifically performed to estimate, on the day before a patient died, that individual patient's chance of surviving for 2 months. A patient with metastatic lung cancer on the day before death had a median chance of 0.17 of living for 2 more months.[11] This finding underscores the clinical uncertainty that ICU physicians must deal with in making plans of care with patients and families. Decision making that hinges on certain death will often occur too late for optimal support of the dying person and their family. Clinicians should attempt to describe a typical trajectory of ICU care that ends in survival and one that ends in death to help patients and/or surrogate decision makers understand the kinds of decisions they will likely face. This method of identifying in advance possible in making decisions points can give patients or their surrogate decision makers time to weigh options and discuss their concerns with the medical team.

Patient perception of likelihood of survival influences preferences for resuscitation
In the SUPPORT study, patients were prospectively asked to estimate their chance of survival, and patients with lung and colon cancer tended to overestimate their survival.[4] These overestimates may have led them to overstate their preferences for life-extending therapy such as mechanical ventilation. Patients who thought they were going to live for at least 6 months were more likely to favor life-extending therapy over comfort care than patients who were less optimistic (but more realistic) about their prognosis. This study suggests that a realistic understanding of prognosis affects patient choices about life-extending

therapy. Failure of an ICU team to challenge a patient's unrealistic hope about survival may lead to patient preferences for life-extending ICU therapies that result in burdensome care.

Implications of New or Experimental Therapy

"Salvage" chemotherapy

Salvage chemotherapy generally refers to "beyond first-line" chemotherapy, but this term has no standard meaning in the oncology lexicon. It may refer to either chemotherapy given with palliative (noncurative) intent or chemotherapy given with curative intent (for example, stem cell transplantation for relapsed lymphoma). The studies noted above, (especially that by Groeger et al.[3]) have identified salient variables involved in predicting survival after ICU admission associated with salvage chemotherapy, and these include disease status (i.e., remission or relapse). There are no studies that specifically examine the relationship of beyond first-line anticancer therapies to the use of ICU care. It sometimes happens that a patient or physician may believe that continued anticancer therapy may prolong survival, however briefly. Yet anticancer therapy administered to critically ill patients near death may be more likely to hasten death because toxicity for these patients is severe. ICU clinicians and oncologists should be careful not to offer "salvage" chemotherapy as a way to avoid discussing death with patients and their families.

Research protocols and their influence on end-of-life care

There are no studies examining the influence of experimental anticancer treatment protocols on end-of-life care. However, it is notable that 85% of patients enrolled in phase I studies identified possible therapeutic benefit as the most important factor in their decision to proceed, even though historical data indicate that < 5% of patients derive therapeutic benefit from a phase I study.[12] Patient trust in their primary oncologist was the second most important factor (15%) in deciding to participate in a phase I study. These findings underscore the importance of addressing patient hope and expectation in addition to objective prognostic data when discussing end-of-life issues with cancer patients and their families in the ICU.

Cancer-Specific Complications and Their Palliative Management

In this section, specific ICU scenarios are highlighted. It is hoped that palliative management can be improved by identifying points to anticipate and communicate to a patient and/or family during the decision-making process, as well as common symptoms and issues that require assessment and treatment.

Respiratory failure, especially after marrow or stem cell transplant

The paradigmatic example is death from cytomegalovirus (CMV) pneumonitis after an allogeneic marrow transplant. The prognosis for these patients is extremely poor (for some patients, survival is unprecedented[9]), and physicians should not consider a trial of mechanical ventilation to be routine. Before intubation, patients and family members should engage in a discussion that includes information about chances of survival, and how death would be managed if the patient is intubated versus not intubated. It may be useful to clearly state that foregoing intubation can be seen as a way to ensure a certain type of death, rather than as a gesture of giving up. Unlike some patients with acute respiratory disease syndrome (ARDS), these patients usually have a relentlessly progressive hypoxia, and untreatable hypoxia should be specifically identified as a marker of immanent death. Dyspnea is the most important symptom to manage, usually with continuous infusion opioids. Therapy should include sedation and/or anxiolytics as needed, psychological preparation of the family and ICU staff, and timing of discontinuation of ventilatory support to ensure easy availability of support staff.

Tumor lysis syndrome

Most commonly observed after initial chemotherapy for high-grade lymphoma, this syndrome is characterized by renal failure, hyperuricemia, and hyperkalemia. Tumor lysis syndrome causes death most often via uncontrollable electrolyte abnormalities leading to arrhythmias. Physicians should discuss the possible need for dialysis, cardioversion, and anticancer treatment failure. Electrolyte abnormalities that persist despite dialysis should be specifically identified as a marker of immanent death. Palliative management should include discontinuation of intravenous hydration to prevent discomfort from edema and respiratory secretions, monitoring and treatment for delirium, and psychological support for the family.

Venoocclusive disease of the liver

This complication of stem cell or marrow transplantation often results in ICU care because of the need for management to prevent or treat hepatorenal syndrome (the usual cause of death for these patients). Patients may develop a bilirubin level in excess of 20 mg/dl, but the point at which renal failure develops can be quite variable. The development of renal failure should be specifically identified as a marker of immanent death. In addition, patients and families should be informed that cognitive capacity usually becomes more compromised as patients near death. Palliative management should include discontinuation of intravenous hydration, monitoring and treatment for delirium, and a plan for use of lab tests, antibiotics, and transfusion of blood products. Bilirubin values are not a reliable guide to the timing of death.

Interleukin-2-related hemodynamic complications

High-dose interleukin-2 (IL-2) for treatment of advanced renal cell carcinoma and melanoma can be associated with a capillary leak syndrome characterized by low systemic vascular resistance (SVR), high cardiac output, and hypotension. In contrast to management of sepsis, the use of dopamine is routine in these settings and intravenous saline is limited to reduce the potential for pulmonary edema. The IL-2 syndrome is uncommonly fatal, but it may be if sepsis or renal failure are superimposed. Palliative management should include a plan for handling vasopressors, which physicians may regard as routine IL-2-related supportive care.

All-trans retinoic acid syndrome

Patients with acute promyelocytic leukemia treated with all-trans-retinoic acid (ATRA), which is used as a leukemic differentiation agent, may develop hyperleukocytosis with a diffuse capillary leak syndrome characterized by skin rash, pulmonary infiltrates, and hypotension. Treatment involves high-dose steroids and sometimes blood pressure support with pressors. Death from this syndrome is uncommon, but it can evolve into multiorgan system failure, especially if the patient was concurrently treated with anti-leukemia chemotherapy. Palliative management should include development of a plan to manage or withdraw mechanical ventilation, a plan to withdraw pressors, treatment of dyspnea, and treatment of bleeding in patients with ongoing disseminated intravascular coagulation secondary to acute promeylocytic leukemia.

Superior vena cava syndrome

The prognosis for superior vena cava (SVC) syndrome varies with the underlying cancer diagnosis. Superior vena cava syndrome from lymphoma or small cell lung cancer that is previously untreated may respond dramatically to chemotherapy. However, for other types of cancer, response is usually less than dramatic—short-term survival is common but long-term survival is uncommon. Although patients are sometimes admitted to ICUs for observation, these patients should not automatically receive emergent radiotherapy. In most cases, a diagnostic procedure can be performed that will direct specific anticancer therapy. Palliative management may include opioids for dyspnea or pain related to upper body swelling, management of anxiety, and discussion of care plans involving successful anticancer treatment or unsuccessful anticancer treatment.

Pericardial tamponade

Malignant pericardial tamponade is most often associated with solid tumors and is usually a marker for widespread cancer. The prognosis for patients is about 30 days. However, substantial symptomatic improvement can occur after pericardial drainage, which can be performed by percutaneous needle drainage or surgical creation of a pericardial window. These procedures are invasive but can provide dramatic symptomatic relief, and they merit consideration for most patients.

References

1. Gerain J, Sculier JP, Malengreaux A, Rykaert C, Themelin L. Causes of deaths in an oncologic intensive care unit: a clinical and pathological study of 34 autopsies. *Eur J Cancer* 1990;26:377–381.
2. Schapira DV, Studnicki J, Bradham DD, Wolff P, Jarrett A. Intensive care, survival, and expense of treating critically ill cancer patients [see comments]. *JAMA* 1993; 269:783–786.
3. Groeger JS, Lemeshow S, Price K, Nierman DM, White P Jr, Klar J, Granovsky S, Horak D, Kish SK. Multicenter outcome study of cancer patients admitted to the intensive care unit: a probability of mortality model. *J Clin Oncol* 1998;16:761–770.
4. Weeks JC, Cook EF, O'Day SJ, Peterson LM, Wenger N, Reding D, Harrell FE, Kussin P, Dawson NV, Connors AF Jr, Lynn J, Phillips RS. Relationship between cancer patients' predictions of prognosis and their treatment preferences [see comments]. *JAMA* 1998;279:1709–1714.
5. Delvecchio Good MJ, Good BJ, Schaffer C, Lind SE. American oncology and the discourse on hope. *Cult Med Psychiatry* 1990;14:59–79.
6. Kodish E, Post SG. Oncology and hope. *J Clin Oncol* 1995;13:1817.
7. Groeger JS, White P Jr, Nierman DM, Glassman J, Shi W, Horak D, Price K. Outcome for cancer patients requiring mechanical ventilation. *J Clin Oncol* 1999; 17:991–997.
8. Blot F, Guiguet M, Nitenberg G, Leclercq B, Gachot B, Escudier B. Prognostic factors for neutropenic patients in an intensive care unit: respective roles of underlying malignancies and acute organ failures. *Eur J Cancer* 1997;33:1031–1037.
9. Rubenfeld GD, Crawford SW. Withdrawing life support from mechanically ventilated recipients of bone marrow transplants: a case for evidence-based guidelines [see comments]. *Ann Intern Med* 1996;125:625–633.
10. Faber-Langendoen K. Resuscitation of patients with metastatic cancer. Is transient benefit still futile? [see comments]. *Arch Intern Med* 1991;151:235–239.
11. Lynn J, Harrell F Jr, Cohn F, Wagner D, Connors AF Jr. Prognoses of seriously ill hospitalized patients on the days before death: implications for patient care and public policy. *New Horiz* 1997;5:56–61.
12. Decoster G, Stein G, Holdener EE. Responses and toxic deaths in phase I clinical trials. *Ann Oncol* 1990;1:175–181.
13. Snow RM, Miller WC, Rice DL, Ali MK. Respiratory failure in cancer patients. *JAMA* 1979;241:2039–2042.
14. Peters SG, Meadows JAD, Gracey DR. Outcome of respiratory failure in hematologic malignancy. *Chest* 1988;94:99–102.
15. Crawford SW, Schwartz DA, Petersen FB, Clark JG. Mechanical ventilation after marrow transplantation. Risk factors and clinical outcome. *Am Rev Respir Dis* 1988;137:682–687.

16. Brunet F, Lanore JJ, Dhainaut JF, Dreyfuss F, Vaxelaire JF, Nouira S, Giraud T, Armaganidis A, Monsallier JF. Is intensive care justified for patients with haematological malignancies? *Intensive Care Med* 1990;16:291–297.
17. Faber-Langendoen K, Caplan AL, McGlave PB. Survival of adult bone marrow transplant patients receiving mechanical ventilation: a case for restricted use. *Bone Marrow Transplant* 1993;12:501–507.
18. Epner DE, White P, Krasnoff M, Khanduja S, Kimball KT, Knaus WA. Outcome of mechanical ventilation for adults with hematologic malignancy. *J Investig Med* 1996;44:254–260.

Chapter 24

Congestive Heart Failure

JONATHAN
SACKNER-BERNSTEIN

*C*ongestive heart failure is caused by the inability of the heart to pump blood sufficiently to meet the body's metabolic demands. Clinically, it manifests as symptoms of dyspnea and/or fatigue, and the natural history is one of gradual progression, leading to disability and death. There are many causes; ischemic heart disease dominates in the developed countries, although hypertension and valvular disease (including rheumatic heart disease) also lead to this syndrome.[1] Heart failure is associated with an increased risk of sudden death, but in most cases, the natural history features frequent hospitalizations and progressive symptoms prior to death.[2] Congestive heart failure is growing in incidence, especially in advanced age,[1] is the leading reason for hospitalization in those over 65 years of age in the United States, and is a major cause of death.[1,2] It is no surprise, therefore, that congestive heart failure is both a costly disease to society, with an estimated $23 billion spent on hospitalizations alone in 1991,[3] and a devastating one for patients and their families, with a prognosis similar to that of many cancers.[4]

As the heart failure syndrome progresses, patients are at risk for recurrent hospital admissions, frequently to the ICU. Increased monitoring, intravenous medications, and mechanical circulatory and respiratory support intensify the costs of these hospitalizations. In general, volume overload and low cardiac output states can be successfully treated, but inevitably, the disease will prove refractory, if not during one admission, certainly at a later one. The frequent and early successes alter expectations of physicians and patients, creating the illusion that these exacerbations can be reversed consistently and quickly. However, these patients do face the inevitable prospect of death, with each subsequent heart failure hospitalization signifying an increased risk of death.[5] Unfor-

311

tunately few physicians counsel patients effectively[6] and few patients are prepared for decisions about end-of-life care.[7,8]

This chapter will focus on specific issues surrounding ICU care of patients with congestive heart failure. As it is not possible to define the criteria for limiting treatments in these patient, the chapter will focus on potential therapeutic options, with the perspective that the decision to limit care, based on the circumstances of the individual patient, will direct the level of aggressiveness and appropriateness of each of the strategies outlined.

Prognostic Issues in the ICU

The decision to limit care for the patient in the ICU is the result of an exhaustive process. First and foremost is the search for a reversible cause of the heart failure syndrome (Table 24–1). In the absence of such a therapeutic option, the decision to limit treatments should be based upon statistically and clinically robust prognostic tools. Unfortunately, such tools are not available for patients in the ICU with advanced heart failure, for two primary reasons. First, the databases that exist typically include patients who are different from those commonly admitted to the ICU; ambulatory patients who are transplant eligible are enrolled, which limits the population to those under 65 year of age.[9-11] Even the models that are validated in ambulatory patients[9] may not be directly applicable to the patients in the ICU, as they do not include patients on inotropic support, those with multi-organ system failure, or those over 65 years of age—common characteristics of patients admitted to the ICU. Additionally, these databases use an endpoint of death or urgent transplant, not whether survivors were satisfied with their quality of life 6 months after initial evaluation. Thus, despite the robust statistical power of these models, they are not clinically relevant to the decision to limit care in the ICU patient. Second, all of these prognostic assessments are based upon an initial evaluation, and as

Table 24–1. Reversible causes of heart failure

Etiology	Therapeutic Strategy
Acute myocarditis	No immunosuppression, supportive care
Coronary artery disease with hibernating myocardium	Viability study prior to revascularization
Valve disease	Stabilize as prelude to surgery
Metabolic abnormalities	Correct underlying deficiency
Hypothyroidism	
Beriberi (thiamine deficiency)	
Carnitine deficiency	
Selenium deficiency	

clinicians we know that the response to therapies is a strong predictor of the clinical course. For example, it would be no surprise that a patient who responds to dobutamine with a brisk diuresis and reversal of azotemia should fare better than one who does not respond to dobutamine, milrinone, nitroprusside, or intra-aortic counter pulsation. However, if these patients looked the same at the time of admission to the ICU, we would conclude from published literature that their prognoses would be equivalent, yet we know that this would not be the case. Determination of the appropriateness of limiting treatments could be enhanced if we had data that account for the response over time. These data become available as a result of the National Institutes of Health (NIH) sponsored trial designed to evaluate the utility of Swan-Ganz–guided therapy for patients admitted to the ICU with heart failure (Escape), initiated in 1999.

With this limitation in the literature, it would seem reasonable to apply lessons learned elsewhere as factors that could gauge the likelihood of recovery for patients in the ICU. A potential and powerful predictor of outcome in these patients is the presence of multi-organ system failure, in particular the degree of dysfunction and number of organ systems involved. Older patients are consistently at higher risk, and it would seem reasonable to assume this to be the case for heart failure. Ambulatory patients with hyponatremia are at higher risk of death,[12] and it appears likely that this is so in critically ill patients as well. Factors that would seem predictive of a worse outcome are listed in Table 24–2.

These shortcomings amplify the difficulty of the decision-making process to limit treatments. Several questions must be asked that cannot be based on large datasets. Does the patient believe that the effects of an intervention are worthwhile, especially if current quality of life is poor, the likelihood of response is remote, and the outcome is a markedly limited lifestyle? How comfortable are the family and health care providers with a patient deciding to "give up"? How can we present these possibilities simply enough for critically ill patients and their families to understand, while giving a balanced and realis-

Table 24–2. Proposed prognostic variables in ICU patients with exacerbation of congestive heart failure

Cardiogenic shock

Multi-organ system failure
 (as a function of the degree of organ failure and the number of systems failing)

Unresponsive to therapy within first 24–48 hours

Persistent hyponatremia

Refractory arrhythmias

Advanced age

Myocardial ischemia

tic perspective? One question for which we know the answer is that of when to start the discussion about end-of life care: it is never too early, and rarely easy.

Issues in Limiting Treatment in the ICU

The natural history of heart failure creates the impression that all exacerbations can be effectively treated. For example, patients with mild to moderate heart failure can experience frequent episodes of clinical decompensation, generally manifest as volume overload, which may lead to hospitalization,[2] but these can be treated rapidly and effectively with the use of potent intravenous diuretics and, occasionally, intravenous inotropes or vasodilators (Table 24–3). Because improvements can be observed within hours of the initiation of therapy, the physicians caring for the patient are viewed as omnipotent. In the case of a patient in the ICU with advanced disease, this scenario may have occurred several times during previous hospitalization. Thus the expectation develops that the highly trained cardiologist will once again be able to reverse the condition and rescue the patient from their perilous state. In fact, there are many tools to accomplish this task, including diuretics, inotropes and vasodilators. Standard ICU modalities including mechanical ventilatory support and dialysis are complemented by mechanical/surgical approaches to support the failing left ventricle. These tools add to the perception of the patient *and the cardiologist* of the power and resources available. If success is a matter of using the right tool aggressively enough, then the cardiologist will not see a need to discuss end-of-life issues. However, a patient hospitalized with a heart failure exacerbation is subsequently at higher risk of death[5] and should be targeted for discussion of resuscitation preferences and other end-of-life care issues. These factors contribute to the relatively low rate of do-not-resuscitate (DNR) orders for patients treated by cardiologists compared with those treated by other specialists.[6] For these reasons, physicians must manage both their own expectations and those of the patient and family.

Not infrequently, management of these patients involves a choice between improving the heart failure or creating an additional problem. This dilemma creates a situation of disease swapping—the trading of one problem for an-

Table 24–3. Steps in management of heart failure in the ICU, divided by the primary clinical manifestation of the clinical presentation. As therapy progresses to subsequent level, discussion about end of life care should intensify

Volume Overload	Hypotension
IV diuretics	IV pressors
IV inotropes	IV inotropes
IV vasodilators	Mechanical support
Mechanical support	

other. In sicker patients and those with comorbidities that affect vital organs, such as renal dysfunction in diabetics or pulmonary disease in tobacco users, this is particularly true. Patients with advanced disease admitted to an ICU with clinical decompensation frequently develop dysfunction of noncardiovascular organs. This typically occurs in patients with poor end-organ perfusion due to low cardiac output with significant volume overload, where azotemia and pulmonary edema are prominent abnormalities. Diuretics would improve volume status and dyspnea, but they may exacerbate azotemia. Positive inotropic agents could improve end-organ perfusion, reverse azotemia, and improve symptoms, but they increase the risk of arrhythmias such as ventricular tachycardia. Although vasodilator therapy does not produce arrhythmias and may improve end-organ perfusion while it reduces ventricular filling pressure and dyspnea, it does little to address the underlying volume overload. Thus, a trade-off emerges—progressive renal insufficiency or severe dyspnea due to volume overload, which may lead to consideration of dialysis. However, the manner in which such options are presented may determine the choice made by a patient. For example, a patient told that imminent death is certain unless dialysis is commenced immediately will likely choose dialysis. But if the patient is told that, although dialysis is the only way to improve dyspnea, it would be only a temporary and minimal improvement, and it is uncomfortable and associated with a risk of life-threatening infections and a marked limitation in independence, perhaps the patient would opt out of this intervention. Both descriptions could appear coercive, thus they need to be framed within the preferences of the individual patient to permit informed decision making. The greatest problem with this type of situation occurs when no firm decision is made, leaving the patient with severe dyspnea and compromised renal function, thus likely to die without palliation of the symptoms of dyspnea.

Recent reports have shown that mechanical assistance therapy for the failing heart is safe and effective when used in patients who are waiting for a heart transplant.[4,13] As is the case with the literature on predictive models for patients with heart failure, the experience with these devices is limited to use in a select population of patients whose conditions differs from that of most patients seen in the ICU with heart failure. A trial has been undertaken to evaluate the safety and effectiveness of this rescue therapy in patients older than 65 years.[4] Recently, much attention has been paid to left ventriculoplasty surgery, also know as the Batista procedure, or ventricular reduction surgery.[14] This surgery is primarily for patients without coronary artery disease (CAD) who have markedly dilated ventricles, in whom a segment of the lateral wall of the left ventricle is excised in an effort to reduce left ventricular volume and normalize wall stress. Simultaneously, a modified mitral valvuloplasty is performed to reduce mitral regurgitation. The initial favorable reports have not been corroborated, therefore, this surgery should not be considered part of the management of patients with heart failure.

Several studies are investigating the utility of implantable cardioverter defibrillators (ICDs) in patients with heart failure. Recent studes have defined a subset of patients with heart failure at risk of sudden death, and ICD implantation rates in these groups have increased markedly. Many cardiologists expect the ongoing studies to increase the proportion of patients with ICDs to increase, making the issue of device management one of increasing importance. For example, a patient with an ICD who has decided not to receive resuscitative efforts should have the device turned off. Further, the management of the ICD needs to be discussed with patients and their families. If a choice between the mode of death needs to be made, many patients feel comfortable turning off the ICD so that a sudden event would be terminal, as opposed to a more prolonged course of progressive symptoms.

Pharmacologic therapy of decompensated heart failure has focused on the use of positive inotropic agents, especially dobutamine and milrinone. Although these agents produce measurable hemodynamic changes within minutes of initiation, they increase the risk of death during long-term use. For this reason, the product insert for these agents has recently been scrutinized by the U.S. Food and Drug Administration (FDA) and is undergoing revision to indicate that use of positive inotropic agents needs to be limited. However, patients who have severe symptoms of dyspnea who do respond to inotropic therapy may be offered continuous administration, even while at home. This palliative therapy, in addition to intravenous morphine, can markedly reduce the symptoms in advanced cases. Unfortunately, reimbursement for this strategy can be difficult to obtain for patients who are not awaiting transplant, and repeated pulmonary artery catheterizations are required for Medicare approval. Despite this barrier, the use of positive inotropes and intravenous morphine are integral parts of palliative therapy, even after patients and physicians commit to limit curative therapy.

Conclusion

Therapeutic modalities for patients in the ICU with advanced heart failure are numerous and generally effective, but eventually, the disease will prove refractory. These early and frequent successes alter the expectations of cardiologists treating patients with congestive heart failure, enforcing a barrier that hinders end-of-life discussions and planning. Each of the new therapies holds great promise, but with a potential cost that may be difficult to communicate to a patient and family. The techniques and skills outlined elsewhere in this book are crucial to effective communication when a patient reaches the end stages of this disease and rescue therapies are changed to palliative therapies.

The management of congestive heart failure in the ICU is demanding because of the volume of patients and the complexity of medical management. Communication regarding the prognosis and the life-threatening nature of this disorder needs to be a primary focus of the overall management plan, especially in the compensated, ambulatory state. With effective communication and the development of tools specific to the decision-making process of limiting treatments in the ICU, humane treatment and palliation plans can be effectively implemented.

References

1. Senni M, Tribouilloy CM, Rodeheffer RJ, Jacobsen SJ, Evans JM, Bailey KR, Redfield MM. Congestive heart failure in the community: trends in incidence and survival in a 10-year period. *Arch Intern Med* 1998;159:29–34.
2. McMurray JJV, Petrie MC, Murdoch DR, Davie AP. Clinical epidemiology of heart failure: public and private health burden. *Euro Heart J* 1998;19(Suppl P):9–16.
3. O'Connell JB, Bristow MR. Economic impact of heart failure in the United States: time for a different approach. *J Heart Lung Transplant* 1994;13(4):S107–S112.
4. Goldstein DJ, Oz MC, Rose EA. Implantable left ventricular assist devices. *N Engl J Med* 1998;339:1522–1533.
5. Pfeffer MA, Braunwald E, Moye LA, Basta L, Brown EJ, Cuddy TE, Dans BR, Geltman EM, Goldman S, Flaker GC. Effect of captopril on mortality and morbidity in patients with left ventricular dysfunction after myocardial infarction. *N Engl J Med* 1992;327:669–677.
6. Wachter RM, Luce JM, Hearst N, Lo B. Decisions about resuscitation: inequities among patients with different diseases but similar prognoses. *Ann Intern Med* 1989;111:525–532.
7. Krumholz HM, Phillips RS, Hamel MB, Tano JM, Bellamy P, Broste SK, Cariff RM, Vidaillet H, Davis RB, Muhlbaier LH, Connors AF, Lynn J, Goldman L. Resuscitation preferences among patients with sever congestive heart failure. Results for the SUPPORT project. *Circulation* 1998;98:648–655.
8. Kennedy GT, Crawford MH. Resuscitation issues in patients with severe congestive heart failure. *Congestive Heart Failure* 1998;Sept/Oct:33–36.
9. Aaronson KD, Schwartz JS, Chen TM, Wong KL, Goin JE, Mancini DM. Development and prospective validation of a clinical index to predict survival in ambulatory patients referred for cardiac transplant evaluation. *Circulation* 1997;95:2660–2667.
10. Deng MC, Gradaus R, Hammel D, Weyand M, Gunther F, Kerber S, Haverkamp W, Roeder N, Breithardt G, Scheld HH. Heart transplant candidates at high risk can be identified at the time of initial evaluation. *Transplant Int* 1996;9:38–45.
11. Morley D, Brozena SC. Assessing risk by hemodynamic profile in patients awaiting cardiac transplantation. *Am J Cardiol* 1994;73:379–383.
12. Lee WH, Packer M. Prognostic importance of serum sodium concentration and its modification by converting-enzyme inhibition in patients with severe chronic heart failure. *Circulation* 1986;73:257–267.
13. McCarthy PM, Smedira NO, Vargo RL, Goormastic M, Hobbs RE, Starling RC, Young JB. One hundred patients with the heart mate left ventricular assist device: evolving concepts and technology. *J Thorac Cardiovasc Surg* 1998;115:904–912.
14. Suma H, Isomura T, Horii T, Sato T, Kikuchi N, Iwahashi K, Hosokawa J. Two-year experience of the Batista operation for non-ischemic cardiomyopathy. *J Cardiol* 1998;32:269–276.

Chapter 25

Chronic Obstructive Pulmonary Disease

JOHN E. HEFFNER

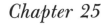

*C*hronic obstructive pulmonary disease (COPD) presents considerable challenges and unique opportunities for physicians who care for critically ill patients at the end of life. This disease is the fourth leading cause of death in the United States, afflicting 30 to 35 million Americans, one-half of whom have symptomatic disease.[1] Patients with symptomatic disease follow a progressive course over several decades, experiencing a more rapid loss of lung function than age-matched, nonsmoking individuals. This gradual and predictable deterioration of lung function provides an opportunity for patients and their physicians to anticipate the general nature of future respiratory health events and initiate timely advance care planning.

Once patients develop moderate to severe COPD, however, their clinical course is punctuated by unpredictable, acute exacerbations of airway disease. Each of these exacerbations can cause life-threatening respiratory failure and may require intubation and mechanical ventilation. Episodes of respiratory failure challenge physicians to determine whether patients will recover and resume their baseline respiratory function, recover with more severe functional limitations, fail to wean from mechanical ventilation and require long-term ventilatory support, or die during hospitalization. Treating all patients aggressively at the outset of their ICU hospital stay neglects the possibility that respiratory failure in some patients represents the terminal phase of COPD, when aggressive life support may offer little opportunity of short-term survival and a dubious postrecovery quality of life. The prediction of which patients will receive sufficient benefit from life-supportive care to warrant its institution represents a major challenge to critical care physicians.

Predicting Outcomes

As an aggregate, patients with acute respiratory failure due to an acute exacerbation of COPD have a relatively good probability of survival to hospital discharge compared with patients who have other causes of respiratory failure. Multiple observational studies indicate that 66% to 94% of patients with COPD and a variety of comorbid conditions admitted with respiratory failure with or without the need for intubation survive their hospital stay.[2,3] More than 90% of patients are expected to survive if their respiratory failure occurs as a result of an acute exacerbation of COPD rather than a comorbid condition, such as congestive heart failure.[4] Survival to hospital discharge ranges from 60% to 74% in hospitalized patients with COPD who require intubation and mechanical ventilation for respiratory failure.[5]

An episode of respiratory failure, does however, identify a subgroup of patients who have a poor long-term survival. Patients with COPD admitted with respiratory failure with or without a need for intubation have an overall 2-year survival of 51%.[3] Patients who require intubation and mechanical ventilation for respiratory failure have a 1-year survival that ranges between 19% and 42%.[2]

The probability of acquiring greater functional limitations after an episode of respiratory failure is less well defined. Experience indicates, however, that some patients rapidly regain their baseline function while others experience more severe levels of dyspnea and decreased functional capacity after hospital discharge.

Several studies have examined how clinical factors that are assessable at the time of admission can be used to identify the subgroup of patients with COPD who will not survive an episode of acute respiratory failure. Examined factors include (1) clinical features of the acute respiratory failure, (2) baseline lung function, (3) existence of comorbid conditions, (4) quality of life factors, and (5) initial response to critical care support.

Clinical features of acute respiratory failure have poor predictive ability in identifying patients who will fail to benefit from ICU care.[2] The severity of arterial blood gas abnormalities, metabolic derangements, or hemodynamic instability has limited predictive accuracy to direct decision making for the individual patient. Results of acute illness scoring systems, such as Acute Physiology and Chronic Health Evaluation (APACHE) II and the Simplified Acute Physiology Score (SAPS), also have poor predictive abilities for patients with COPD and respiratory failure.[6] Most of the available studies that examine this factor are compromised by spectrum bias with poor control for comorbid conditions. Multivariate models, however, do not sufficiently improve the predictive ability of clinical factors available at the time of admission to allow their use in clinical practice.[7]

Baseline levels of functional impairment correlate better with clinical outcome than acute changes in physiology.[5,8,9] Models have not been derived, however, that incorporate measures of baseline function with other clinical factors.

The survivor effect wherein patients with more advanced disease may survive respiratory failure despite severe underlying airway disease may further limit the predictive value of baseline lung function.

Some but not all studies indicate that comorbid disorders, such as congestive heart failure, pulmonary thromboemboli, pneumonia, and gastrointestinal hemorrhage, have a greater impact on survival of patients with COPD during an episode of respiratory failure than the nature of the respiratory failure itself.[7,10] No model exists, however, that incorporates the presence and severity of comorbid conditions in predicting the outcome of hospitalized patients with acute exacerbations of COPD.

It is difficult to incorporate quality of life into decision making to provide life-supportive care for patients with COPD at the outset of acute respiratory failure. Physicians tend to underestimate the quality of their patients' lives compared to patients' self-perceptions.[11] In one study, elderly patients ventilated for any cause of respiratory failure considered their quality of life satisfactory and did not regard themselves as burdens on community health care resources.[12]

Limited data suggest that the probability of survival of patients with COPD diminishes as mechanical ventilation becomes prolonged. Insufficient data exist, however, to develop a reliable predictor of survival from duration of intubation. For other etiologies of respiratory failure, duration of intubation has not proven to correspond with probability of survival.

No studies provide a profile of the patient with COPD complicated by acute respiratory failure for whom life-supportive care would be futile. In this patient population, decisions to withhold intubation and mechanical ventilation most often derive from patients' perceptions of their preexisting quality of life and the relative benefits and burdens of life-supportive interventions rather than from clinicians' ability to define futility.

Communicating with Patients and Families

The discussion above indicates that most but not all patients with respiratory failure due to an acute exacerbation of COPD will survive but that survival and the risk of worsened functional impairment after recovery are difficult to predict. In managing patients with moderate to severe COPD complicated by acute respiratory failure, critical care physicians need to blend their imperfect prognosticating abilities with patients' life goals, values, end-of-life wishes, and self-perceived quality of life so that individual patients will have the greatest opportunity to receive the most appropriate end-of-life care.

Patients with COPD appear to have established opinions regarding the acceptability of life-supportive care, which vary depending on clinical circumstances. In a questionnaire study of patients with chronic lung disease who were enrolled in pulmonary rehabilitation,[13] patients were less likely to state an interest in accepting life-supportive care when their baseline or anticipated postrecovery activity levels were poor or if the probability of survival was low. Unfortunately, most of these patients did not communicate these wishes to their physicians and did not think that their physicians understood their end-of-life wishes. Moreover, less than one-half of these patients had completed formal advance directives.

Most patients with COPD, however, indicate a willingness to discuss end-of-life issues and receive explicit information regarding the nature of life-supportive care.[13] Although they would prefer to receive this information as an outpatient during periods of stable health, they are willing to participate in their end-of-life decision making during hospitalizations for acute events. In discussing treatment options with patients and their families, critical care physicians should adopt an explicit approach to quantify anticipated outcomes and at the same time convey the uncertainties and imprecision of medical predictions (Table 25–1). Also, the nature of life-supportive care should be described so that patients and their families can make informed decisions. Life-supportive care can be presented like

Table 25–1. Components of discussing life-supportive care with patients and families during episodes of respiratory failure

Advance planning

Does the patient have established opinions regarding the acceptability of life-supportive care that apply to this clinical circumstance?
Has the patient decided that life-supportive care is unacceptable in all clinical circumstances because of poor baseline functional capacity?

Rationale for life-supportive care

Why is life-supportive care needed?

Alternatives to care

Are their alternatives to life-supportive care?
Is there time to reassess the patient for evidence of improvement before initiating life-supportive care?
What alternatives exist if the patient fails to wean from mechanical ventilation?
Can care be later withdrawn?
Are long-term resources available for managing prolonged ventilatory support?

Anticipated outcomes

What are the best estimates for survival and postrecovery functional capacity?
What is the level of precision of these estimates?

Nature of life supportive care

What components of life-supportive care are being considered?
What do patients experience during initiation of care such as translaryngeal intubation, mechanical ventilation, and tracheotomy?
What are the anticipated benefits and risks of life-supportive care?

any other health care intervention in which the reasons for health care recommendations, alternative approaches, potential benefit from each alternative, risks in terms of complications and suffering, and probability of outcome are discussed. Patients with respiratory failure due to exacerbations of COPD are particularly suitable for these discussions because most require predictable elements of life-prolonging care that include airway management, ventilatory support, weaning protocols, and treatment with sedatives and analgesics.

Available data indicate that patients with chronic lung disease wish to participate with their physicians in explicit discussions of the nature of life-supportive interventions that they may later require.[13] Although many physicians shield their patients from such discussions because they don't want to evoke fear, depression, hopelessness, and anxiety in their patients, most patients do not consider these discussions anxiety provoking, or they wish to participate even if some anxiety is experienced. A clear understanding of health care interventions underlies the patient's ability to provide informed consent.

In discussing life-supportive interventions, physicians can emphasize their limited ability to predict clinical outcomes from ICU care. Patients and families can more effectively incorporate this uncertainty into their decision making if they understand that life-prolonging care can be withdrawn later if it fails to provide anticipated benefits. Patients also benefit from the knowledge that effective approaches do exist to manage dyspnea, pain, and suffering during the withdrawal of life support.

Impact of New Technologies and Patient Care Resources on End-of-Life Care

For patients with COPD, management issues during episodes of respiratory failure have pivoted around the decision to perform translaryngeal intubation and initiate mechanical ventilation. The advent of noninvasive positive pressure ventilation (NPPV) provides an alternative approach to ventilatory support that decreases mortality in subgroups of patients with acute respiratory failure due to COPD.[14] This new technology requires that physicians clearly describe to patients the different approaches that exist to initiate ventilatory support. Patients may mistakenly frame their life-supportive decisions around a belief that they do not want to "die on a ventilator," not realizing that options exist that they may find more acceptable. Patients also need to be informed that NPPV can be used as a component of palliative care, to manage dyspnea for patients who refuse life-prolonging care and expect to die during their hospitalization.[15]

Patients who present with respiratory failure in the terminal phase of COPD may need information about a potential benefit from lung volume reduction surgery (LVRS) before they can make decisions about the withholding or withdrawal of life-supportive care. In highly selected patients with emphysema, LVRS has been demonstrated to provide significant short-term improvement in functional status and spirometric test values.[16] It remains unclear whether LVRS can be applied to the general population of patients with advanced COPD. The long-term duration of improved pulmonary function demonstrated with LVRS and its overall impact on mortality remain unknown. The National Emphysema Treatment Trial is an ongoing study that addresses these questions. At present, LVRS is not considered salvage therapy for patients with COPD who face end-of-life decisions.

Although 40% of lung transplants are performed in patients with COPD, transplantation surgery is not a treatment option for patients with advanced COPD who are considering the acceptability of life-supportive care. Only 1000 lung transplants are performed worldwide each year, and patients typically wait on transplant lists for 18 to 24 months before surgery is performed.[16] Rigorous selective criteria exclude most patients with COPD who present with acute respiratory failure.

The advent of long-term acute care (LTAC) facilities impacts life support decision making for patients with advanced COPD. Studies indicate that patients who require prolonged ventilatory support benefit from a transfer to LTAC units from acute care facilities when they achieve clinical stability.[17] The location, nature, and funding requirements for LTAC units should be a component of discussions with patients and their families when the withholding or withdrawal of life support is being considered.

Disease-Specific Complications and Palliative Care

Dyspnea represents a major complication during the terminal phase of COPD.[18] It occurs in 29% to 90% of dying patients regardless of their underlying condition.[19] Almost all of the patients with COPD monitored in the Study to Understand Prognoses and Preferences for Outcomes and Risks of Treatment (SUPPORT) experienced dyspnea during the last few days of life.[20] Patients who elect not to undergo intubation for an episode of respiratory failure are at risk of suffering from profound shortness of breath. unless they are carefully monitored and aggressively managed with appropriate palliative care.

Among nonpharmacologic measures available to reduce dyspnea, supplemental oxygen provides marginal benefit. A recent controlled study failed to demonstrate reduced dyspnea in cancer patients who were given oxygen compared to patients managed with compressed air.[21] Although supplemental oxygen by simple delivery systems is a traditional measure in palliative care for hypoxic patients, uncomfortable masks that ensure adequate inspired oxygen saturations but interfere with communication or cause facial discomfort are unlikely to provide meaningful improvements to warrant their use. An electric fan directed toward the patient's face produces a stream of cold air that can diminish the severity of dyspnea.[22,23]

The terminal phase of respiratory failure may produce marked increases in work of breathing and hypercapnia that can induce severe dyspnea. Limited data suggest that NPPV via a face mask can lessen dyspnea while still allowing patients to communicate with their families during mask removal.[15] Patients or family members can apply the NPPV mask intermittently as needed when symptoms worsen. Continuous positive airway pressure (CPAP) has not been shown to relieve dyspnea in spontaneously breathing patients with COPD.[24,25]

Among the pharmacologic approaches, continued specific therapy of the underlying airway disease with inhaled bronchodilators and corticosteroids is indicated. Beta-agonist drugs should be dosed carefully so as to avoid the discomforts of adrenergic side-effects.

Systemic opioids provide the most effective palliative relief of severe dyspnea by altering the perception of breathlessness, decreasing ventilatory response to hypoxia and hypercapnia, and reducing oxygen consumption. During the terminal phase of COPD, opioids are considered by ethicists and legal authorities to be acceptable for managing dyspnea when these agents are given for symptom relief without the intention of hastening death (principle of "double effect"). It is acceptable to provide opioids if dyspnea relief is the primary intention and if an accelerated death is an anticipated but unintended consequence. Some critical care experts observe, however, that dyspnea in terminal patients with advanced lung disease is so severe that lethal doses of opioids may be required to relieve discomfort.[18] In such circumstances, relief of dyspnea may require a hastening of death, which intertwines intended and unintended consequences, so that the principle of double effect may no longer apply.[26] In our experience, however, most patients experience relief of dyspnea at opioid doses that do not extinguish respiratory drive. Clearly, more effective approaches to controlling dyspnea without depressing ventilatory drive are needed for terminal patients with COPD.

Table 25–2 provides dosing information for opioid agents used in the palliative care of dyspnea. Oral opioids provide unreliable relief of dyspnea for patients with COPD[27] and produce considerable adverse side-effects.[28] Nebulized opioids may diminish dyspnea without affecting ventilatory drive,[29,30] although a recent report indicates that respiratory depression can occur.[31] Profound dyspnea usually requires parenteral morphine. Doses should be adjusted to anticipate dyspnea rather than administered on an as-needed basis.

Benzodiazepines have failed to demonstrate advantages over use of placebo in relieving dyspnea in ambulatory patients with advanced COPD.[32] During the terminal phase of the disease, however, they may assist the dying patient if dyspnea is accompanied by anxiety.[19] Because they cloud consciousness, their use is reserved for severe dyspnea during the final days of life. Chlorpromazine has been reported to lessen dyspnea that is unresponsive to opioids and benzodiazepines.[33]

Patients with COPD frequently experience an intractable cough at the end of life, which can aggravate dyspnea, cause musculoskeletal pain, and fracture ribs. Opioids are the most effective cough-suppressive agents (Table 25–2). Some patients may respond to nebulized anesthetics (Table 25–2).[34] Expectorants and mucolytics have no demonstrated value for lessening cough.

During the last hours of life, retained secretions produce a "death rattle,"

Table 25–2. Agents used to manage symptoms related to chronic obstructive pulmonary disease at the end of life

Indication	Drug	Commonly used dosage
Dyspnea	*Morphine*	
	Oral	5–10 mg q4 hr
	Per rectum	5–10 mg q4 hr
	IV, SQ, or IM	Titrate to relieve dyspnea
	Nebulized	5 mg in 2 ml normal saline q4 hr with hand-held nebulizer
	Benzodiazepines	
	Lorazepam, oral, sublingual, IV	1–2 mg q1–4 hr
	Diazepam, oral, IV	2.5–25 mg daily
	Midazolam, SQ	5–10 mg SQ then 10–30 mg continuous SQ infusion for 2 days
	Chlorpromazine IV	12.5 mg iv q4–6 hr
	Chlorpromazine, per rectum	25 mg q4–6 hr
Cough	*Opioids*	
	Codeine, oral	30–60 mg q4 hr
	Morphine, IV	2.5–5 mg q4 hr
	Inhaled anesthetics	
	Bupivacaine, 0.25%	5 mg q4–6 hr
Retained secretions	*Anticholinergic agents*	
	Scopolamine, SQ	0.4 to 0.6 mg q4–6 hr
	Scopolamine transdermal patch	q72 hr
	Hyoscyamine, SQ	0.25–0.5 mg q4–6 hr
	Atropine, SQ	0.4 mg q4–6 hr

IM, intramuscular; IV, intravenous; SQ, subcutaneous.

which distresses families but usually goes unnoticed by patients. Because oropharyngeal and nasopharyngeal suctioning causes patient discomfort, retained secretions can be treated most effectively with anticholinergic agents (Table 25–2).

Conclusion

Regardless of the underlying disease or condition, terminal dyspnea represents a potential source of suffering for patients as they pass through the end of life. Patients with advanced COPD comprise a unique population who live for years in the shadow of dyspnea, and these patients become all too familiar with its capacity for engendering a special form of agony. They also learn from experience during the later stages of their disease that therapeutic approaches for alleviating chronic dyspnea are woefully inadequate. Such patients develop intimate fears that they will some day slowly "suffocate to death." As patients with COPD progress in the severity of their disease, they benefit from perceptive caregivers who anticipate, recognize, and confront these special fears. Comprehensive care can then emerge from an early and ongoing dialogue with caregivers regarding end-of-life issues, advance planning, and the nature of life-sustaining interventions and their probable outcomes, and the promise of palliative care for alleviating the terminal manifestations of airway disease.

References

1. Petty TL. Definitions, causes, course, and prognosis of chronic obstructive pulmonary disease. *Respir Care Clin North Am* 1998;4:345–358.
2. Heffner JE. Chronic obstructive pulmonary disease—ethical considerations of care. *Clin Pulm Med* 1996;3:1–8.
3. Connors AF, Dawson NV, Thomas C, Harrell FE, Desbiens N, Fulkerson WJ, Kussin P, Bellamy P, Goldman L, Knaus WA. Outcomes following acute exacerbations of severe chronic obstructive lung disease. The SUPPORT investigators. *Am J Respir Crit Care Med* 1996;154:959–967.
4. Martin TR, Lewis SW, Albert RK. The prognosis of patients with chronic obstructive pulmonary disease after hospitalization for acute respiratory failure. *Chest* 1982; 82:310–314.
5. Portier F, Defouilloy C, Muir JF. Determinants of immediate survival among chronic respiratory insufficiency patients admitted to an intensive care unit for acute respiratory failure. *Chest* 1992;101:204–210.
6. Knaus WA. Prognosis with mechanical ventilation: the influence of disease, severity of disease, age and chronic health status on survival from an acute illness. *Am Rev Respir Dis* 1989;140:S8–S13.
7. Kaelin RM, Assimacopoulos A, Chevrolet JC. Failure to predict six-month survival of patients with COPD requiring mechanical ventilation by analysis of simple indices. *Chest* 1987;92:971–978.
8. Jessen O. Tracheostomy and artificial ventilation in chronic lung disease. *Lancet* 1967;2:9–12.
9. Menzies R, Gibbons W, Goldberg P. Determinants of weaning and survival among patients with COPD who require mechanical ventilation for acute respiratory failure. *Chest* 1989;95:398–405.
10. Rieves RD, Bass D, Carter RR, Griffith JE, Norman JR. Severe COPD and acute respiratory failure. Correlates for survival at the time of tracheal intubation. *Chest* 1993;104:854–860.
11. Uhlmann RF, Pearlman RA. Perceived quality of life and preferences for life-sustaining treatment in older adults. *Arch Intern Med* 1991;151:495–497.
12. McLean RF, McIntosh JD, Kung GY, Leung DM, Byrick RJ. Outcome of respiratory intensive care for the elderly. *Crit Care Med* 1985;13:625–629.
13. Heffner JE, Fahy B, Hilling L, Barbieri C. Attitudes regarding advance directives among patients in pulmonary rehabilitation. *Am J Respir Crit Care Med* 1996; 154:1735–1740.
14. Hess D, Medoff B. Mechanical ventilation of the patient with chronic obstructive pulmonary disease. *Respir Care Clin North Am* 1998;4:439–473.
15. Meduri GU, Fox RC, Abou-Shala N, Leeper KV, Wunderink RG. Noninvasive me-

chanical ventilation via face mask in patients with acute respiratory failure who refused endotracheal intubation. *Crit Care Med* 1994;22:1584–1590.

16. Edelman JD, Kotloff RM. Surgical approaches to advanced emphysema. *Respir Care Clin North Am* 1998;4:513–539.

17. Gracey DR, Viggiano RW, Naessens JM, Hubmayr RD, Silverstein MD, Koenig GE. Outcomes of patients admitted to a chronic ventilator-dependent unit in an acute-care hospital. *Mayo Clinic Proc* 1992;67:131–136.

18. Hansen-Flaschen J. Advanced lung disease: palliation and terminal care. *Clin Chest Med* 1997;18:645–655.

19. Rousseau P. Nonpain symptom management in terminal care. *Clin Geriatr Med* 1996;12:313–327.

20. Lynn J, Teno JM, Phillips RS, et al. Perceptions by family members of the dying experience of older and serioulsy ill patients. *Ann Intern Med* 1997;126:97–106.

21. Booth S, Kelly M, Cox N, Adams L, Guz A. Does oxygen help dyspnea in patients with cancer? *Am J Respir Crit Care Med* 1996;153:1515–1518.

22. Friedman S. Facial cooling and perception of dyspnea [letter]. *Lancet* 1987;2:1215.

23. Schwartzstein R, Lahive K, Pope A, Weinberger SE, Weiss JW. Cold facial stimulation reduces breathlessness induced in normal subjects. *Am Rev Respir Dis* 1987; 136:58–61.

24. Fessler HE, Brower RG, Permutt S. CPAP reduces inspiratory work more than dyspnea during hyperinflation with intrinsic PEEP. *Chest* 1995;108:432–440.

25. Christensen HR, Simonsen K, Lange P, Clemensten P, Kampmann JP, Viskum K, Heideby J, Koch U. PEEP-masks in patients with severe obstructive pulmonary disease: a negative report. *Eur Respir J* 1990;3:267–272.

26. Quill T. The ambiguity of clinical intentions. *N Engl J Med* 1993;329:1039–1040.

27. Woodcock AA, Gross ER, Gellert A, Shah S, Johnson M, Geddes DM. Effects of dihydrocodeine, alcohol, and caffeine on breathlessness and exercise tolerance in patients with chronic obstructive lung disease and normal blood gases. *N Engl J Med* 1981;305:1611–1616.

28. Boyd KJ, Kelly M. Oral morphine as symptomatic treatment of dyspnoea in patients with advanced cancer. *Palliat Med* 1997;11:277–281.

29. Farncombe M, Chater S, Gillin A. The use of nebulized opioid for breathlessness: a chart review. *Palliat Med* 1994;8:306–312.

30. Zeppetella G. Nebulized morphine in the palliation of dyspnoea. *Palliat Med* 1997; 11:267–275.

31. Jedeikin R, Lang E. Acute respiratory depression as a complication of nebulised morphine. *Can J Anaesth* 1998;45:60–62.

32. O'Donnell DE. Breathlessness in patients with chronic airflow limitation. Mechanisms and management. *Chest* 1994;106:904–912.

33. McIver B, Walsh D, Nelson K. The use of chlorpromazine for symptom control in dying cancer patients. *J Pain Symptom Manage* 1994;9:341–345.

34. Hsu DH. Dyspnea in dying patients. *Can Fam Physician* 1993;39:1635–1638.

Chapter 26

Decisions to Limit Intensive Care in Patients with Coma

EELCO F.M. WIJDICKS

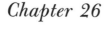eurologists are often involved in decisions to limit life support, partly because of the high prevalence of neurologic catastrophes in critically ill patients receiving intensive care. Neurologic conditions are common in studies on the withholding or withdrawal of life support in critically ill patients. In a survey of withholding care in 1719 patients admitted to ICUs in San Francisco, 66 of 115 (57%) patients had intracranial lesions.[1] Studies looking at neurologic circumstances in which specific forms of life support have been withdrawn are scarce and have poorly documented knowledge, biases, and clinical reasoning.

One may argue that in a patient with an obvious neurologic ictus, a neurologic consultation is imperative to document the severity of coma, to delineate it from other states of altered consciousness, and to confirm the cause of coma. In this chapter, conditions accompanied by a very high certainty of neurologic devastation are discussed. This devastation may prompt discussion with family members who may have uninformed and unrealistic expectations if the critical illness has been under control. Palliative care for patients with neurologic conditions is discussed as well.

General Considerations

Neurologic complications can be overwhelmingly devastating, and when they occur in an evolving critical illness, family members may demand that all supportive medical efforts be stopped. Coma is typically defined as a sleep-like state in which the patient's eyes are closed and there is no motor response to pain other than primitive reflexes. Related disorders of consciousness that should be recognized by any physician because of the implications for outcome are listed in Table 26–1.

Withdrawal of life support in patients with neurologic complications has unique features. First, accurate prediction of outcome remains very difficult except in well-defined disorders with established poor outcomes. For these conditions (Table 26–2), most neurologists would feel very comfortable, after adequate observation, with withdrawal of life support. These conditions are not likely to conflict with the professional judgment of the attending intensive care specialist. Second, patient autonomy cannot be addressed, because the structural lesion of the brain affects any expression of the patient's wishes. In these circumstances, a surrogate decision maker is imperative.

For the vast majority of family members, sustained medical care creates a situation in which one is constantly reminded of what the person once was, and this may be more devastating than acute tragic death. Many family members clearly understand the demoralizing effect on caregivers, the waste of resources, and that high-technologic care is unnecessary.

Any decision about cessation of life-sustaining therapy is based, however, on the patient's autonomy, which in comatose patients is represented by substituted judgment. This was clearly stated by Angell in an editorial on vegetative state: "the judgment about whether to keep such patients alive, once the medical facts are established, requires no medical expertise."[2]

Causes of Coma in the ICU

Coma in critically ill patients is commonly a reflection of progressive organ failure and thus, in most instances, is a terminal event. Many causes of coma are often incorrectly attributed to a metabolic encephalopathy, but in these patients other insults are more likely. In our review of patients with a new-onset stroke in the ICU, a large proportion had an ischemic or hemorrhagic stroke, an affliction that would have been labeled "toxic-metabolic encephalopathy."[3] Acute loss of consciousness with the emergence of pupillary changes and pathologic motor responses often reflects an intracerebral hematoma (e.g., due to coagulopathy or ruptured mycotic aneurysm) with herniation.[4] Poor outcome (severely disabled state, persistent vegetative state, or death) is expected in patients with a hematoma of large volume (≥ 50 ml), age more than 70 years, decreased level of consciousness at ictus, intraventricular extension, or mass effect on computed tomography (CT) scan.[3,4] These comatose patients have virtually no chance of recovery to a functional state unless other systemic factors are depressing the level of consciousness. The mechanism does not influence outcome, but the location may be crucial, because pontine and cerebellum hematomas are associated with poor outcome when coma emerges.[5] Aggressive neurosurgical intervention can be futile, particularly when intraventricular hemorrhage, acute hydrocephalus, and some brain stem reflexes, especially the cornea reflex, are absent.

Table 26–1. Neurologic conditions that produce unresponsiveness

Condition	Self-awareness	Sleep–Wake Cycles	Motor Function	Experiences Suffering	Respiratory Function	EEG	Prognosis for Neurologic Recovery
Persistent vegetative state[a]	Absent	Intact	No purposeful movement; no visual tracking	No	Normal	Polymorphic delta and theta; sometimes slow alpha	Traumatic PVS (1-year outcome): PVS, 15% of patients; dead, 33%; GR, 7%; MD, 17%; SD, 28% Nontraumatic PVS (1-year outcome): PVS, 32% of patients; dead, 53%; GR, 1%; MD, 3%; SD, 11%
Brain death	Absent	Absent	None or only reflex spinal movements	No	Absent	Electrocerebral silence	None
Locked-in syndrome	Present	Intact	Quadriplegia; pseudobulbar palsy; preserved vertical eye movements	Yes	Normal	Normal or mildly abnormal	Without thrombolytic treatment, recovery unlikely; patients remain quadriplegic
Akinetic mutism	Present	Intact	Paucity of movement	Yes	Normal	Nonspecific slowing	Recovery very unlikely but depends on cause

EEG, electroencephalogram; GR, good recovery; MD, moderately disabled; PVS, persistent vegetative state; SD, severely disabled.

[a]Adults only.

From Wijdicks EFM.[4] By permission of Mayo Foundation, as adapted from Medical aspects of the persistent vegetative state: the Multi-Society Task Force on PVS statement of a multi-society task force. *N Engl J Med* 1994;330:1499–1508.

Table 26–2. Neurologic conditions with no hope for recovery

Pontine stage of uncal herniation[15]

Coma and multiple intracranial hemorrhages associated with thrombolysis[4]

Coma and myoclonus status epilepticus[6]

Pontine hemorrhage with hyperthermia[5]

Basilar artery occlusion with coma and apnea[15,16]

Ischemic stroke causing coma in critically ill patients occurs after discontinuation of anticoagulation for a procedure, after cardiovascular surgery, and, rarely, as a result of marked hypotension. If it is associated with coma, the most likely implication is a large middle cerebral artery occlusion or basilar artery occlusion. Prognosticators of poor outcome in carotid territory ischemic stroke are brain swelling and mass effect, gaze palsy and early pupillary asymmetry, and evidence of diencephalic herniation (small unreactive pupils, loss of oculocephalic responses, abnormal motor responses to pain). In the posterior circulation, a locked-in syndrome, cerebellar infarction with brain stem compression and obstructive hydrocephalus, or evidence of bilateral thalamic infarcts indicates a poor outcome.[4]

Outcome prediction in multitrauma associated with head injury is also complex. Patients with a postresuscitation Glasgow coma score of 3 after stabilization have a poor outcome, irrespective of mass lesions or shift on CT scan. Elderly patients ($\geq$ 65 years old) do poorly, and comatose patients in this age category have only a 10% chance of survival and a 4% chance of independent living.[4] Absent pupillary responses and extensor or absent motor responses to pain are potent predictors of poor outcome, irrespective of age or intracerebral lesion.

Hypoxic–ischemic encephalopathy, whether from cardiac resuscitation or from shock, remains a common cause of coma in any ICU. A confident decision on withdrawal of support cannot be made within 72 hours after resuscitation or within 3 days of observation and careful exclusion of possible confounders, such as sedative agents. Myoclonus status epilepticus (brief, constant jerking in limbs and face, often after touch, sound, or tracheal suctioning) has been associated with a poor outcome, and its appearance immediately after resuscitation may influence the level of care[6] (Table 26–3). Absence of bilateral cortical response or somatosensory evoked potentials and a burst suppression pattern on electroencephalography are additional helpful laboratory guides for a poor prognosis.[7]

Discussion with Family

It would be naive to try to capture the complexity of the encounter with the family in a few paragraphs. Neurologists need to guide a sensitive dialogue to an understanding of what they believe are the patient's best interests.[8] Physi-

Table 26–3. Outcome of myoclonic status epilepticus in survivors of cardiac arrest

Reference	Patients n	Surviving to hospital dismissal n
Snyder et al.[17]	4	1
Celesia et al.[18]	13	1
Krumholz et al.[19]	19	0
Jumao-as and Brenner[20]	15	0
Wijdicks et al.[6]	40	0
Young et al.[21]	18	1
Total	109	3 (3%)

Data from Wijdicks EF, Young GB. Myoclonus status in comatose patients after cardiac arrest [letter]. *Lancet* 1994;343:1642–1643.

cians should convey respect and humility to family members who are faced with such complexities and frustrations. One should nonetheless discuss with the family the rationale for continued mechanical ventilation, nutrition, and fluids to maintain a permanently unconscious existence. It is important to use well-defined categories of outcome, summarized in Table 26–4. Futility is undisputed in only a few well-defined conditions, such as brain death (death by neurologic criteria)[9] and a vegetative state of any cause except traumatic brain injury.

Table 26–4. Glasgow Outcome Scale

Good recovery	Patients have the capacity to resume normal occupational and social activities and lead a productive life, although they may have minor physical or mental deficits or complaints.
Moderate disability	Patients are independent and can resume almost all activities of daily living. They are disabled, however, because they can no longer participate in a variety of social and work activities.
Severe disability	Patients can no longer resume most previous personal, social, and work activities. Communication skills are limited, and behavioral and emotional responses are abnormal. Patients are partially or totally dependent on others.
Vegetative state	No evidence of awareness of self or environment and inability to interact with others.
	No evidence of sustained reproducible, purposeful, or voluntary behavioral responses to visual, auditory, tactile, or noxious stimuli.
	No evidence of language comprehension or expression.
	Intermittent wakefulness manifested by sleep–wake cycles.
	Preserved hypothalamic and brain-stem autonomic functions to permit survival with nursing and medical care.
	Variable preserved cranial nerves and spinal reflexes.
	Bowel and bladder incontinence.

Medical opinion may be divided on specific disorders.[10] Problems of diagnosis, the unmeasurable and unpredictable powers of recovery and erratic judgment of physicians, and, perhaps most difficult, the inherent differences in value judgments about the quality of life and the will to enjoy life add to the complexity of determining a patient's level of care.[11] Several neurologic conditions are so devastating that no hope for recovery exists (see Table 26–2); there is a less than 5% chance that the patient will survive the consequences of coma (systemic complications, particularly infections), and no patients have been reported with improvement beyond a severely disabled state (full nursing care, absence of any productive output, and lack of social relationship).

Withdrawal of Life Support

Mechanical ventilation and endotracheal intubation are most commonly considered for withdrawal of support dictated by a neurologic catastrophe. Brain death is considered death by neurologic criteria, and withdrawal is initiated if the family refuses donation. Extubation in patients with coma, however, seldom leads to rapid respiratory arrest. The degree of herniation and brain stem dysfunction predicts respiratory drive. Pontine stages of herniation result in rapid tachypnea interrupted by apnea or, more typically, Cheyne-Stokes breathing. Noisy and rattling breathing may be a source of great distress for families. If repositioning is unsuccessful, glycopyrrolate can be used or scopolamine (Hyoscine) given subcutaneously. Scopolamine relaxes the smooth muscles, and both drugs dry up the secretions of the exocrine glands.[12,13]

Seizures may reoccur in patients when pharmaceutical agents are withdrawn, but this can be anticipated by administering 300 to 600 mg of fosphenytoin intramuscularly several hours before extubation. The family should be explicitly told that this drug is now used for palliation. We have not been successful with any of the antiepileptic drugs in treating myoclonus status epilepticus and have proceeded with paralytic agents for 1 to 2 days before withdrawal of support, because myoclonus disappears within 24 hours in most patients. Paralytic agents should only be used when the patient's comfort has been ensured with other medication.

Terminal sedation ought to be permissible and part of palliation. The administration of opiates for palliation is ethical and legal in all U.S. states. In one study, the average amounts of benzodiazepines and opiates were diazepam at 2.2 mg/hr and morphine sulfate at 3.3 mg/hr in the 24 hours before withdrawal of life support, and 9.8 mg/hr and 11.2 mg/hr, respectively, in the 24 hours thereafter. No evidence exists that these drugs may hasten death.[14] When stages of herniation have been reached (extensor motor responses, light-fixed pupils), the use of sedation is without any rationale. For patients who suffer from intractable headaches and lighter stages of coma, low doses of midazolam or opiates may be effective.

References

1. Smedira NG, Evans BH, Grais LS, Cohen NH, Lo B, Cooke M, Schecter WP, Fink C, Epstein-Jaffe E, May C. Withholding and withdrawal of life support from the critically ill. *N Engl J Med* 1990;322:309–315.
2. Angell M. After Quinlan: the dilemma of the persistent vegetative state. *N Engl J Med* 1994;330:1524–1525.
3. Wijdicks EFM, Scott JP. Stroke in the medical intensive care unit. *Mayo Clin Proc* 1998;73:642–646.
4. Wijdicks EFM. Neurology of Critical Illness Philadelphia: FA Davis, 1995.
5. Wijdicks EFM, St Louis E. Clinical profiles predictive of outcome in pontine hemorrhage. *Neurology* 1997;49:1342–1346.
6. Wijdicks EFM, Parisi JE, Sharbrough FW. Prognostic value of myoclonus status in comatose survivors of cardiac arrest. *Ann Neurol* 1994;35:239–243.
7. Madl C, Kramer L, Yeganehfar W, Eisenhuber E, Icranz A, Ratheiser K, Zauner C, Schneider B, Grimm G. Detection of nontraumatic comatose patients with no benefit of intensive care treatment by recording of sensory evoked potentials. *Arch Neurol* 1996;53:512–516.
8. Franklin C. Decisions about life support: being responsible and responsive. *Crit Care Med* 1998;26:8–9.
9. Wijdicks EF. Determining brain death in adults. *Neurology* 1995;45:1003–1011.
10. The Society of Critical Care Medicine Ethics Committee. Attitudes of critical care medicine professionals concerning foregoing life-sustaining treatments. *Crit Care Med* 1992;20:320–326.
11. Truog RD, Brett AS, Frader J. The problem with futility. *N Engl J Med* 1992; 326:1560–1564.
12. Bennett MI. Death rattle: an audit of Hyoscine (scopolamine) use and review of management. *J Pain Symptom Manage* 1996;12:229–233.
13. Watts T, Jenkins K, Back I. Problem and management of noisy rattling breathing in dying patients. *Int J Palliat Nurs* 1997;3:245–252.
14. Wilson WC, Smedira NG, Fink C, McDowell JA, Luce JM. Ordering and administration of sedatives and analgesics during the withholding and withdrawal of life support from critically ill patients. *JAMA* 1992;267:949–953.
15. Plum F, Posner JB. The Diagnosis of Stupor and Coma, 3rd ed. Philadelphia: FA Davis, 1980.
16. Wijdicks EF, Scott JP. Outcome in patients with acute basilar artery occlusion requiring mechanical ventilation. *Stroke* 1996;27:1301–1303.
17. Snyder BD, Hauser WA, Loewenson RB, Leppik IE, Ramirez-Lassepas M, Gumnit RJ. Neurologic prognosis after cardiopulmonary arrest: III. Seizure activity. *Neurology* 1980;30:1292–1297.
18. Celesia GG, Grigg MM, Ross E. Generalized status myoclonicus in acute anoxic and toxic-metabolic encephalopathies. *Arch Neurol* 1988;45:781–784.
19. Krumholz A, Stern BJ, Weiss HD. Outcome from coma after cardiopulmonary resuscitation: relation to seizures and myoclonus. *Neurology* 1988;38:401–405.
20. Jumao-as A, Brenner RP. Myoclonic status epilepticus: a clinical and electroencephalographic study. *Neurology* 1990;40:1199–1202.
21. Young GB, Gilbert JJ, Zochodne DW. The significance of myoclonic status epilepticus in postanoxic coma. *Neurology* 1990;40:1843–1848.

Chapter 27

Special Concerns for Infants and Children

WALTER M. ROBINSON

$\mathcal{T}$he death of a child in the pediatric ICU is an important but relatively rare occurrence. The total number of deaths from all causes in all locations under the age of 14 is 15,000 per year, with the major causes of mortality being accidents, congenital malformations, and malignant neoplasm.[1] In the United States, the incidence of children needing intensive care is approximately 200 per 100,000. Intensive care for children is generally segregated by age, with neonates being treated in separate intensive care nurseries and those born healthy and older children being cared for in pediatric ICUs. There are similarities but also some important differences in the management of death in the different locations.

Dying in the Neonatal ICU

Admission to the intensive care nursery is most commonly the result of premature birth, but it may also be for stabilization following a term birth with noted congenital anomalies. The practice of withholding resuscitation in the delivery room has slowly declined, with a preference for taking the infant to the intensive care nursery for an initial period of evaluation.[2] A recent study indicates the when the preferences of the parents of premature infants are not known, or when there is great uncertainty as to outcome for a premature infant born in the delivery room, physicians will institute resuscitation at that time, in preparation for transfer to the neonatal ICU. If, however, the preferences of the parents are known, at least for infants of between 23 and 26 weeks gestation, the parents' preferences are the major determination of the treatment performed in the delivery room.[3] While the practice of withdrawing or withholding life support from severely ill newborns was first reported in 1973, the intervening decades have seen substantial controversy over this practice, culminating in the establishment of the so called Baby Doe rules.[4] These Federal rules require that physicians must treat all infants with life-threatening illnesses unless one of three situations pertains: the infant is chronically and irreversibly comatose; the treatment would prolong dying, or would be ineffective in ameliorating or correcting the life-threatening condition faced by the infant; or the treatment would be "virtually futile." Although there has been considerable controversy over the meaning and application of these rules,[5] a consensus has slowly emerged that the rules are not as restrictive as first interpreted.

Prognostic scoring in the neonatal ICU

Until recently, the most common method of prognostication for infants in the neonatal ICU was based on gestational age or birth weight.[6] While there is indeed an association between birth weight and/or gestational age and mortality, the usefulness of these factors as prognostic tools is limited by the fact that most deaths of premature infants occur in the first 2 days of life.[7] The ability of birth weight or gestational age to predict mortality beyond this time is severely limited. As a result, several scales for prediction of mortality have been suggested, most of which are modeled along the lines of the Acute Physiology and Chronic Health Evaluation (APACHE) system used in adult intensive care. Two scales have recently been put forward, each with their own acronym: SNAP (Score of Neonatal Acute Physiology) and CRIB (Clinical Risk Index for Babies). The SNAP[8] is based on the most severe physiologic impairment present in the first 24 hours of life, and the CRIB[9] uses birth weight, gestational age, maximum and minimum FiO_2, maximum base deficit, and presence or absence of any congenital malformations. Because neither of theses prognostic indices can be used before 12 hours of life, a third scale (sometimes called the Berlin scale, after the location of the physicians developing the scale) has been suggested which can be used on admission to the neonatal ICU.[10] In practice, neonatologists may use a variety of factors, culled from several different sources, to estimate outcome for premature infants.[11-13] Because of the difficulty of using these scales in routine care, modification of the scales has been suggested for use at 3 days of life.[14]

Although there may be a general perception that very premature infants are overtreated, the causes of such overtreatment are difficult to assess. As Doron and colleagues aptly put it, parents blame physicians,[15] and physicians blame parents.[16,17] Despite these perceptions, neonatal care has been remarkably successful overall: while mortality rates have declined, rates of severe handicap have not increased,[18,19] which suggests that the improved survival is not at the expense of increased disability. As Stolz and McCormick state, "these results suggest that the majority of even the tiniest premature infants achieve functional outcomes, and that the major increases in survival have not resulted in proportionate increases in severe morbidity."[20]

The debate over the provision of treatment of premature infants and perceptions of under- and overtreatment will strongly influence decisions to withhold or withdraw support in the neonatal ICU. If the outcome of treatment of very premature infants is regarded negatively, then neonatologists are more likely to withhold or withdraw life support.[21] The converse may be true as well, as the calls to restrict care on the basis of birth weight appear to be based on pessimistic views of the outcome for these infants.[22,23] Attempts to use prognostic scales or birth weight and gestational age thresholds (except for gestational age less than 24 weeks) to define "futile" care, and thus to withhold in a systematic manner access to neonatal intensive care, are misguided. The use of such restrictions will only reinforce the already pernicious racial and economic biases present in access to neonatal care and infant survival[24,25] and will not accrue significant resource savings without denying care to infants who would otherwise survive.[20]

Modes of death in the neonatal ICU

Withdrawal of life-sustaining treatment is the most common mode of death in the neonatal ICU (see Table 27–1).[2] In one large 1997 study, 73% percent of the deaths were attributable to the withdrawal or withholding of life-sustaining treatment. Infants with extreme prematurity and/or severe neurologic damage had the highest likelihood of having life-sustaining care withheld. In all cases of withholding treatment, intubation and mechanical ventilation were the treatments withheld; and for all infants for whom treatment was withdrawn, intubation and mechanical ventilation were the treatments withdrawn.[2]

Deciding to withdraw support

The most frequently cited reasons given by neonatologists for the withdrawal of life-sustaining treatment in the 1997 study was the belief of the physician

Table 27–1. Characteristics of death in the neonatal ICU

1. Life-sustaining therapy is more often withdrawn than withheld; DNR orders are written in less than one-quarter of withdrawals.

2. Aggressive delivery room treatment does not preclude withdrawal of life-sustaining therapy once the child's condition is better assessed.

3. Withdrawal of life-sustaining therapy is the most common mode of death among all birth weights, not just those less than 1 kg.

4. The primary reason for withdrawal of life-sustaining therapy is the belief that further therapy is futile in the face of impending death; in less than one-quarter of deaths did intensivists believe quality-of-life concerns were decisive.

Adapted from Wall and Partridge, 1997,[2] with permission.

that continued treatment was futile in the face of imminent death of the patient; this reason was given in approximately three-fourths of the cases.[2] Quality of life concerns were less important, with physicians citing them as the primary reason for withdrawal in less than one-quarter of the cases. Quality-of-life considerations were more likely to be cited by physicians for infants with specific conditions, such as intraventricular hemorrhage.

For parents of critically ill neonates who are considering withdrawal of support, communication with the physicians and nurses is essential.[26–28] Although it may be difficult for some physicians to discuss withdrawal of life-sustaining treatment, avoidance of close family contact as the infant's condition worsens will only make the discussion more difficult. Physicians and nurses must maintain the connections of caring and compassion with families throughout the ICU stay; if families sense that the care team is withdrawing emotional support, this will make withdrawal of life support even more difficult for families and caregivers alike.[29]

Care during and after withdrawal

Despite the development of pain assessment tools for acutely ill neonates, there still is little consensus on the appropriate management of pain in the neonatal ICU.[30] There is, however, no question that the response to acute pain in neonates can be modulated by the use of opiates,[31,32] and the use of opiates to manage the symptoms of dying should be encouraged. In one recent study,[33] the median dose of morphine sulfate used was in the range of 0.1 to 0.2 mg/kg, although experience suggests that this is a dose range appropriate for postsurgical analgesia in the neonate, and that higher doses are likely to be required to treat terminal dyspnea or pain. Opiates were administered to 65% of infants who had life-sustaining therapy withdrawn.[33] Although the data were limited, this report did not show a significant difference in the time to death following ventilator discontinuation between infants receiving opiates and infants who were not treated with opiates. These findings suggest that when used in appropriate doses, opiates do not significantly depress the respiratory drive of infants who are being removed from ventilators. Because this report was limited to study at a single academic hospital, its findings should be viewed with caution; more research is needed on the treatment of symptoms at the end of life in neonates.

The withdrawal of ventilator therapy should be planned in such a way that parents may be able to hold their dying infants, with the minimal amount of interference from monitors, catheters, intravenous lines, or endotracheal tubes (see Table 27–2). In contrast to the practice in many adult ICUs, the endotracheal tube is often removed along with the ventilator in neonates; this is done both for the comfort of the infant (since oral secretions with agonal respirations appear to cause less distress in infants) and for the comfort of the parents while holding the child near the time of death. In the report cited

Table 27–2. Rules of thumb for withdrawal of life sustaining care in neonates

1. Encourage parents to hold the dying child, there should be as little interference as possible from catheters, monitors, intravenous lines, and endotracheal tubes.

2. A quiet room away from the center of the nursery should be used for the family during and after the dying process.

3. Staff should respect the wishes of the parents to be alone, but should remain close by to address any signs of distress in the infant.

4. Neonates, even very premature ones, can perceive pain; opiate analgesia should be used to effectively treat any terminal symptoms during withdrawal.

above, the median time until death following ventilator withdrawal for neonates was in the range of 20 minutes;[33] parents should be prepared for the time course of events, but they should know that each situation is different. If at all possible, a quiet room away from the activity of the nursery should be provided so that the family can hold the dying infant.[34] While staff should respect the parents' wishes to be alone during this time, there should be a plan in place to respond quickly to the infant's discomfort should the need arise. Many parents will have formed a strong bond with the caregivers in the nursery, and may wish to have one or more members of the staff present. Staff should be prepared to take on this role, and staff bereavement practices should take this into account, as discussed in Chapters 13 and 14.

Dying in the Pediatric ICU

The range of patients in the pediatric ICU is broad, but they all share some common characteristics: most are accompanied by worried parents, few families have made any prior decisions to limit care, and very few patients are competent to make their own medical decisions (Table 27–3).

Prognostic scales

Prognostic scales have been developed and validated for the unique aspects of pediatric intensive care. The Pediatric Risk of Mortality (PRISM) scale functions in much the same way as the adult APACHE scales, taking into account

Table 27–3. Characteristics of death in the pediatric ICU

1. Very few, if any, patients will have an advance directive prior to entering the ICU, nor will restriction of therapy have been considered by parents prior to admission.

2. The primary mode of death in the pediatric ICU is withdrawal of a ventilator.

3. For patients who die in the pediatric ICU, the length of stay prior to death is usually 2–3 days.

illness severity as measured by a combination of bedside and laboratory measures.[35] The PRISM score is a useful research tool, for it allows the comparison
of patients across time and, within limits, across ICUs. However, PRISM scores
are a population-based measure and, like all prognostic scales, have limited use
in prediction of individual patient outcomes. Scoring systems such as the
PRISM should therefore not be used as a justification to withhold ICU admission to a child based on the expectation of death during the ICU stay (i.e., that
the stay in the ICU would be futile), since the scales cannot measure the
outcome for any particular child and do not take into account the response to
therapy.

Making the decision to withdraw support

Several factors contribute to the very strong "rule of rescue" in pediatric intensive care. First, death during childhood is always viewed as premature, for it
represents a loss of potential; it is the death of a dream as well as the death of a
child. Neither the culture of medicine nor the culture at large has a socially or
psychologically sanctioned meaning for the death of a child; the common understanding of having "lived a long life" cannot be invoked, and a child's death
evokes a sense of unfairness. Second, a child cannot declare what path suits the
child's interests; the parents and clinicians must decide for the child. In doing
so, caregivers will be affected by both future and present interests in a way that
is substantially different from that with an adult. There can be a tendency in
pediatrics to discount the current suffering of a child because of the great
potential loss of future life; the same tendency is not seen as powerfully in the
treatment of the elderly. These two factors combine to create and maintain a
powerful motivation to continue curative treatment in a child and to regard
even very small chances of recovery as acceptable.

The trajectory of the child's illness strongly influences any decisions made
concerning life-sustaining treatment in the ICU (Table 27–4).[36] The particular
stresses on the family of a child admitted to an ICU for an acute injury will be
different from those of parents whose child had a chronic illness. The family of
an acutely injured child will usually feel a greater sense of shock, and they may
well have feelings of guilt for failing to protect their child against the injury.[29]
For the parents of the chronically ill child, admission to the ICU may be a
frank reminder of the lethality of the child's diagnosis. Parents show many
methods of coping with the severe illness of a child, one common method
being to "never give up hope."[34] In some cases, parents and physicians may
translate "never giving up hope" into a drive for more and more aggressive
therapy, even as the chance of cure for that therapy dwindles. In this situation,
one approach is to openly discuss the difficulty for both the parents and caregivers of holding onto hope for recovery and feeling sorrow at the grim prognosis. Caregivers may try to rechannel the hope of a family toward a hope for
peace or comfort instead of recovery. It may also help to acknowledge that

Table 27–4. Rules of thumb for withdrawal of life-sustaining therapy in the pediatric ICU

1. Consider the trajectory of the child's illness in making decisions about limitation of therapy; chronically ill children and their families may have needs and concerns that are different from those of acutely ill children.

2. The decision to limit therapy must be made on a shared basis with the family, and the family should be integrated into the comfort plan for the dying child.

3. Analgesia and sedation should be given according to symptoms, and a specific plan to monitor and manage any increase in symptoms should be established.

4. Quiet areas should be established, with opportunities for the parent to hold the child and for all the family to visit; staff should remain nearby to address symptoms.

comfort measures themselves do not decrease the chance of the hoped-for miracle of recovery.

In discussing the decision to change the goals of care, good communication with the family is essential.[37] Integration of the family into the care of the child will make communication easier by encouraging a shared caring for the child's illness. Families can be essential in helping a child cope with the stress of intensive care, and this focus on the experience of the child can often lead to greater insight on the part of both families and caregivers.[38-40] Various methods, from liberal visitation to "family rounds" to structured family discussion times can be used to improve communication. This should help when a difficult decision must be made about redirecting the goals of care.

Modes of death in pediatric ICUs

The decision to limit life-sustaining therapy in the pediatric ICU is made relatively early in the ICU stay. Children for whom life-sustaining therapy is eventually withheld or withdrawn have a median total length of stay in the pediatric ICU of 2 to 3 days, although the variability in length of stay is quite large, with some patients staying in the unit as long as 100 days.[41,42] The usual cause of death in the pediatric ICU is respiratory (rather than cardiac) failure; withdrawal of the ventilator is the most common mode of death.[41-44] For example, in a single pediatric ICU in Salt Lake City in 1993, 32% of all deaths followed the withdrawal of a ventilator, with only 19% of deaths following a failed attempt at cardiopulmonary resuscitation.[42] In a 1997 study of 100 consecutive deaths in three pediatrics ICUs in Boston, 65% of pediatric deaths were accompanied by withdrawal of the ventilator.[43]

Care during and after the withdrawal of life support

In the literature there is only limited discussion of the specific practices used during ventilator withdrawal in children. Burns et al. report that in the great majority of cases, the child is simply extubated, but some children undergo a "terminal wean" of the ventilator.[43] In their case series, analgesics were being given to 81% of children before ventilator withdrawal and the dosage of analgesic was increased in 62% of children at the time the ventilator was removed. Benzodiazepines were given in 76% of children and the dosage was increased in 49% of children as the ventilator was withdrawn. Barbiturates were added in 11% of children and 26% of children were receiving neuromuscular blocking agents at the time of withdrawal.[43]

The use of neuromuscular blocking agents deserves further comment. Depending on the agent used, the route of excretion or the speed of metabolism may be adversely affected by organ system failure in the child. While it is usual practice to stop administration of these agents once the decision to withdraw life support is made, neuromuscular function is not always intact before support is withdrawn. In the setting of end-organ failure, the time required to reestablish muscle function may be prolonged; in some cases, full muscle function may not return for days, if at all. The question as to how the pediatric intensivist ought to proceed in such cases has yet to be settled. Some clinicians will withdraw ventilatory support even without return of muscle function; others will decide to wait until at least some function has returned. If the decision is made to proceed in spite of continued neuromuscular blockade, careful attention must be paid to adequate sedation and analgesia, as the usual signs and symptoms of terminal respiratory distress will be masked. If the decision is to wait until muscle function has returned, clinicians should have repeated discussions among themselves and with the family to explain the reasoning behind the wait and to formulate a plan for comfort measures during the wait. This period of waiting can be extremely stressful for both the family and caregivers, requiring good communication and planing.

When ventilatory support is withdrawn and after the death of the child, the parents should be encouraged to hold the child or to spend time alone with the child's body. A humanizing gesture is to provide a rocking chair in which to hold the child. Rocking the child may help parents maintain the deep connection between them and their child, especially after a period of distancing that can accompany high-technology treatment. At the time of death, the parents will often have strong, positive memories of the child's infancy, and holding the child may help parents cope by returning to a time of safety and comfort. Some parents will want to bathe and dress the child for the last time, others will not. Remembrances of the child—a lock of hair, or some special toy, for example—may be very important to family members.

Autopsy requests

Autopsy requests in pediatrics are essential, and there is good evidence that the autopsy may reveal previously unknown information for the parents and clinicians.[45,46] The findings of an autopsy may be particularly useful to parents who are grieving the loss of a child.[47] In acute traumatic injuries, parents may be left with lingering unease about the severity of the injury, and autopsy findings can confirm that the child's injuries were too extreme to support continued life. For the family of a child dying of chronic illness, there may be doubts as to the extent of progression of the child's illness; an autopsy finding in this instance can confirm that the illness had progressed to a fatal stage. Follow-up visits to discuss the results of an autopsy should be integrated into a bereavement program for families. Some families, especially those having children with cancer or with genetic diagnoses, may have discussed autopsy at an earlier time. In all cases, the request for an autopsy should be made by someone familiar to the family and the child; in cases of chronic illness, the child's primary pediatrician may be the best person to discuss this subject.

The stress of caring for a dying child on physician and nurses should be acknowledged through open discussion among the staff while setting the goals of care.[48] Medical and nursing staff may unintentionally start to withdraw emotional support from families once the child's survival is viewed as unlikely. This phenomenon, often called "compassion fatigue," can be lessened by instilling an environment of open communication among staff and providing staff-directed bereavement activities (for strategies to support grief and bereavement among staff, see Chapter 14).

References

1. Guyer B, Strobino D, Ventura S. Annual summary of vital statistics. *Pediatrics* 1996;98:1007–1010.
2. Wall S, Partridge J. Death in the intensive care nursery: physician practice of withdrawing and withholding life support. *Pediatrics* 1997;99:64–70.
3. Doron M, Veness-Meehan K, Margolis L, Holoman E, Stiles A. Delivery room resuscitation decisions for extremely premature infants. *Pediatrics* 1998;102:574–582.
4. Duff R, Campbell A. Moral and ethical dilemmas in the special care nursery. *New Eng J Med* 1973;289:890–894.
5. Services Department of Health and Human Services. Child abuse and neglect prevention treatment programs: final rule. *Fed Register* 1985;50:1478–1492.
6. Tyson J, Younes N, Verter J, Wright L. Viability, morbidity, and resource use among newborns of 501- to 800-g birth weight. *JAMA* 1996;276:1645–1651.
7. Meadow W, Reimshisel T, Lantos J. Birthweight specific mortality for extremely low birth weight infants vanishes by four days of life: epidemiology and ethics in the neonatal intensive care unit. *Pediatrics* 1996;97:636–643.
8. Richardson D, Gray J, McCormick M, Workman M, Goldmann D. Score for neonatal acute physiology: a physiologic severity index for neonatal intensive care. *Pediatrics* 1993;91:617–623.
9. Tarnow-Mordi W, et al. The CRIB (Clinical Risk Index for Babies) score: a tool for assessing intital neonatal risk and comparing preformance of neonatal intensive care units. *Lancet* 1993;342:193–198.
10. Maier R, Rey M, Metze B, Oblanden M. Comparison of mortality risk: a score for very low birth weight infants. *Arch Dis Child Fetal Neonat Ed* 1997;76:F146–F151.

11. Candee D, Sheehan J, Cook CD, Husted SD, Bargen M. Moral reasoning and decisions in dilemma of neonatal care. *Pediatr Res* 1982;16:846–850.

12. Poses M, Bekes C, Winkler REA. Are two (inexperienced) heads better than one (experienced) head? *Arch Intern Med* 1990;150:1874–1878.

13. Stevens S, Richardson D, Gray J, Goldmann DA, McCormick MC. Estimating neonatal mortality risk: clinicians' judgements. *Pediatrics* 1994;93:945–950.

14. Fowlie P, Tarnow-Mordi W, Gould C, Strang D. Predicting outcome in very low birth weight infants using an objective measure of illness severity and cranial ultrasound scanning. *Arch Dis Child Fetal Neonat Ed* 1998;78:F175–F178.

15. Silverman W. Overtreatment of neonates: a personal retrospective. *Pediatrics* 1992; 90:971–976.

16. Sanders M, Donohue P, Oberdorf MA, Rosenkrantz T, Allen M. Perceptions of the limit of viability: neonatologists' attitudes towards extremely premature infants. *J Perinatol* 1995;15:494–502.

17. Rosenthal E. As more tiny infants live, choices and burdens grow. *New York Times* September 29 Section A 1991:1.

18. McCormick M, Brooks-Gunn J, Workman-Daniels K, Turner J, Peckham G. The health and development status of very-low birth weight children at school age. *JAMA* 1992;267:2204–2208.

19. Hack M, Taylor H, Klein N, Eiben R, Schatschneider C, Mercuri-Minich N. School age outcomes in children with birth weights under 750 g. *N Engl J Med* 1994; 331:753–759.

20. Stolz J, McCormick M. Restricting access to neonatal intensive care: effect on mortality and economic savings. *Pediatrics* 1998;101:344–348.

21. Sanders M, Donohue P, Oberdorf M, Rosenkrantz T, Allen M. Impact of the perception of viability on resource allocation in the neonatal intensive care unit. *J Perinatol* 1998;18:347–351.

22. Paneth N. Tiny babies—enormous costs. *Birth* 1992;19:154–161.

23. Hack M, Fanaroff A. Outcomes of extremely immature infants—a perinatal dilemma. *N Engl J Med* 1993;329:1649–1650.

24. McCormick M, Barfield W, Stolz J. About benefits and costs: pick on someone your own size. *Sci Am Sci Med* 1995;2:4.

25. Hadorn D. The problem of discrimination in health care priority setting. *JAMA* 1992;268:1454–1459.

26. Persault C, Collinge J, Outerbridge E. Family support in the neonatal intensive care unit. *Dimens Heath Serv* 1979;56:16–20.

27. Mahan C. The family of the critically ill neonate. *Crit Care Update* 1983;10:24–28.

28. Perlman N, Freedman J, Abramovitch R, Whyte H, Kirplani H, Perlman M. Informational needs of parents of sick infants. *Pediatrics* 1991;88:512–518.

29. Waller D, Todres I, Cassem N. Coping with poor prognosis in the pediatric intensive care unit. *Am J Dis Child* 1979;133:1121–1124.

30. McLaughlin C, Hull J, Edwards W, Cramer C, Dewey W. Neonatal pain: a comprehensive survey of attitudes and practices. *J Pain Symptom Manage* 1993;8:7–16.

31. Pokela M. Pain relief can reduce hypoxemia in distressed neonates during routine treatment procedures. *Pediatrics* 1994;93:379–383.

32. Boreus L. Pain in the newborn—pharmacodynmaic aspects. *Dev Pharmacol Ther* 1990;15.

33. Partridge J, Wall S. Analgesia for dying infants whose life support is withdrawn or withheld. *Pediatrics* 1997;99:76–79.
34. Whitfield J, Siegal R, Glicken A, Harmon R, Powers L, Goldson E. The application of hospice concepts to neonatal care. *Am J Dis Child* 1982;136:421–424.
35. Pollack M, Ruttiman U, Getson P. The Pediatric Risk of Mortality (PRISM) Score. *Crit Care Med* 1988;16:1110–1116.
36. Rothstein P. Psychological stress in families of children in a pediatric intensive care unit. *Pediatr Clin North Am* 1980;27:613–619.
37. Todres I, Earle J, Jellineck M. Enhancing communication: the physician an the family in the pediatric intensive care unit. *Pediatr Clin North Am* 1994;41:1395–1404.
38. Fiser D, Stanford C, Dorman D. Services for parental distress reduction in the pediatric ICU. *Crit Care Med* 1984;126:504–508.
39. Hanson M, Young D, Carden F. Psychological evaluation and support in the pediatric intensive care unit. *Pediatr Ann* 1986;15:60–65.
40. Green M. Parent care in the intensive care unit. *Am J Dis Child* 1979;113:119–123.
41. Mink R, Pollack M. Resuscitation and withdrawal of therapy in pediatric intensive care. *Pediatrics* 1992;89:961–963.
42. Vernon D, Dean J, Timmons O, Banner W, Allen-Webb E. Modes of death in the pediatric intensive care unit: withdrawal and limitation of supportive care. *Crit Care Med* 1993;21:1798–1802.
43. Burns J, Outwater K, Geller M. Ventilator withdrawal at the end of life. *Pediatrics* 1997;100:456.
44. Ackerman A. Death in the pediatric intensive care unit. *Crit Care Med* 1993; 21:1803–1805.
45. Beckwith J. The value of the pediatric postmortem examination. *Pediatr Clin North Am* 1989;36:30–36.
46. Stanbouley J, Kahn E, Boxer R. Correlation between clinical diagnoses and autopsy findings in critically ill children. *Pediatrics* 1993;92:248–251.
47. Riggs D, Weibley R. Autopsies and the pediatric intensive care unit. *Pediatr Clin North Am* 1994;41:1383–1390.
48. Jellinek M, Todres I, Catlin E, Cassem E, Salzman A. Pediatric intensive care training: confronting the dark side. *Crit Care Med* 1993;21:775–779.

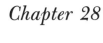

Chapter 28

Special Concerns
for the Very Old

JUDITH E. NELSON
DAVID M. NIERMAN

Approximately 60% of all patients admitted to adult ICUs in the United States are 65 or older, even though this age group comprises less than 15% of the total population.[1] Over the next several decades, this group is expected to grow more than any other in the population as a whole, with particularly rapid expansion of the subgroup of the "oldest old"— individuals over age 85.[2] Current estimates from the Census Bureau project that by 2030, the number of persons aged 65 or over will more than double, from approximately 33 million in 1995 to nearly 70 million, while the 85 and older subgroup is projected to increase from 3.6 million in 1995 to almost 8.5 million by 2030, and over 18 million by 2050.[2] At the same time, the range of aggressive surgical and medical interventions available to an increasingly elderly population continues to expand, with the likelihood of a concomitant rise in complications requiring intensive care. We must expect more elderly patients in our ICUs and be prepared to address special concerns relating to their care during critical illness, including attention to end-of-life issues.

Prognostication of Outcome

Among clinicians, the perception is prevalent that older patients derive less benefit from intensive care than younger ones. It is also widely felt that for the elderly, the burden of aggressive, invasive interventions in an ICU may be less tolerable, both to patients and caregivers. While these views may not be stated openly or explicitly and may not even be consciously recognized, they undoubtedly inform and contribute to day-to-day decisions about initiating and continuing ICU care of elderly individuals in the United States and elsewhere.[3–5] A growing literature documents that even after adjustment for prognoses and preferences for life-extending care, older patient age is associated with a greater tendency on the part of health care providers to withhold aggressive treatments, including ventilator support and other intensive care interventions, dialysis, and surgery.[4,6–9] Often, however, these decisions lack support in data collected and analyzed by rigorous methods and are based instead on limited studies without adequate controls, on anecdotal experience, and/or the insidious influence of ageism that continues in our medical system and the larger society.[4,10,11]

In the current context of rising health care costs, aging of the population, and growing pressure for cost containment, concerns about the utility of intensive care for older patients have prompted proposals to exclude persons over a specified age from scarce and expensive ICU resources.[12,13] Proponents of this approach argue that open and systematic rationing would be justified in both economic and ethical terms and preferable to covert rationing on an individual basis by the "gatekeepers" of ICUs.[13] To date, however, no professional organization or governmental authority in the United States has endorsed age-based allocation of intensive care. Recently, the American Thoracic Society stated that "ICU admissions or continued ICU care must not be denied to a patient who otherwise meets established thresholds for medical need and benefit solely on the basis of extremes of age."[14] On the other hand, the Society of Critical Care Medicine has discouraged admission to the ICU of "[v]ery elderly individuals who are failing to thrive due to irreversible, chronic illness."[15]

Impact of age on ICU outcome

Informed decision making by patients and providers, as well as rational allocation of resources, requires knowledge of existing evidence—and its limitations—with respect to the effectiveness and burdens of intensive care for elderly patients with critical illness. Although there are no randomized, controlled trials of modern ICU interventions in any age-group, numerous descriptive studies conducted in the United States and elsewhere[16–32] provide relevant data of differing quality, as summarized in Table 28–1 and other reviews of the literature.[10,33,34] Taken together, and read critically, these studies suggest that age by itself is not the major determinant of the utility of critical care for elderly patients and/or not a valid single criterion for refusing initial access to ICUs or continued use of ICU interventions. While there is some conflict within the literature and ICU and hospital mortality tend to rise with increasing age, studies controlling for severity of illness and/or previous health and functional status have generally found age as such to be a less important, or even insignificant, predictor of outcome.[10,19,24,33] In a recent study of outcomes after intensive care in Japan, age per se did not influence survival, but was associated with poorer functional status in 1-year survivors.[35] No model predicting outcome specifically for elderly patients receiving intensive care has been prospectively tested. Three major predictive models, Acute Physiology and Chronic Health Evaluation (APACHE), Mortality Prediction Model (MPM), and Simplified Acute Physiology Score (SAPS), include age as a variable, but its impact on the prediction of outcome is comparatively small in all of these.[34] A stronger, negative influence of advancing age has been observed in some studies of patients requiring mechanical ventilation,[31,36,37] but none supports categorical exclusion of elderly patients based on age alone, and a recent prospective study by Ely et al. found no difference between elderly patients and others in duration of mechanical ventilation, length of stay in the ICU or the hospital, or mortality rate, after adjustment for severity of illness. Among older patients with critical illness, the need for prolonged mechanical ventilation,[37–39] renal replacement,[36,37] and resuscitation from cardiopulmonary arrest[40,41] have been associated with poorer outcome, although reasonable hospital survival has been reported after rapid resuscitation from out-of-hospital cardiac arrest due to ventricular fibrillation.[42]

Limitations of prognostic data

Interpretation and generalization from existing data require caution, for two important reasons: the heterogeneity of the elderly population, and the preselection bias introduced in attaining such data.

Heterogeneity of elderly population

Studies of intensive care generally fail to recognize distinctions that have been carefully drawn in the geriatrics literature among different elderly age cohorts, each of which has special medical, psychological, and social characteristics and needs. Whereas geriatricians emphasize unique features of the "young old" (65–74), the "middle old" (75–84), and the "oldest old" (85 and over),[10] age criteria for inclusion in most ICU studies are less precise, and outcomes of ICU care have been reported in general terms for groups of "elderly" patients defined as broadly as patients over the age of 55 years. Nor are definitions consistent from study to study, making cross-study conclusions and comparisons more difficult.

Preselection bias

Another limitation of present data arises from preselection bias.[43] Many older patients are never referred for ICU evaluation because they, their family members, and/or their physicians decide not to pursue an aggressive course. Others are presented to ICUs but denied admission because the prognosis is thought to be unfavorable, based on age and/or other factors. Since the size and nature of this larger population of critically ill elderly patients remaining outside of ICUs have not (to our knowledge) been defined, it is impossible to know whether patients admitted to ICUs have provided a representative sample for the outcomes research conducted to date. It is likely, however, that existing

Table 28–1. Outcome of intensive care for the elderly: mortality

Reference and country	Patient type		Elderly patients (n)	Mortality percent		
	ICU	Age range (years)		ICU	in hospital[a]	Post-discharge[a]
Campion et al., 1981[16] USA	MICU/CCU	65–74	624	8	14	33 (6–18 months)
		≥75	560	10	16	43 (6–18 months)
LeGall et al., 1982[17] France	Multi	≥70	40	—	—	69 (1 year)
Fedullo and Swinburne, 1983[18] USA	MICU	70–79	61	26	41	—
		80–89	23	30	34	—
Nicolas et al., 1987[19] France	Med/Surg, 7 hospitals	>65	191	37	—	—
Sage et al., 1987[20] USA	Med/Surg	>65	134	—	12	28 (18 months)
Chalfin and Carlon, 1990[21] USA	Med/Surg (cancer hospital)	65–74	324	27	36	—
		≥75	163	17	30	—
Ridley et al., 1990[22] Scotland	MICU	65–74	102	29	—	38 (18–42 months)
		75–84	39	21	—	49
		≥85	3	0	—	67
Wu et al., 1990[23] USA	MICU	≥75	130	17	51	—
Mahul et al., 1991[24] France	Med/Surg, 4 hospitals	>70	295	20–29 (4 hospitals)	—	49 (1 year)
Mayer-Oakes et al., 1991[25] USA	MICUs, 3 hospitals	65–74	104	—	30	45 (6 months)
		≥75	153	—	38	49

Study	Type	Age	N			
Chelluri et al., 1992[26] USA	All adult	≥85	34	26	38	—
Heuser et al., 1992[27] USA	All adult, 78 hospitals	≥65	2208	—	8	—
Kass et al., 1992[28] USA	Med/Surg	≥85	105	30	—	64 (1 year)
Chelluri et al., 1993[29] USA	All adult (excluded cancer patients with "poor prognosis")	65–74	43	21	40	58 (1 year)
		≥75	54	31	39	63
Rockwood et al., 1993[30] Canada	Multi, 2 hospitals	>65	406	16	—	49 (1 year)
Cohen and Lambrinos, 1995[31] USA	All beds for MV patients, 243 NY hospitals	70–74	5613	—	51	—
		75–79	5874	—	56	—
		80–84	4910	—	62	—
		85–89	3145	—	67	—
		90+	1812	—	75	—
Djaini and Ridley, 1997[32] England	ICU	>70:	474	19:	—	47 (1 year)
		70–74		12	—	—
		75–79		17	—	—
		80–84		26	—	—
		≥85		34	—	—

CCU, cardiac care unit; Med/Surg, medical/surgical ICU; MICU, medical ICU; Multi, multidisciplinary ICU; MV mechanically ventilated.

*Cumulative results.

reports for groups of preselected patients are "best-case" scenarios, whereas outcomes of unselected patients, such as those described in trauma series[44,45] and those drawn disproportionately from nursing home and chronic care populations, are far less favorable.

The "oldest old"—patients over 85 years

A limited number of studies have separately examined outcomes of intensive care for the "oldest old," or patients over the age of 85.[24,26,28,32] Intuitively, this group might be expected to be particularly frail, having the lowest physiologic reserves and poorest prognoses during critical illness. But those who survive to the ninth decade of life may actually be a select population of the physiologically fittest individuals, with greater tolerance for the stresses of critical illness than their "unselected" younger counterparts. Most studies show that, as has been found for more broadly defined groups of elderly patients, in-hospital mortality for the oldest old is comparable to that of younger patients with similar severity of illness and premorbid status. For example, in a retrospective study by Chelluri et al., of 34 patients over 85 years of age admitted to medical/surgical ICUs,[26] representing about 1% of the total number of patients admitted to these ICUs during the study period, hospital survival was 62% and almost the same as that of a similar population of medical ICU patients in all adult age-groups. In our own institution, where there is no formal policy regarding age as a criterion for ICU decision making but it is undoubtedly taken into consideration on a case-by-case basis, recent data revealed surprisingly favorable rates of ICU and hospital survival for patients over 85 years of age who received care in our ICUs: among 222 very elderly patients admitted during a recent 1-year period, 77% survived their hospitalization (D.M. Nierman, unpublished data, 1998). Interestingly, among patients with various malignancies treated in a major U.S. cancer center's ICU, Chalfin and Carlon[21] actually found overall hospital mortality to be lower in the group of patients 75 years of age and older than in patients aged 65 to 74, or even those aged 19 to 64. In The Netherlands, Tran et al.[46] found that multiple organ system failure occurred less often and mortality was lower in octogenerians than in patients 71–80 years of age in a medical ICU.

Functional recovery

For many patients, for their families, and for intensive care providers, the most important information relates not to short-term endpoints, such as ICU and hospital mortalities, but to longer-term outcomes, including functional status and quality of life as well as mortality after hospital discharge. These data are less well developed and more difficult to aggregate or summarize because of the variety of measures used, the heterogeneity of patients to whom these measures have been applied, and the small size of some samples.[16,17,20,24,26,30,36,47-52]

Studies evaluating the functional status and quality of life of elderly survivors of intensive care are presented in Table 28–2. Among those assessing functional status, Campion et al.[16] reported activity levels for over 1800 patients at 1 year after discharge from medical or coronary care units at Massachussetts General Hospital. In the oldest age-group (75 and older), nearly 90% of patients had been admitted from home, and approximately 60% were capable at baseline of at least mild exertion. At follow-up, about 90% of these patients were again residing at home, and 50% could perform mild or (rarely) more strenuous physical activity. In a study of 295 patients aged 70 years and older at 1 year after discharge from French ICUs, Mahul et al.[24] found that for almost 80% of these patients, the functional status was either as good as or better than it had been before admission to the ICU. Other investigators have also found that at 1 year after discharge from ICUs, the majority of elderly patients who survive have attained or exceeded their premorbid status.[17,48] Roche et al.[53] recently reported functional outcomes of medical, cardiac, and surgical ICU patients in a Veterans Administration medical center: 6-month mortality in this group, from which patients who were comatose or unable to communicate in the ICU were excluded, was 22% for patients between 65 and 74 years of age and 14% for patients older than 75; approximately half of the patients returned to their baseline function or improved by 6 months after intensive care, regardless of age. Baseline functional status, rather than abnormal physiologic status on admission to the ICU as measured by APACHE II, was the main determinant of functional recovery. On the whole, these data suggest that the majority of elderly survivors of intensive care, like younger counterparts, can be expected to return to their baseline level of function, with the latter serving as an important predictor of functional recovery.

Futile Treatment

Some investigators have concluded that cardiopulmonary resuscitation (CPR) of elderly patients is futile in certain circumstances. In a study by Murphy et al.[40] of more than 500 patients aged 70 and over in an urban area, the rate of hospital survival for patients resuscitated out of the hospital was less than 1%. In this study and others,[41,54] hospital survival after CPR also approached zero, regardless of whether the arrest occurred in or outside of the hospital, for patients with unwitnessed arrests, nonventricular arrhythmias, resuscitation without rapid response (generally 5 minutes or less), and/or acute or chronic dysfunction of multiple organ systems. Nevertheless, at least brief attempts to resuscitate have generally been considered justified and not futile, even outside the hospital setting, for patients without significant comorbidities who are found in ventricular fibrillation.[42] With respect to interventions other than CPR, several investigators [37,39] have found that among elderly patients requiring prolonged mechanical ventilation and particularly those with cancer and/or

Table 28–2. Outcome of intensive care for the elderly: functional status, quality of life

Reference and country	Patient type		Elderly patients (n)	Measures/follow-up period	Results
	ICU	Age range (years)			
Campion et al., 1981[16] USA	MICU/CCU	65–74	624	Physical activity at 6–18 months vs. pre-ICU	In both elderly groups, no change in % home at f/u vs. baseline
		≥75	560		Lifestyle with mild or more exertion: 65–74 years, 76% (baseline); 70% (f/u) ≥75 years, 68% (baseline); 50% (f/u) Sedentary lifestyle: 65–74 years, 11% (baseline); 26% (f/u) ≥75 years, 18% (baseline); 43% (f/u)
LeGall et al., 1982[17] France	Med/Surg	≥50	67	Functional status 3 months pre-ICU, 1 year post-ICU	49% of survivors ≥50 years: no change at 1 year; 51% had worse function
		≥70	18		Functional outcome influenced by age + no. of organ failures
McClean et al., 1985[36] Canada	Multi-RICU	≥75	14	Functional status, attitudes re: QOL and ICU, 12–24 months post-ICU	43% with activity level at f/u ≥ baseline 85% QOL worthwhile 77% would repeat ICU if indicated
Sage et al., 1987[20] USA	Med/Surg	≥65	59	SIP uniscale, at 18 months post-ICU	90% self-rated as "acceptably" or "extremely" healthy Slightly (not significantly) lower adjusted SIP and uniscale for ICU survivors vs. elderly controls
Zaren and Hedstrand, 1987[47] Sweden	Med/Surg	≥65	199	Functional status at 1 year post-ICU vs. 3 months pre-ICU	80% of patients independent at home vs. 90% at baseline Poor baseline function, ICU LOS ≥1 week, MV, predicted worse functional outcome

Study	Setting	Age	N	Outcome	Results
Zaren and Bergstrom, 1989[48] Sweden	Med/Surg	≥65	350	Functional status at 1 year post-ICU vs. 3 months pre-ICU	73% of patients' functional status at 1 yr ≥ baseline; MV but not ICU LOS associated with worse functional outcome
Mundt et al., 1989[49] USA	Med/Surg	≥70	262	Functional status in physical, psychologic, and social domains at 6 months post-ICU	Most had worse functional status, but more contact with family; 72% of previously working patients still working
Ridley and Wallace, 1990[50] Scotland	Multi	≥60	40	PQOL, Katz's ADL, other functional capacity 1–3 years post-ICU	82% of patients had same or improved status; 7% deteriorated
Mahul et al., 1991[24] France	Med/Surg, 4 hospitals	≥70	106	Residence and functional status at 1 year post-ICU	88% at home, 70% independent at 1 year; 80% functional status ≥ baseline; No clinical parameters at ICU admission predicted functional outcome
Chelluri et al., 1992[26] USA	Med/Surg	≥85	21	Residence and level of activity; attitudes re: QOL and ICU	86% of patients from home; 43% independent; 62% discharged to home, 5% to rehab hospital; 8/10 QOL = good or fair; 9/10 would receive ICU care again
Mata et al., 1992[51] Spain	Med/Surg	61–75 ≥76	155 33	Function and PQOL at ICU admission and 1 year post-ICU	50% worse function, 50% same or better function vs. baseline; Lower function not mirrored by lower subjective perception of QOL; 1-year QOL influenced by baseline QOL, age, illness severity

(continued)

Table 28-2.—Continued

Reference and country	Patient type ICU	Age range (years)	Elderly patients (n)	Measures/follow-up period	Results
Chelluri et al., 1993[29] USA	ICU	≥65	38	Katz's ADL, PQOL, CES-D at 1 year post-ICU	All 65- to 74-year-olds from home back at home at 1 year; 85% pts ≥75 years at home at 1 year 84% independent ADLs at 1 year vs. 94% at baseline No decline in PQOL from baseline; no difference in PQOL compared to community elderly controls CES-D same as controls 71% willing to repeat ICU if indicated
Rockwood et al., 1993[30] Canada	Multi, 2 hospitals	>65	175	Health status, functional capacity, attitudes re: ICU at 1 year post-ICU	Majority independent in ADL Compared to control elderly in community, same proportion perceived health as good to very good despite worse function 70% satisfied with health status 54% had health status ≥5 years before ICU 66% had health status ≥ contemporaries
Konopad et al., 1995[52] Canada	Med/Surg	66–76 >75	46 175	Spitzer's QOL at ICU admission and 1 year post-ICU	Activity level and ADL worse for all age-groups Patients >75 years perceived health status as better 82% of 66 to 75-year-olds, 71% of patients >75 years home at 1 year

ADL, activities of daily living; CCU, cardiac care unit; CES-D, Center of Epidemiologic Studies-Depression Score; f/u, follow-up; LOS, length of stay; Med/Surg, medical/surgical ICU; MICU, medical ICU; Multi, multidisciplinary ICU; MV, mechanical ventilation; PQOL, perceived quality of life; QOL, quality of life; RICU, respiratory ICU; SIP, Sickness Impact Profile.

nonpulmonary organ system dysfunction, hospital survival was low and post-discharge quality of life among survivors was poor, while care of these patients was costly. In these studies, however, survival exceeded the extremely low levels that have been most often used to define futile treatment.

Special Communication Issues

Sensory deficits and cognitive impairment

The critically ill elderly patient presents special communication issues. Many if not most of these patients are simply unable to communicate with the ICU staff, or even with their own loved ones. While obstacles to communication are often present for ICU patients of all ages,[55] older patients are likely to have more severe problems. Preexisting sensory deficits of vision, hearing, and speech are more common[10] and can further complicate the already difficult task of communicating effectively about complex matters during the crisis of critical illness. Cognition may also have been impaired chronically and, in any event, is likely to deteriorate in the ICU because of the acute illness, the pharmacologic treatments that have unpredictable but typically more extreme effects in the elderly, and stresses imposed by the ICU environment. Older patients often experience delirium during hospitalization for serious illness.[56] Even in the absence of cognitive impairment, often there is still a "vast gulf between lay and professional understandings of human physiology and the role of technology" and about multiple aspects of life-sustaining treatment, such that neither patients nor families can participate in an informed, meaningful dialogue about appropriate goals of intensive care.[57]

Goal setting in the context of chronic illness and/or functional impairment

Communication about ICU care in general and about end-of-life issues in particular involves discussion and definition of appropriate treatment goals. For the elderly patient with critical illness, these goals may be more difficult to define,[10] particularly for the professional caregivers. Intensivists are trained to perform dramatic resuscitative efforts, to use sophisticated technology to reverse even the most serious illness and achieve definitive cure. Such clearly successful outcomes, however, may be especially elusive in caring for older patients, who suffer more often from chronic diseases that will continue after intensive care and that may be incompletely understood by physicians lacking expertise in geriatric medicine. In many cases, it is the doctor, and not the patient or surrogate, who may have to make the most significant adjustment of orientation, shifting the objectives of aggressive treatment from clear-cut cure to return to a baseline of impaired but subjectively acceptable function. In other cases, family expectations may be unrealistic. A "disjunction between institutionalized technology use and deep concern about overtreatment," also termed "ethical dissonance," has been identified as a barrier to appropriate clinical decision making and communication as well as to the emotional well-being of caregivers, particularly with respect to the critically ill patient of advanced age.[57] Effective communication about the utility of initiating or continuing intensive care for an elderly patient requires close and ongoing consideration of age-specific benefits and burdens.

Family dynamics

Dynamics within the families of older patients may also affect both the process and content of communication. When the critical illness has an unexpected and rapid onset, decision making by the family may require an abrupt reversal of long-standing roles, with children now assuming authority and responsibility for a parent who traditionally has been the dominant figure in the family. In other situations, the surrogate for the patient is a spouse who is also elderly, who faces the potential or real loss of a lifetime companion, and who may be particularly vulnerable because of physical, social, and economic needs. Among patients themselves, dislike of dependency and fear of becoming burdensome to family members are influences that must be investigated and openly discussed in the course of communication about continuing or limiting intensive care. More often than for other age-groups, elderly patients, especially those without children, may have no identifiable surrogate, having outlived family and friends and/or lived in increasing social isolation. Decisions regarding these patients, when they lack capacity and advance directives, are particularly delicate and require the most careful and unbiased appraisal of the patient's interest as well as appropriate contact with ethics committees and legal authorities.

Determining patient preferences

Given that very few elderly patients with critical illness are capable of direct involvement in communication and decision making,[58] considerable effort is often required to discern their preferences for initiation and/or continuation of intensive care. Usually, these have not been discussed in advance with either the family or the physician, although data indicate that older patients are willing to do so if the opportunity is provided.[59,60] While there is recent evidence that more patients are preparing advance directives,[61] these patients are still the minority. Moreover, a significant proportion of directives that are prepared are never identified or included in the medical record,[62] and even those that are available often fail to address the complex issues that arise during the course of critical illness. Unfortunately, the preferences of elderly patients for life-supporting treatment are poorly predicted by surrogates, including their closest relatives and long-standing primary doctors.[63,64]

Age-related changes in perception of life quality

An important observation made in multiple studies is that most older people perceive and determine quality of life differently from younger people. In general, the elderly are more satisfied with the quality of their lives, despite chronic illness or functional impairment.[10,33,52] They typically see their quality of life as better than that seen by younger, healthy persons presented with the same situation hypothetically, and better than when viewed by their physicians. In addition, as shown by the Hospitalized Elderly Longitudinal Project (HELP) investigators,[65] elderly patients may value the time spent in their current state of health, even if they see their health as suboptimal, more than they value excellent health if that means a shorter life. In our own ICUs, recent data indicate that even among the "oldest old" survivors of critical care (85 + years), the quality of life 1 to 2 years after the ICU experience is acceptable to the majority, including those living in skilled nursing facilities (D.M. Nierman, unpublished data, 1998).

Preferences of elderly patients for life-supporting treatment

When presented with a hypothetical choice between "a course of treatment that focuses on extending life as much as possible, even if it means having more pain and discomfort," or "a plan of care that focuses on relieving pain and discomfort as much as possible, even if that means not living as long," 37% of seriously ill, hospitalized patients aged 70–79 and 27% aged 80 or older wanted life-extending care, as compared to 61% of patients 50 years of age or younger.[4] Physicians often underestimated the desire of older patients for aggressive care (79% of the time for patients 80 years of age and older), were less likely to want life-extending care for themselves if they were in an older patient's situation rather than in a younger patient's situation, and were more likely to withhold life-sustaining treatments because of their misperceptions of the preferences of the elderly. Torian et al.[66] found that 85% of patients in an acute care geriatric unit wished to have CPR, even though they had multiple medical comorbidities and generally poor functional status and had been counseled about the benefits and limitations of CPR. As a group, most elderly individuals interviewed in outpatient settings have expressed a preference for resuscitation in the event of an arrest and in the absence of severe neurologic impairment[67,68] or imminent death from terminal illness.[59] Their understanding of the nature and expected outcomes of CPR, however, is usually poor,[59,67] and a strong tendency to overestimate the likelihood of a successful outcome has been observed.[43,69–71] Some,[69,71] but not all,[67] studies indicate that after interventions to educate them about CPR techniques and outcomes, fewer elderly individuals would opt for resuscitation. Older patients' preferences for life-sustaining treatment are not necessarily limited by their perceptions of the current quality of their lives.[71,72]

With respect to intensive care interventions other than CPR, Danis et al.[68] found that in the context of a hypothetical terminal illness, 76% of elderly patients wanted intensive care, 86% wanted "artificial respiration," and 69% wanted tube feeding. Recently, Murphy and Santilli[73] reported that among 287 persons with a mean age of 77 years who were interviewed during routine office visits to a geriatrics clinic, 88% would opt for short-term mechanical ventilation if the duration were brief (several days to a week) and the chance of recovery were reasonably good (estimated at 20%–50%), whereas less than 4% wanted "long-term" mechanical ventilation of an unspecified duration. Sixty-five percent of these patients wanted "short-term" tube feeding, but less than 5% would choose it for the "long term," as in the situation of advanced neuro-degenerative disease. Such data, gathered in outpatient settings, may not reflect decisions that would be made at the time of critical illness, when the prospect of ICU care is immediate and, even in similar life circumstances, preferences for end-of-life care may not be stable over time.[68]

Conclusions and Recommendations

Older patients are a unique, growing, and particularly vulnerable group. As health care providers and society struggle to define appropriate guidelines for allocating costly services such as ICU treatment, the wishes and needs of the elderly, and the benefits and burdens that can reasonably be expected for them, their families, and our health care system will need to be investigated further and considered carefully. For those who provide ICU care on a day-to-day basis, conflicts may arise between treatment preferences of individual elderly patients or their surrogates and perceived or real demands of the local institution and community and/or the larger society. Vindication of patient autonomy, which remains an important obligation for caregivers, requires knowledge and interpretation of existing information about meaningful outcomes of intensive care for the elderly, including the impact of age and other variables on short- and longer-term mortalities and on post-ICU functional status and quality of life. In appropriate cases, the expertise of specialists in geriatric medicine should be engaged. Relevant information will need to be communicated in understandable terms to the patients and their families, taking into account the special challenges of communication to and about patients of advanced age. Familiarity with existing evidence about general preferences of elderly patients is helpful and, to the extent these data reflect the choices of competent patients in similar circumstances, may actually be more useful than the substituted judgments of family or physician surrogates, which are frequently discordant with decisions by the patients themselves. Every effort should be made, in an open and unbiased manner, to ascertain the individual patient's own views and choices, in situations where this is possible. Importantly, caregivers must conduct continuing, thorough, and honest self-examination for age-based biases and/or inappropriate projection onto patients of their own beliefs and values, including standards of life quality. Available evidence indicates that the elderly also have a powerful instinct for survival and that their will to live, even in the face of diminished function and comparatively poor health, is often at least as strong, perhaps stronger, than that of younger counterparts. The ongoing challenge for providers of intensive care will be to determine, in an evidence-based and unbiased way, whether the burdens of a trial of intensive care are justified by potential benefits for an individual elderly patient and to recalculate the burdens and benefits, in a similarly objective way, as the trial proceeds and the critical illness unfolds. The elderly should not "as a final rite of passage, need to proceed through the gates of technology,"[74] but neither should ICU doors be closed to selected older patients, even in the oldest old group, who can improve through the use of critical care to a subjectively acceptable state of health and quality of life. Further research relating to outcomes of and preferences for intensive care in this specific age-group and to the symptom experience of older patients during ICU treatment can be expected to facilitate decision making and clinical care in this difficult area of critical care practice.

References

1. Groeger JS, Guntupalli KK, Strosberg M, Halpern N, Raphaely RC, Cerra F, Kaye W. Descriptive analysis of critical care units in the United States: Patient characteristics and intensive care unit utilization. *Crit Care Med* 1993;21:279–291.
2. U.S. Census Bureau. Projections of the Population, by Age and Sex: 1995–2050. Washington, DC. U.S. Government Printing Office, 1996.
3. Cook DJ, Guyatt GH, Jaeschke R, Reeve J, Spanier A, King D, Molloy W, Willan A, Streiner DL. Determinants in Canadian health care workers of the decision to withdraw life support from the critically ill. *JAMA* 1995;273:703–708.
4. Hamel MB, Teno JM, Goldman L, Lynn J, Davis RB, Galanos AN, Desbiens N, Connors AF Jr, Wenger N, Phillips RS. Patient age and decisions to withhold life-sustaining treatments from seriously ill, hospitalized adults. *Ann Intern Med* 1999; 130:116–125.
5. Knaus WA, Le Gall JR, Wagner DP, Loirat P, Cullen DJ, Glaser P, Mercier Philippe, Nikki P, Snyder J, LeGall Jr, Draper EA, Campos RA, Kohles MK, Granthil C, Nicolas F, Shin B, Wattel F, Zimmerman JE. A comparison of intensive care in the U.S.A. and France. *Lancet* 1982;2:642–646.
6. Castillo-Lorente E, Rivera-Fernandez R, Vasquez-Mata G. Limitation of therapeutic activity in elderly critically ill patients. *Crit Care Med* 1997;25:1643–1648.
7. Hamel MB, Phillips RS, Teno JM, Lynn J, Galanos AN, Davis RB, Connors AF Jr, Oye RK, Desbiens N, Reding DJ, Goldman L. Seriously ill hospitalized adults: do we spend less on older patients? *J Am Geriatr Soc* 1996;44:1043–1048.
8. Hakim RB, Teno JM, Harrell FE Jr, Knaus WA, Wenger N, Phillips RS. Factors associated with do-not-resuscitate orders: patients' preferences, prognoses, and physicians' judgments. SUPPORT Investigators. Study to Understand Prognoses and Preferences for Outcomes and Risks of Treatment. *Ann Intern Med* 1996;125:284–293.

9. Hanson LC, Danis M. Use of life-sustaining care for the elderly. *J Am Geriatr Soc* 1991;39:772–777.

10. Adelman RD, Berger JT, Macina LO. Critical care for the geriatric patient. *Clin Geriatr Med* 1994;10:19–30.

11. Butler R. Age-ism: another form of bigotry. *Gerontologist* 1969;9:243–246.

12. Callahan D. Old age and new policy. *JAMA* 1989;261:905–906.

13. Callahan D. Controlling the costs of health care for the elderly—fair means and foul. *N Engl J Med* 1996;335:744–746.

14. American Thoracic Society. Fair allocation of intensive care unit resources. *Am J Respir Crit Care Med* 1997;156:1282–1301.

15. Society of Critical Care Medicine Ethics Committee. Consensus statement on the triage of critically ill patients. *JAMA* 1994;271:1200–1203.

16. Campion EW, Mulley AG, Goldstein RL, Barnett GO, Thibault GE. Medical intensive care for the elderly. *JAMA* 1981;246:2052–2056.

17. Le Gall JR, Brun-Buisson C, Trunet P, Latournerie J, Chantereau S, Rapin M. Influence of age, previous health status, and severity of acute illness on outcome from intensive care. *Crit Care Med* 1982;10:575–577.

18. Fedullo AJ, Swinburne AJ. Relationship of patient age to cost and survival in a medical ICU. *Crit Care Med* 1983;11:155–159.

19. Nicolas F, Le Gall JR, Loirat P, Alperovitch A, Villers D. Influence of patients' age on survival, level of therapy and length of stay in intensive care units. *Intensive Care Med* 1987;13:9–13.

20. Sage WM, Hurdst CR, Silverman JF, Bortz WM. Intensive care for the elderly: outcome of elective and nonelective admissions. *J Am Geriatr Soc* 1987;35:312–318.

21. Chalfin DB, Carlon GC. Age and utilization of intensive care unit resources of critically ill cancer patients. *Crit Care Med* 1990;18:694–698.

22. Ridley SA, Jackson R, Findlay J, Wallace P. Long term survival after intensive care. *BMJ* 1990;301:1127–1130.

23. Wu A, Rubin HR, Rosen MJ. Are elderly people less responsive to intensive care? *J Am Geriatr Soc* 1990;38:621–627.

24. Mahul P, Perrot D, Tempelhoff G, Gaussorgue SP, Jospe R, Ducreux JC, Dumont A, Motin J, Auboyer C, Robert D. Short-and long-term prognosis, functional outcome following ICU for elderly. *Intensive Care Med* 1991;17:7–10.

25. Mayer-Oakes SA, Oye RK, Leake B. Predictors of mortality in older patients following medical intensive care: the importance of functional status. *J Am Geriatr Soc* 1991;39:862–868.

26. Chelluri L, Pinsky MR, Grenvik A. Outcome of intensive care of the "oldest-old" critically ill patients. *Crit Care Med* 1992;20:757–761.

27. Heuser MD, Case LD, Ettinger WH. Mortality in intensive care patients with respiratory disease. *Arch Intern Med* 1992;152:1683–1688.

28. Kass JE, Castriotta RJ, Malakoff F. Intensive care unit outcome in the very elderly. *Crit Care Med* 1992;20:1666–1671.

29. Chelluri L, Pinsky MR, Donahoe MP, Grenvik A. Long-term outcome of critically ill elderly patients requiring intensive care. *JAMA* 1993;269:3119–3123.

30. Rockwood K, Noseworthy TW, Gibney RTN, Konopad E, Shustack A, Stollery D, Johnston R, Grace M. One-year outcome of elderly and young patients admitted to intensive care units. *Crit Care Med* 1993;21:687–691.

31. Cohen IL, Lambrinos J. Investigating the impact of age on outcome of mechanical ventilation using a population of 41,848 patients from a statewide database. *Chest* 1995;107:1673–1680.
32. Djaiani G, Ridley S. Outcome of intensive care in the elderly. *Anaesthesia* 1997; 52:1130–1136.
33. Chelluri L, Grenvik A, Silverman M. Intensive care for critically ill elderly: mortality, costs, and quality of life. *Arch Intern Med* 1995;155:1013–1022.
34. Chalfin DB. Outcome assessment in elderly patients with critical illness and respiratory failure. *Clin Chest Med* 1993;14:583–589.
35. Short TG, Buckley TA, Rowbottom MY, Wong E, Oh TE. Long-term outcome and functional health status following intensive care in Hong Kong. *Crit Care Med* 1999;27:51–57.
36. McLean RF, McIntosh JD, Kung GY, Leung DMW, Byrick R. Outcome of respiratory intensive care for the elderly. *Crit Care Med* 1985;13:625–629.
37. Swinburne AJ, Fedullo AJ, Bixby K, Lee DK, Wahl GW. Analysis of outcome after treatment with mechanical ventilation. *Arch Intern Med* 1993;153:1657–1662.
37a. Ely EW, Evans GW, Haponik EF. Mechanical ventilation in a cohort of elderly patients admitted to an intensive care unit. *Ann Intern Med* 1999;131:96–104.
38. Cohen IL, Lambrinos J, Fein A. Mechanical ventilation for the elderly patient in intensive care. *JAMA* 1993;269:1025–1029.
39. Elpern EH, Larson R, Douglass P, Rosen RL, Bone RC. Long-term outcomes for elderly survivors of prolonged ventilator assistance. *Chest* 1989;96:1120–1124.
40. Murphy DJ, Murray AM, Robinson BE, Campion EW. Outcomes of cardiopulmonary resuscitation in the elderly. *Ann Intern Med* 1989;111:199–205.
41. Taffet GE, Teasdale TA, Luchi RJ. In-hospital cardiopulmonary resuscitation. *JAMA* 1988;260:2069–2072.
42. Longstreth WT, Cobb LA, Fahrenbruch CE, Copass MK. Does age affect outcomes of out-of-hospital cardiopulmonary resuscitation? *JAMA* 1990;264:2109–2110.
43. Clarke DE, Goldstein MK, Raffin TA. Ethical dilemmas in the critically ill elderly. *Clin Geriatr Med* 1994;10:91–101.
44. Goins WA, Reynolds HN, Nyanjom D. Outcome following intensive care unit stay in multiple trauma patients. *Crit Care Med* 1991;19:339–345.
45. Cullinane DC, Morris JA Jr. The impact of age and medical comorbidities on the outcome following severe trauma. *J Intensive Care Med* 1999;14:86–94.
46. Tran DD, Groeneveld ABJ, Van Der Meulen J, Nauta JJ, Van Schijndel RJMS, Thijs LG. Age, chronic disease, sepsis, organ system failure, and mortality in a medical intensive care unit. *Crit Care Med* 1990;18:474–479.
47. Zaren B, Hedstrand U. Quality of life among long-term survivors of intensive care. *Crit Care Med* 1987;15:743–747.
48. Zaren B, Bergstrom R. Survival compared to the general population and changes in health status among intensive care patients. *Acta Anaesthesiol Scand* 1989;33: 6–12.
49. Mundt DJ, Gage RW, Lemeshow S, Pastides H, Teres D, Avrunin JS. Intensive care unit patient follow-up. *Arch Intern Med* 1989;149:68–72.
50. Ridley SA, Wallace PGM. Quality of life after intensive care. *Anaesthesia* 1990; 45:808–813.
51. Vasquez Mata G, Rivera Fernandez R, Gonzalez Carmona A, Delgado-Rodriguez

M, Torres Ruiz JM, Raya Pugnaire AR, Aguayo de Hoyos E. Factors related to quality of life 12 months after discharge from an intensive care unit. *Crit Care Med* 1992;20:1257–1262.

52. Konopad E, Noseworthy TW, Johnston R, Shustack A, Grace M. Quality of life measures before and one year after admission to an intensive care unit. *Crit Care Med* 1995;23:1653–1659.

53. Roche VML, Kramer A, Hester E, Welsh CH. Long-term functional outcome after intensive care. *J Am Geriatr Soc* 1999;47:18–24.

54. Bachman JW, McDonald GS, O'Brien PC. A study of out-of-hospital cardiac arrest in northeastern Minnesota. *JAMA* 1986;256:477–483.

55. Gilligan T, Raffin TA. Physician virtues and communicating with patients. *New Horiz* 1997;5:6–14.

56. Francis J, Martin D, Kapoor WN. A prospective study of delirium in hospitalized elderly. *JAMA* 1990;263:1097–1101.

57. Kaufman SR. Intensive care, old age, and the problem of death in America. *Gerontologist* 1998;38:715–725.

58. Quill TE, Bennett NM. The effects of a hospital policy and state legislation on resuscitation orders for geriatric patients. *Arch Intern Med* 1992;152:569–572.

59. Shmerling RH, Bedell SE, Lilienfeld A, Delbanco TL. Discussing cardiopulmonary resuscitation. *J Gen Intern Med* 1988;3:317–321.

60. Wagner A. Cardiopulmonary resuscitation in the aged. *N Engl J Med* 1984; 310:1129–1130.

61. Hammes BJ, Rooney BL. Death and end-of-life planning in one midwestern community. *Arch Intern Med* 1998;158:383–390.

62. Morrison RS, Olson E, Mertz KR, Meier DE. The inaccessibility of advance directives on transfer from ambulatory to acute care settings. *JAMA* 1995;274:478–482.

63. Uhlmann RF, Pearlman RA, Cain KC. Physicians' and spouses' predictions of elderly patients' resuscitation preferences. *J Gerontol* 1988;43:M115–M121.

64. Seckler A, Meier DE, Mulvihill M. Substituted judgement: how accurate are proxy predictions? *Ann Intern Med* 1991;115:92–98.

65. Tsevat J, Dawson NV, Wu AW, Lynn J, Soukup JR, Cook EF, Vidaillet H, Phillips RS. Health values of hospitalized patients 80 years or older. *JAMA* 1998;279:371–375.

66. Torian LC, Davidson EJ, Fillit HM, Fulop G, Sell LL. Decisions for and against resuscitation in an acute geriatric medicine unit serving the frail elderly. *Arch Intern Med* 1992;152:561–565.

67. Schonwetter RS, Teasdale TA, Taffet G, Robinson BE, Luchi RJ. Educating the elderly: cardiopulmonary resuscitation decisions before and after intervention. *J Am Geriatr Soc* 1991;39:372–377.

68. Danis M, Garrett J, Harris R, Donald LP. Stability of choices about life-sustaining treatments. *Ann Intern Med* 1994;120:567–573.

69. Murphy DJ, Burrows D, Santilli S. The influence of the probability of survival on patients' preferences regarding cardiopulmonary resuscitation. *N Engl J Med* 1994; 330:545–549.

70. Miller DL, Jahnigen DW, Gorbien MJ, Simbartl L. Cardiopulmonary resuscitation: how useful? *Arch Intern Med* 1992;152:578–582.

71. Schonwetter RS, Walker RM, Kramer DR, Robinson BE. Resuscitation decision making in the elderly. *J Gen Intern Med* 1993;8:296–300.

72. Danis M, Patrick DL, Southerland LI, Green ML. Patients' and families' preferences for medical intensive care. *JAMA* 1988;260:797–802.
73. Murphy DJ, Santilli S. Elderly patients' preferences for long-term life support. *Arch Fam Med* 1998;7:484–488.
74. Gordon M, Cheung M. DNR policy and CPR practice in geriatric long-term institutional care. *Can Med Assoc J* 1991;145:209–212.

Index